ANALYSIS OF AGGREGATES AND PARTICLES IN PROTEIN PHARMACEUTICALS

ANALYSIS OF AGGREGATES AND PARTICLES IN PROTEIN PHARMACEUTICALS

Edited by

Hanns-Christian Mahler
F. Hoffmann-La Roche Ltd., Basel, Switzerland

Wim Jiskoot
Leiden University, Leiden, The Netherlands

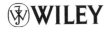WILEY

A JOHN WILEY & SONS, INC., PUBLICATION

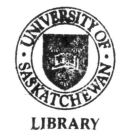

Published by John Wiley & Sons, Inc., Hoboken, New Jersey.
Published simultaneously in Canada.

For general information on our other products and services or for technical support, please contact our Customer Care Department within the United States at (800) 762-2974, outside the United States at (317) 572-3993 or fax (317) 572-4002.

Wiley also publishes its books in a variety of electronic formats. Some content that appears in print may not be available in electronic formats. For more information about Wiley products, visit our web site at www.wiley.com.

Library of Congress Cataloging-in-Publication Data:

Analysis of aggregates and particles in protein pharmaceuticals / edited by Hanns-Christian Mahler, Wim Jiskoot.
    p. ; cm.
Includes bibliographical references.
ISBN 978-0-470-49718-0 (cloth)
  I. Mahler, Hanns-Christian. II. Jiskoot, Wim.
  [DNLM: 1. Pharmaceutical Preparations—analysis. 2. Chemistry Techniques, Analytical—methods. 3. Proteins—pharmacokinetics. QV 25]
  LC classification not assigned
  615.1′9—dc23

                               2011026192

Printed in the United States of America

10 9 8 7 6 5 4 3 2 1

To my beloved son, Conrad Louis,
and my wonderful wife, Christiane
—Hanns-Christian Mahler

" . . . a dream that became a reality and
spread throughout the stars"
—Capt. Kirk

CONTENTS

CONTRIBUTORS

MARKUS BLUEMEL, Analytical Research and Development of the Process Science and Production Department, Novartis Pharma AG, Basel, Switzerland

MARIOLA BOZOVA, Analytical Research and Development of the Process Science and Production Department, Novartis Pharma AG, Basel, Switzerland

KEVIN BRAECKMANS, Laboratory of General Biochemistry and Physical Pharmacy, Ghent University, Ghent, Belgium

SHAWN CAO, Process and Product Development, Amgen Inc., Thousand Oaks, California, USA

JOHN F. CARPENTER, Department of Pharmaceutical Sciences, University of Colorado Denver, Aurora, Colorado, USA

BARRY CHERNEY, Division of Therapeutic Proteins, U.S. Food and Drug Administration, Rockville, Maryland, USA

TAPAN K. DAS, BioTherapeutics Pharmaceutical Sciences, Pfizer, St. Louis, Missouri, USA

BARTHÉLEMY DEMEULE, Late Stage Pharmaceutical Development, Genentech, Inc., South San Francisco, California, USA

JOHN DEN ENGELSMAN, Analytical Development and Validation, Schering Plough Research Institute, Oss, The Netherlands

MANUEL DIEZ, Analytical Research and Development of the Process Science and Production Department, Novartis Pharma AG, Basel, Switzerland

REZA ESFANDIARY, Department of Pharmaceutical Chemistry, University of Kansas, Lawrence, Kansas, USA

ROBERTO FALKENSTEIN, Bioprocess Development, Purification, Pharma Technical Development Biologics Europe, Roche Diagnostics GmbH, Penzberg, Germany

STEFAN FISCHER, Late-Stage Pharmaceutical and Processing Development, Pharmaceutical and Device Development, Pharma Technical Development Biologics Europe, F. Hoffmann-La Roche Ltd, Basel, Switzerland

KURT FORRER, Analytical Research and Development of the Process Science and Production Department, Novartis Pharma AG, Basel, Switzerland

WOLFGANG FRIESS, Department of Pharmacy, Pharmaceutical Technology and Biopharmaceutics, Ludwig-Maximilians-University Munich, Munich, Germany

PATRICK GARIDEL, Pharmaceutical Development, Process Science/Biopharmaceuticals, Boehringer Ingelheim Pharma GmbH & Co. KG, Biberach an der Riss, Germany

ANDREA HAWE, Division of Drug Delivery Technology, Biologics Formulation Group, Leiden University, Leiden, The Netherlands

STEFAN HEPBILDIKLER, Bioprocess Development, Purification, Pharma Technical Development Biologics Europe, Roche Diagnostics GmbH, Penzberg, Germany

ANDREA HERRE, Biopharmaceuticals, Quality Control and Materials Testing, Boehringer Ingelheim Pharma GmbH & Co. KG, Biberach an der Riss, Germany

YIJIA JIANG, Process and Product Development, Amgen Inc., Thousand Oaks, California, USA

WIM JISKOOT, Division of Drug Delivery Technology, Biologics Formulation Group, Leiden University, Leiden, The Netherlands

LENE JØRGENSEN, Department of Pharmaceutics and Analytical Chemistry, University of Copenhagen, Copenhagen, Denmark

FABIAN KEBBEL, Pharmaceutical Development, Process Science/Biopharmaceuticals, Boehringer Ingelheim Pharma GmbH & Co. KG, Biberach an der Riss, Germany

WERNER KLICHE, Biopharmaceuticals, Quality Control and Materials Testing, Boehringer Ingelheim Pharma GmbH & Co. KG, Biberach an der Riss, Germany

ATANAS KOULOV, Analytical Research and Development of the Process Science and Production Department, Novartis Pharma AG, Basel, Switzerland

WOLFGANG KUHNE, Bioprocess Development, Purification, Pharma Technical Development Biologics Europe, Roche Diagnostics GmbH, Penzberg, Germany

MARKUS LANKERS, rap.Id Particle Systems GmbH, Berlin, Germany

THORSTEN LEMM, Bioprocess Development, Purification, Pharma Technical Development Biologics Europe, Roche Diagnostics GmbH, Penzberg, Germany

JUN LIU, Late Stage Pharmaceutical Development, Genentech, Inc., South San Francisco, California, USA

HANNS-CHRISTIAN MAHLER, Pharmaceutical and Device Development, Pharma Technical Development Biologics Europe, F. Hoffmann-La Roche Ltd, Basel, Switzerland

CHARLES RUSSELL MIDDAUGH, Department of Pharmaceutical Chemistry, University of Kansas, Lawrence, Kansas, USA

LINDA NARHI, Process and Product Development, Amgen Inc., Thousand Oaks, California, USA

JOHN S. PHILO, Alliance Protein Laboratories, Thousand Oaks, California, USA

ROBERT A. POOLE, Division of Drug Delivery Technology, Biologics Formulation Group, Leiden University, Leiden, The Netherlands

MIRIAM PRINTZ, Department of Pharmacy, Pharmaceutical Technology and Biopharmaceutics, Ludwig-Maximilians-University Munich, Munich, Germany

RAHUL S. RAJAN, Process and Product Development, Amgen Inc., Thousand Oaks, California, USA

HANS ROGL, Bioprocess Development, Purification, Pharma Technical Development Biologics Europe, Roche Diagnostics GmbH, Penzberg, Germany

AMY S. ROSENBERG, Division of Therapeutic Proteins, U.S. Food and Drug Administration, Rockville, Maryland, USA

EVA ROSENBERG, Bioprocess Development, Purification, Pharma Technical Development Biologics Europe, Roche Diagnostics GmbH, Penzberg, Germany

STEVEN J. SHIRE, Late Stage Pharmaceutical Development, Genentech, Inc., South San Francisco, California, USA

RONALD SMULDERS, Analytical Method and Validation, Merck Manufacturing Division, Oss, The Netherlands

MARCO VAN DE WEERT, Department of Pharmaceutics and Analytical Chemistry, University of Copenhagen, Copenhagen, Denmark

OLIVER VALET, rap.Id Particle Systems GmbH, Berlin, Germany

HANS VOS, Biological and Sterile Product Development, Schering plough Research Institute, Oss, The Netherlands

GERHARD WINTER, Department of Pharmacy, Pharmaceutical Technology and Biopharmaceutics, Ludwig-Maximilians-University Munich, Munich, Germany

FRANK ZETTL, Bioprocess Development, Purification, Pharma Technical Development Biologics Europe, Roche Diagnostics GmbH, Penzberg, Germany

HUI ZHAO, Analytical Research and Development of the Process Science and Production Department, Novartis Pharma AG, Basel, Switzerland

RALF ZIPPELIUS, Pharma Biotech Production, Roche Diagnostics GmbH, Penzberg, Germany

PREFACE

Protein pharmaceuticals are increasingly used to treat life-threatening and chronic diseases, such as several forms of cancer and inflammation, viral infections, metabolic disorders, and central nervous system diseases. The pharmaceutical quality of these important products is the key to their safety and efficacy. To assess and assure the high quality of protein pharmaceuticals during their development, production, and use, science- and risk-based comprehensive analytical and process strategies are required.

With respect to the quality of protein pharmaceuticals, especially protein aggregation, particles have recently received increased interest from industry, academia, and regulators as some aggregates may have biological consequences, such as immunogenicity, altered bioactivity, or altered pharmacokinetics. In a protein pharmaceutical, aggregates would include all protein assemblies larger than the smallest naturally occurring, active subunit (e.g., monomer). Protein aggregates can differ in structure, size, "solubility," reversibility, and type of bond, as further explained in the Glossary. Particles are defined as *undissolved species*—other than gas bubbles—that are unintentionally present in the product. Particles can be subdivided according to their size and can be proteinaceous or nonproteinaceous (see Glossary).

This book covers a broad range of analytical methods to detect and characterize the entire spectrum of protein aggregates and particles that may be present in a protein pharmaceutical. Moreover, it provides examples of how these methods can be applied during process and formulation development. An introduction to the topic of aggregates and particles, especially with regard to their potential immunogenicity, is given in Chapter 1. Chapters 2–4 deal with analytical methods related to "soluble" aggregates, based on separation, light scattering, and some emerging techniques. Chapters 5–7 deal with so-called insoluble aggregates and particles. Methods to measure subvisible particles are discussed first, followed by a discussion on visible particles. Finally, some emerging methods to measure insoluble matter are discussed. Chapters 8–12 deal with spectroscopic techniques that may help to characterize aggregates and particles, to better elucidate their structure, as well as to identify and differentiate proteinaceous and nonproteinaceous particles. Specific chapters are devoted to UV–vis, fluorescence, infrared and Raman spectroscopy, and microscopic methods. In Chapter 13, various methods are discussed and compared in the overall context of aggregate analysis. Finally, Chapters 14 and 15 are dedicated to discussing approaches to tackle aggregates and particles encountered during protein purification and formulation development.

This book not only provides a comprehensive overview of methods to analyze protein aggregates and particles but also includes case studies to illustrate challenges in this area. Technical and nontechnical scientists from analytics, process development, formulation development, quality control and quality assurance, regulatory sciences, manufacturing and project management, as well as interested parties from industry, academia, and regulatory authorities will benefit from this book. In addition, the book can serve as reference for students in the field of protein pharmaceuticals.

WIM JISKOOT
HANNS-CHRISTIAN MAHLER

Leiden, The Netherlands
Basel, Switzerland
October 2011

GLOSSARY

Protein Aggregates All protein assemblies larger (e.g., dimer, hexamer, ... million-mer, ...) than the smallest naturally occurring, active subunit (e.g., monomer).

Protein aggregates can differ in

1. Structure (native, denatured, or partially denatured)
2. Size (small to large; nanometer to millimeter range)
3. "Solubility"[1]
   (a) *Soluble aggregates* are aggregate species that are small enough to enter the column of a chromatographic separation or that cannot be filtered or centrifuged with predefined separation processes
   (b) *Insoluble aggregates* are aggregate species that can be filtered or centrifuged and thus typically escape chromatographic separation without further sample preparation
4. Reversibility (i.e., irreversible aggregates vs reversible aggregates/self-association)
5. Type of bond: covalent (S–S mediated or non-S–S mediated) versus noncovalent aggregates.

Particles Undissolved species—other than gas bubbles—that are unintentionally present in the product. These may include foreign particles or protein particles.

Foreign Particles Particles that are not intrinsic to the product and therefore typically are not proteinaceous. Examples include particles derived from contaminations of primary packaging (e.g., glass particles in vials), insects or insect parts, and contaminations derived from manufacturing process (e.g., cellulose fiber from cleaning wipes, metal parts from pumps, etc.).

---

[1]Categorizing an aggregate as being "soluble" or "insoluble" depends on the method and conditions used (e.g., chromatographic column, eluent, filter size, filter material, centrifugation time and speed, etc.).

Protein Particles   Protein aggregates that are sufficiently large to be detected "visually" or by using detection methods for "subvisible" particles. A protein particle may also be defined as a *large insoluble aggregate*.

Visible Particles   Insoluble matter that can be visualized by respective inspection aids and means such as light, rotation, magnification lenses, and adequate background. Visibility may depend on a number of factors. Visibility can be in the range of about 75–150 μm (arbitrary boundary) and larger. Visible particles may include foreign particles or protein particles.

Subvisible Particles   Insoluble matter that cannot be easily visualized, which falls into the category of "particles" (i.e., larger than may be 1 μm but not yet visible, i.e., 75–150 μm; arbitrary boundaries). Subvisible particles may include foreign particles or protein particles.

Submicrometer Particles   Insoluble matter between about 0.1 and 1 μm (arbitrary boundaries). Submicrometer particles may include foreign particles or protein particles.

1 The Critical Need for Robust Assays for Quantitation and Characterization of Aggregates of Therapeutic Proteins

JOHN F. CARPENTER

Department of Pharmaceutical Sciences, University of Colorado Denver, Aurora, Colorado, USA

BARRY CHERNEY and AMY S. ROSENBERG

Division of Therapeutic Proteins, U.S. Food and Drug Administration, Rockville, Maryland, USA

1.1 INTRODUCTION

Since the commercialization of monoclonal antibodies and recombinant therapeutic proteins in the 1980s, millions of lives have been saved or improved by these unique medicines. As with all therapeutics, assurance of product quality is key to providing a consistent clinical performance related to both safety and effectiveness. These assurances are more challenging with therapeutic proteins than with small molecular entities because of their heightened susceptibility to degradation via physical or chemical means, the dependency for their activity on often complex three-dimensional conformation, the complicated manufacturing processes needed for their production, and their propensity to induce immune responses, relative to small molecular entities. Indeed, extensive development and formulation studies to obtain a product that has appropriate stability during production, shipping, storage, and delivery to the patients are undertaken for each protein therapeutic. Robust, high resolution analytical methods are essential to meet the requirement to ensure product quality and for the development of the appropriate means to stabilize the protein.

Analysis of Aggregates and Particles in Protein Pharmaceuticals, First Edition.
Edited by Hanns-Christian Mahler, Wim Jiskoot.
© 2012 John Wiley & Sons, Inc., Published 2012 by John Wiley & Sons, Inc.

Degradation of therapeutic proteins by one or multiple means (e.g., heat, light, agitation, and long-term storage in aqueous solution) causes a loss of product quality and, critically, may cause adverse effects on safety and efficacy. Among degradation products of therapeutic proteins that have adverse effects on safety and efficacy are protein aggregates [1,2]. Aggregates include assemblies of protein molecules ranging from dimers to those large enough (e.g., ≥ 0.5 μm) to be classified as subvisible particles to larger, visible particles. Typically, oligomeric protein aggregates that are small enough to remain in solution are referred to as *soluble aggregates* and/or *high molecular weight species*. Assemblies of protein molecules large enough to be pelleted during centrifugation or filtered out of solution are often termed *insoluble aggregates*. Aggregate assemblies large enough to be detected and quantified with particle-counting instruments are usually called *subvisible particles*. If they are large enough to be seen with the unaided eye, particles are referred to as *visible*.

There are many challenges regarding the choice of analytical methods for assessment of protein aggregates and evaluation of the data from such methods. First, the methods employed must cover the extremely large size range of aggregates, usually requiring several methods to provide rigorous data across this size range [3,4]. Second, analysis of aggregates is challenging because the mass fraction of the aggregates in a sample may be extremely low (e.g., 0.1–1.0%), thus requiring highly sensitive methods. Third, the process of conducting the analysis may change the aggregate composition in a sample. For example, sample dilution during size-exclusion chromatography may cause disaggregation [3]. Thus, it absolutely essential to use orthogonal methods to assure the accuracy and robustness of a given analytical method for protein aggregates [5]. Orthogonal methods are those that use a different operating principle to obtain corroborating data on a given analyte. For example, sedimentation velocity analytical ultracentrifugation (SV-AUC) is routinely used to confirm results from size-exclusion chromatography [2–5].

Besides presenting challenges for analytical methods, aggregates pose a particular concern for patient safety in that they may be potent inducers of immune responses with varying manifestations [1,2]. The spectrum of clinical effects induced by aggregates pertains to a multiplicity of factors including but not limited to their size and valency, whether the key epitopes in the protein are in the native state or degraded, and whether the therapeutic protein product has an endogenous counterpart or is a foreign protein [1,2]. On one end of the spectrum are mild effects including minor alterations of pharmacokinetics, while on the other end of the spectrum are serious clinical effects including frank anaphylactic reactions (IgG or IgE mediated), neutralization of product activity with loss of efficacy, and, for therapeutic counterparts of endogenous proteins, neutralization of both product and endogenous counterpart [1,2]. The latter may result in a factor or cellular deficiency caused by loss of activity of the endogenous protein, if it has a unique function. Immune responses triggered by aggregates may target aggregate-specific (i.e., denatured or cryptic) epitopes, which do not cross react on the native protein, such as was the case in older studies of human serum albumin, intravenous immunoglobulin, and human growth hormone [1,2]. Alternatively, immune responses triggered by aggregates in which the native protein conformation is preserved may neutralize the critical native domains that mediate activity, as is the case for example, for a percentage of patients taking type I interferon therapy [1,2].

Indeed, advantage has been taken of the capacity of a protein, in its native state, to elicit an immune response by constructing or formulating target proteins as particulates in vaccines. Typically, in vaccines, the particulates are formed by adsorbing the protein antigen onto the surface of another material such as a colloidal aluminum salt or other experimental microparticles [6]. Heterogeneous particles may also be present among protein aggregates in therapeutic protein products [6] arising from adsorption of proteins to particles originating from filling pumps, such as stainless steel particles, or from the container closure, such as glass particles [7–9].

There is a preponderance of data in the literature that indicate that aggregates are culprits in causing immune responses to protein therapeutics and vaccine antigens (reviewed in 1,2). Therefore, for protein therapeutics, it is critical to assure that aggregates are at the lowest level practical and to minimize, in particular, the higher MW aggregates with multiple repetitive units, implicated in immune response induction. Meeting this standard requires that manufacturing processes, formulations, storage and shipping conditions, and education of patients and medical personnel administering these drugs are optimized for minimizing aggregate formation and that there are proper, robust, and high resolution assays developed to quantify and characterize protein aggregates for each therapeutic protein.

Developing such assays properly requires substantial knowledge and expertise—with respect to the specific challenges of the assays as well as to the properties of the given protein—because each therapeutic protein has unique physicochemical properties giving rise to different degradation pathways that engender aggregation. For example, even minor sequence changes (e.g., point mutations) or chemical degradation of a few residues in therapeutic monoclonal antibodies can cause different stability and aggregation behaviors [10,11]. For these reasons, it is generally not sufficient to rely on so-called platform analytical methods for a given class of products such as monoclonal antibodies. Of course, the experience and expertise gained with analytical method development for similar proteins can be extremely valuable in guiding work on a new therapeutic protein, and a standard algorithm to method development can guide and substantially shorten the development cycle. But ultimately, analytical methods for each protein product must be "customized" for that particular protein. Shortcuts could lead to problems with reliability and accuracy of analytical methods that could compromise product quality and patient safety.

Therefore, appropriate time and resource investment, in the areas of process understanding and validation, personnel training, equipment, facilities, raw materials qualification, and analytical methods development and validation are required because these are ultimately essential to development of successful manufacturing and commercialization processes. The main methods for analysis of protein aggregates, their development and applications, challenges with their implementation, and the critical technical issues affecting their performance are expertly discussed in this book. These methods fall into the broad categories described below.

1.2 METHODS FOR SIZING AND QUANTIFYING SOLUBLE AGGREGATES

The main analytical method used to quantify and size soluble aggregates is high performance size-exclusion chromatography (HP-SEC) [3–5]. This method is used to characterize protein aggregates during process development for bulk drug substance and for release and stability assessments for drug product as well as during formulation development. Therefore, it is critically important that the values generated by HP-SEC for a given therapeutic protein precisely and accurately reflect the actual values for aggregates in a sample. Meeting this goal is challenging because of the potential for aggregates to dissociate during HP-SEC runs and/or to adsorb to the column media [3–5]. Owing to these problems, orthogonal methods should be employed to assess and assure the accuracy of results from HP-SEC and to guide development of robust HP-SEC methods for a given protein [3–5]. Currently, SV-AUC is a method used for this purpose, but this method also has its own challenges for obtaining robust, reproducible results for protein aggregates. There are also efforts to develop field-flow fractionation as a method to quantify and size soluble aggregates but because of its own particular challenges, this approach has not yet been as widely adopted as SEC-HPLC and SV-AUC.

1.3 METHODS FOR SIZING AND QUANTIFYING PARTICLES

Protein aggregates that are large enough to be considered as particles often constitute a minute mass fraction of the protein molecules in the drug product. Therefore, typically, the amount of protein in particles cannot be quantified based on loss of monomer. Instead, the particles are counted and sized by methods such as light obscuration, microflow imaging, and Coulter counting [12]. Each of these methods has its benefits and drawbacks, and there is a substantial amount of new research in this area [12]. Among the critical points is the need to differentiate between microparticles containing both foreign materials (and to identify the foreign material) and protein and those containing protein alone, as this is essential for identifying causative factors and precluding aggregate formation in subsequent lots. Of course, because proteins readily adsorb to foreign microparticles arising from materials involved in product manufacture and storage (e.g., steel particles from piston pumps and glass particles for storage vessels) [9], it is expected that essentially all particles analyzed will contain at least a fraction of protein molecules.

Special attention is given to visible particles because each lot of parenteral dosage forms (e.g., vials, syringes, or more rarely ampoules) is subjected to 100% visual inspection after manufacturing. This approach requires highly skilled and trained operators. There are now efforts to automate "visible inspection," which presumably could increase throughput.

1.4 METHODS FOR CHARACTERIZING CONFORMATION OF PROTEIN MOLECULES IN AGGREGATES

The conformation of protein molecules in aggregates can affect their biological activity as well as the consequences of immune responses directed to such of aggregates. Characterization of conformation of protein molecules in soluble aggregates can be studied in a mixture or after separation of a given aggregate population. Analysis by methods such as fluorescence spectroscopy (intrinsic, with fluorescence dyes or quenching), UV absorbance and near-UV circular dichroism spectroscopy, binding to conformationally dependent antibodies for tertiary structure, and infrared and far-UV circular dichroism spectroscopy for secondary structure should be considered. A potency assay for biological function may be used, although some proteins aggregated in their native state may lose the capacity to interact productively through their cognate receptors. For protein molecules in particles, in some cases, the particles can be separated from the solution and studied with these same spectroscopic methods [8].

1.5 REGULATORY ISSUES

It is a general principle that product quality attributes that contribute to clinical safety and efficacy must be identified, their levels correlated with clinical experience in patient populations, and specifications set for them to ensure that a favorable clinical performance profile is maintained with each lot of product produced. Of course, consistent with the principles established in the "Quality by Design Initiative," enhanced knowledge of the attribute's impact on the safety and efficacy profile of the product may allow more flexibility in setting specifications. Aggregates are considered a critical attribute in terms of their potential to elicit immune responses and affect product activity, enhancing or diminishing potency. Thus, even in phase I clinical trials, the aggregate content must be characterized and routinely measured for each lot by well-qualified assays and provisional specifications set.

Exploring process and formulation modifications to minimize protein aggregation is crucial during product development. Of course, for products that pose a higher risk to patient safety, such as those for which neutralizing antibodies can neutralize endogenous proteins with unique biological functions, special care must be taken at the earliest stages of product development to accurately detect protein aggregates and to minimize their formation. For licensed products, it is important to ensure that the preferred aggregate assay for routine aggregate assessment, such as HP-SEC, can detect all the aggregate species that are likely to be present in the product, based on a full understanding of the process as it affects aggregation and on product degradation pathways. Therefore, orthogonal methods such as SV-AUC, field-flow fractionation, or other potential methods should be used to verify that any method or set of methods proposed for routine detection of aggregate species is capable of detecting and quantifying the desired range of aggregate species. It may be necessary to evaluate the robustness of the HP-SEC assay by demonstrating its ability to detect all protein aggregates generated under relevant stress conditions. If so confirmed, then HP-SEC may be the sole tool utilized for aggregate detection for routine assessments. However, following significant changes in manufacture, as is routinely done for nearly all protein therapeutics in the course of development, a more extensive comparability study must be performed in which the critical product quality attributes of the post-manufacturing change product are compared with those of the pre-change product by using well-qualified and robust assays. In such cases, aggregate assessment may again warrant orthogonal techniques to evaluate the levels and types of aggregates present in the post-manufacturing change product.

Regarding particulate assessment, the light obscuration test, as defined by USP 30 monograph <788>, requires analysis of particles >10 and >25 µm, leaving a gap in assessment of particles in the 0.1–10 µm subvisible range [6]. Although light obscuration can be used to quantitate particles that are between 2 and 10 µm, other methods such as Resonant Mass Measurement or Nanoparticle Tracking Analysis are currently being developed and evaluated for quantitation of particles that are <2.0 µm in size. The use of novel methods for evaluation of protein particles in the GMP environment will require a concerted effort.

1.6 IMPORTANCE OF THE CURRENT BOOK

Protein aggregates are a critically important class of degradation products in therapeutic proteins. Therefore, robust analytical methods for aggregates are essential for assuring the safety and efficacy of these products and for guiding their development. The current book is an invaluable resource for researchers and managers working on therapeutic proteins. It provides expert reviews of the state-of-the art for the range of analytical methods used for assessment of protein aggregates and the numerous challenges that are unique to each method. Furthermore, the book provides insight into the future of method development and regulatory issues for protein aggregates. With comprehensive coverage of the key issues, this book will be a critical reference for the field for many years.

REFERENCES

1. Rosenberg AS. Effects of protein aggregates: an immunologic perspective. AAPS J 2006;8:E501–E507.

2. Cordoba-Rodriguez R. Aggregates in MAbs and recombinant therapeutic proteins: a regulatory perspective. Biopharm Int 2008;21(11):44–53.

3. Philo JS. Is any measurement method optimal for all aggregate sizes and types? AAPS J 2006;8:E564–E571.

4. Philo JS. A critical review of methods for size characterization of non-particulate protein aggregates. Curr Pharm Biotechnol 2009;10:358–372.

5. Carpenter JF, Randolph TW, Jiskoot W, Crommelin DJA, Middaugh CR, Winter G. Potential inaccurate quantitation and sizing of protein aggregates by size exclusion chromatography: essential need to use orthogonal methods to assure the quality of therapeutic protein products. J Pharm Sci 2010;99:2200–2208.

6. Singh M, Chakrapani A, D O'Hagan. Nanoparticles and microparticles as vaccine delivery systems. Expert Rev. Vaccines 2007;6:797–808.

7. Chi EY, Weickmann J, Carpenter JF, Manning MC, Randolph TW. Heterogeneous nucleation-controlled particle formation of recombinant human platelet-activating factor acetylhydrolase in pharmaceutical formulation. J Pharm Sci 2005;94:256–274.

8. Tyagi AK, Randolph TW, Dong A, Maloney KM, Hitscherich C, Carpenter JF Jr. IgG particle formation during filling pump operation: a case study of heterogeneous nucleation on stainless steel nanoparticles. J Pharm Sci 2009;98:94–104.

9. Bee JS, Chiu D, Sawicki S, Stevenson JL, Chatterjee K, Freund E, Carpenter JF, Randolph TW. Monoclonal antibody interactions with micro- and nanoparticles: adsorption, aggregation, and accelerated stress studies. J Pharm Sci 2009;98:3218–3238.

10. Lu Y, Harding SE, Rowe AJ, Davis KG, Fish B, Varley P, Gee C, Mulot S. The effect of a point mutation on the stability of IgG4 as monitored by analytical ultracentrifugation. J Pharm Sci 2008;97:960–969.

11. Liu D, Ren D, Huang H, Dankberg J, Rosenfeld R, Cocco MJ, Li L, Brems DN, Remmele RL Jr. Structure and stability changes of human IgG1 Fc as a consequence of methionine oxidation. Biochemistry 2008;47:5088–5100.

12. Narhi LO, Jiang Y, Cao S, Benedek K, Shnek D. A critical review of analytical methods for subvisible and visible particles. Curr Pharm Biotechnol 2009;10:373–381.

SECTION I
Methods Used for Detecting, Quantifying, and Sizing of Protein Aggregates and Particles

2 Separation-Based Analytical Methods for Measuring Protein Aggregation

JUN LIU, BARTHÉLEMY DEMEULE, and STEVEN J. SHIRE

Late Stage Pharmaceutical Development, Genentech, Inc., South San Francisco, California, USA

2.1 INTRODUCTION

Aggregation is one of the common degradation routes of protein pharmaceuticals and widely recognized as a critical quality attribute owing to its potential impact on product quality, safety, and efficacy [1–3]. The term *protein aggregates* refers to a broad spectrum of diversified self-associated states of proteins. The mechanisms of protein aggregation are quite complicated, and aggregates can form through different pathways [4,5]. Stressed conditions such as denaturants, organic solvents, high or low temperatures, agitation, freeze–thaw, cavitation, and low or high pH can cause structural alteration in proteins and result in aggregation [4–7]. In addition, chemical modifications, such as deamidation, isomerization, oxidation, fragmentation, and disulfide shuffling, have been shown to be related to protein aggregation in some cases [8]. Protein aggregates, particularly those formed by covalent linkages or strong noncovalent associations between unfolded molecules, are likely to be irreversible after simple dilution and are generally more stable than those formed by relatively weak noncovalent bonds. Stable aggregates are easier to detect as they are less likely to dissociate during the analytical process. Protein aggregates can also be formed because of reversible self-association of native molecules through noncovalent interactions, such as charge–charge, dipole–dipole, and hydrophobic interactions. The multivalent reversible self-association of proteins in their native form has been associated with an increase in solution viscosity, protein gelation, protein crystallization, and phase separation [9–13]. Although aggregates formed by proteins in their native conformation have the potential to generate more antidrug antibodies than those formed by unfolded proteins [14,15], it should be noted that not

Analysis of Aggregates and Particles in Protein Pharmaceuticals, First Edition.
Edited by Hanns-Christian Mahler, Wim Jiskoot.

all the aggregates are the same. Protein aggregates formed by weak reversible self-association can be easily dissociated in human serum owing to significant dilution. Even protein aggregates, which either slowly or never dissociate, may be perfectly safe and harmless. From a quality control point of view, these aggregates may have to be treated differently from those that may cause potential safety issues.

Protein aggregates can be found in all kinds of sizes and shapes (Chapter 1). The size of protein aggregates can be as small as a few nanometers where they are completely soluble to a size of a few micrometers or even millimeters where they become visible particles or precipitates. Because of the complexity of protein aggregation, there is no single analytical method that can cover the entire size range of protein aggregates. The accurate and precise detection and characterization of protein aggregates remain a challenging task, particularly for proteins in formulations or physiologically relevant conditions. Often orthogonal methods are implemented to analyze protein aggregates and to understand the mechanism of protein aggregation [9]. These methods have also been used to qualify and support the validation of size exclusion chromatography (SEC) for product release and stability testing [16].

The common analytical methods for the analysis of protein aggregates include SEC, analytical ultracentrifugation (AUC), field-flow fractionation (FFF), and gel electrophoresis. These methods involve partial or complete separation of the different species and are mainly used to measure the levels of protein aggregates and determine their sizes. Recently, the AUC with a fluorescence detection system (FDS) has also shown promise to measure protein self-association at high concentration directly in formulation buffer or human serum. Thus, for the first time, protein aggregates can be directly measured under physiologically relevant conditions, which may lead to a better understanding of the relationship between protein aggregation and immunogenicity [10]. In this chapter, we review the use of SEC, AUC, FFF, and gel electrophoresis for protein aggregate characterization and quantification. Several examples are presented to address the current practice, progress, and challenges.

2.2 SIZE EXCLUSION CHROMATOGRAPHY

2.2.1 Theory, Instrumentation, and Background

SEC, also known as gel filtration or gel permeation chromatography, is the most commonly used analytical method for the analysis of protein size distribution. The separation of proteins of different sizes is based on their differences in hydrodynamic volume, which is essentially a function of molecular weight (MW), shape, and solution properties. The SEC column is usually packed with cross-linked porous polymer microspheres with pores of various sizes. The species with larger hydrodynamic volumes elute earlier because they are excluded from the smaller pores, whereas the buffer and smaller proteins penetrate into a larger fraction of the pores resulting in longer elution times. Advances in chromatographic media have resulted in the development of column matrices with lower protein adsorption and sufficient mechanical strength [17,18] to prevent the collapse of the pores under the high pressure used in high-performance liquid chromatography (HPLC).

An SEC column is often used in an HPLC system. Samples are automatically injected into the column, and the elution is carried out at a constant flow rate by a high-pressure pump. Each individual peak is measured using different detectors, such as ultraviolet (UV), refractive index (RI), light scattering (LS), and viscometer detectors, for routine analysis and product characterization. The UV and RI detectors are mainly used for determining the concentration or weight percentage of each species. It is generally assumed that the protein aggregates have the same absorptivity or specific RI increment as the monomer; however, this assumption may not hold true if the environment of chromophores has been significantly altered due to self-association or fragmentation. In addition, LS from the large species may also contribute to the measured peak area, especially when the signal is collected at a low wavelength, such as at 214 nm. LS and viscometer detectors are mainly used to determine the size or MW of individual peaks. These methods have proved to be very useful to provide accurate assessment and characterization of different species [11].

2.2.2 Advantages, Challenges, and Key Considerations

SEC methods that are used in virtually every laboratory provide rapid and precise measurements of protein aggregates. The method can also be easily validated, and generic protocols have been developed for particular classes of protein pharmaceuticals, such as monoclonal antibodies, within the control system for product release or stability testing. The separation usually occurs under mild conditions and does not require specific protein binding to the column, thus significantly reducing the risk of protein loss through irreversible binding or protein inactivation. However, the method suffers from a few limitations that need to be carefully assessed. The separation is based on hydrodynamic volume of the different species rather than molecular mass. Therefore, large globular proteins may elute at the same place as smaller elongated or highly glycosylated species. This can result in significant errors in determinations of MW if an MW standard of globular protein is used [12] as it has been shown previously by work on highly pegylated and glycosylated proteins where the extended sugar or polyethylene glycol residues lead to greater hydrodynamic volume and thus greater apparent MW [19]. In addition, different protein molecules may interact very differently with the column matrix, particularly for those proteins with altered structures or under low-salt conditions. The large protein aggregates beyond the upper size limit of the SEC column may be filtered by the column matrix; therefore, it is important to assess sample recovery routinely. To avoid detector saturation and loss of resolution, high-concentration protein solutions are generally diluted even before injection onto the SEC column. This may interfere with the detection and characterization of concentration-dependent reversible aggregates.

The development of the SEC method usually includes selection of column matrix, elution buffers, injection volume/concentration, flow rate, and column temperature. The column matrices are often composed of beads made from cross-linked dextran, polyacrylamide, or agarose. The dextran and polyacrylamide matrices separate proteins of small-to-moderate MWs, while the agarose matrices have larger pores and are more applicable for separation of much larger proteins. The selection of a column matrix and column type should be based primarily on the size distribution of the proteins to be separated. Longer columns and smaller microspheres may increase the resolution of separation; however, a longer column may also increase the dilution, back pressure, and running time of the method. Therefore, these parameters should be carefully evaluated and balanced.

The elution buffer should have a pH compatible with the column matrix and the proteins. To prevent preferential interactions of aggregates with the column matrix, organic solvents or salts are often added to decrease matrix–protein interactions, but a careful study needs to be conducted to ensure that such chemical components do not cause protein aggregation and alter the true size distribution. The elution buffer should not contain chemicals that have significant UV absorption, which may interfere with detection. The mobile phase should be filtered and degassed, since air bubbles or particles can damage the column and significantly increase the baseline noise and interfere with the UV, LS, and RI detection.

To improve resolution, the protein sample should be relatively concentrated and the sample volume kept small (typically 1–5% of the column bed volume). The viscosity of the sample should not be significantly higher than the mobile phase buffer or peak broadening may occur. Higher flow rates will allow a faster separation; however, slower flow rates can result in better resolution of peaks.

To use SEC as an analytical tool for quantification of aggregates and estimation of a formulation's shelf life and physical characteristics, it is imperative to have reproducible measurements. For protein aggregates with dissociation rates on the timescale of the SEC separation, the method could lead to significant underestimation of protein aggregates. The rapid dissociation of a monoclonal antibody (mAb) on dilution can yield varying aggregate levels determined by SEC, depending on the product concentration, time, and temperature of analysis after sample dilution [20]. For slower dissociating protein aggregates, reproducible results can be obtained by optimizing the loading concentration and limiting the sample preparation and running time.

2.2.3 Applications

The SEC method has been widely used for detecting soluble aggregates of protein pharmaceuticals. Figure 2.1 shows an SEC chromatogram of an mAb after storage at 40°C for six months. The sample was eluted in phosphate-buffered saline (PBS) at a flow rate of 0.5 mL/min. The peaks shown in Fig. 2.1a were detected by a UV detector (Agilent Technologies) and in Fig. 2.1b by an online LS detector (Wyatt Technologies). The SEC method resolves both aggregates and fragments. The LS detector provided the MWs of aggregates. The high-molecular-weight species (HMS) have an MW of more than 1,000,000 Da, while

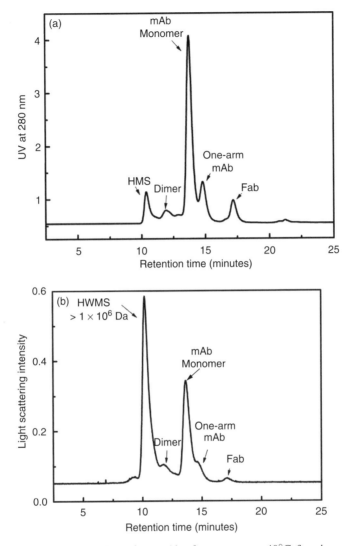

FIGURE 2.1 Size distribution of an mAb after storage at $40°C$ for six months. The SEC study was conducted using a TSK SUPER SW 3000 column (4.6×300 mm) in PBS (100 mM sodium chloride, 0.1 M potassium phosphate at pH 6.8). The chromatogram was collected using (a) a UV detector at 280 nm and (b) an LS detector at $90°$.

the smaller aggregate has an MW corresponding to a dimer. The two fragment peaks have also been identified as Fab and one-armed antibody. These are common degradation products for an mAb in a liquid formulation stored at elevated temperatures over time.

It is well known that the SEC method, in general, is less suitable for analyzing reversible protein aggregates, particularly for samples containing faster dissociating species, because of the significant dilution during the separation process. This limitation has been shown recently using several preparations of concentrated mAb and their fragments [21,22]. The reversible self-association was only detected by off-line LS and AUC at high protein concentration but not by the SEC method. For aggregates undergoing slow dissociation at the timescale of the SEC separation, the method can be optimized to provide useful information about protein aggregates. Examples using Avastin® have shown that the reversible aggregates can be detected under "neat" or undiluted conditions without sample incubation [20]. On the basis of the understanding of the kinetics of aggregate dissociation, an optimized SEC method has been successfully developed to measure protein aggregates for product release and stability testing.

2.3   ANALYTICAL ULTRACENTRIFUGATION

2.3.1   Theory, Instrumentation, and Background

The AUC is a versatile tool and has been the method of choice for studying the reversible self-association of macromolecules [9]. The AUC can be operated in two basic modes: sedimentation velocity and sedimentation equilibrium. Although there is no physical separation of protein species in centrifuge cells during sedimentation equilibrium experiments, sedimentation equilibrium and velocity methods are closely related. Thus, we include the discussion of both methods in this chapter. The sedimentation velocity experiment is usually conducted at relatively high rotor speeds and the centrifuge run only takes a few hours to complete. Each protein species can form a unique boundary and sediment at a characteristic speed under a specified centrifugal force on the basis of its molecular mass and shape. The velocity of the moving boundary determines the sedimentation coefficient, which is defined as the sedimentation velocity divided by the centrifugal field strength. The sedimentation coefficient depends not only on the molecular mass but also on the shape of the molecule. Analysis of the sedimentation coefficient and shape of the moving boundary can yield the size distribution, diffusion coefficient, MW, and even equilibrium constants of interacting species [23]. The sedimentation equilibrium experiment is often operated at lower rotor speeds, and the experiment usually takes a few days to complete. The sedimentation of proteins under the lower centrifugal field is opposed by diffusion and buoyancy, and eventually when they reach equilibrium, a time-independent exponential concentration gradient of the protein is established throughout the centrifuge cell. The concentration gradient at equilibrium can be rigorously described by the first principle of thermodynamic theory and has been widely used to determine the MW, stoichiometry, binding affinity, and virial coefficient of interacting or self-associating proteins [24].

The AUC essentially consists of a high-speed centrifuge with a precise temperature control, a rotor with several cell compartments, and optical systems that measure the concentration of proteins under any speed at a given time and radial position. The protein samples and buffer reference are loaded into parallel channels in a centerpiece that is covered by a quartz or sapphire window on each

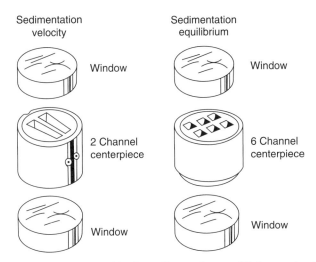

FIGURE 2.2   Typical cell assembly for sedimentation equilibrium and velocity experiments.

side (Fig. 2.2). The concentration of proteins under a centrifugal field along the radial position can be determined at any given time by absorption, interference, and fluorescence optical systems.

The UV/VIS absorption optical system measures protein concentration based on the fact that many macromolecular species such as protein and DNA contain chromophores that absorb incident light in the UV range. The concentration of macromolecules is calculated according to Beer's law. The absorption optical system offers high sensitivity and specificity and can discriminate between molecules with different chromophores. Depending on the step size, the radial scan by the UV/VIS optical system can take up to several minutes. This can have a significant impact on the number of scans acquired during each experiment. The absorption optical system uses a Xenon flash lamp, providing a usable wavelength range between 190 and 800 nm. The accuracy of the wavelength is calibrated with the spectrum of incident light or a wavelength reference cell that contains a holmium oxide filter. The typical accuracy of the wavelength is within ± 3 nm.

The interference optical system measures the protein concentration based on changes in RI. It provides rapid, high-precision data acquisition for samples in a broad range of concentrations [25]. In addition, the interference optical system can be used with molecular species that do not contain chromophores with a significant absorbance in the UV–visible range. The light source for the interference optical system is a 30-mW, 660-nm laser. The interference patterns are recorded digitally on a CCD camera and then converted to a graphical representation of fringe displacement as a function of radial position. The fringe displacement is related to weight concentration through the specific RI, cell optical pathlength, and wavelength. The interference optical system captures data much faster than the current UV/VIS optical system; therefore, it can generate more scans from each run. This should help to improve the reproducibility of data analysis. The fast UV absorbance optical system that is currently being developed overcomes the scan speed limitation and has better sensitivity and wavelength precision [26]. This should significantly improve the results obtained with the UV/VIS optical system.

Both interference and UV/VIS optical system are limited by the large RI gradients formed during sedimentation of high-concentration protein solutions. These gradients result in an effect known as *Wiener skewing* where the light beam is bent, resulting in a decrease of the intensity of the transmitted light [27]. Decreasing the optical pathlength by using thin gaskets or cell centerpieces with pathlengths as narrow as 0.6 mm rather than the standard centerpiece with 1.2 cm pathlength has been used to circumvent this problem [27], but loading of the cells can be complicated and difficult. For sedimentation equilibrium analysis, an alternate technique that uses a preparative ultracentrifuge has been described and used to analyze protein formulations at 100 mg/mL [21,28].

The FDS is the most recent addition to the AUC. The instrument uses a confocal optical configuration comprising a CW solid-state laser with excitation wavelength at 488 nm. The emission is collected above 505 nm using a band pass filter [29]. The fluorescence optical system measures the protein's concentration distribution based on the fluorescence intensity of a fluorescently labeled protein or protein with intrinsic fluorescence. For most of the protein pharmaceuticals, labeling of a protein with a fluorescent dye such as Alexa Fluor 488® is required to obtain an adequate signal. The condition of labeling should be optimized and labeled protein should be characterized to ensure that the protein is not significantly altered. The method has high sensitivity, dynamic range, and specificity and allows for the detection of protein aggregates in more complex matrices such as highly concentrated protein formulations, cell culture media, and human serum. The specificity and sensitivity of an FDS are accomplished by using the fluorescently labeled mAb as a reporter molecule, which is added at low concentration to the unlabeled mAb at a high concentration or complex biological media. Since the fluorescent signal is collected from a narrow layer of sample on the top of the centrifuge cell, the RI gradients formed by high-concentration protein do not interfere with the fluorescent signal. Thus, it can be used for the analysis of highly concentrated protein solutions [30].

2.3.2   Advantages, Challenges, and Key Considerations

With recent advances in hardware and data analysis software, particularly for sedimentation velocity analysis, the AUC has become one of the most widely used orthogonal approaches for measuring and characterizing the size distribution of therapeutic protein aggregates in the biopharmaceutical industry. Sedimentation velocity studies have been used routinely to confirm SEC results. Quantification and identification of major aggregate species have been performed successfully for protein pharmaceuticals [16].

Sedimentation velocity and sedimentation equilibrium are considered as the preferred methods for analyzing reversible self-associating proteins since they have limited sample dilution during the centrifuge run and are compatible with many different buffer conditions. In sedimentation velocity analysis, the boundary formed during the sedimentation will become a reaction boundary in the presence of reversible self-association. The reaction boundary corresponds to not only the individual interacting species but also the redistribution between these species at different concentrations. Analysis of the amplitude and asymptotic shape of the reaction boundary can yield qualitative information on reversible interacting systems [31]. In sedimentation equilibrium analysis, the concentration gradients formed by interacting species at different concentrations for a fixed rotor speed and temperature are governed by their MWs and equilibrium constants. Analysis of the concentration gradient using appropriate mathematical models yields quantitative information about the size and distribution of protein species.

Like many biophysical methods, the AUC also has its own limitations. The method has a low throughput and requires well-trained personnel to conduct the experiment and analyze data. Some excipients, such as sorbitol, at high concentration and high rotor speed may create a significant concentration gradient that can affect the accuracy of quantitation. This will often require additional effort to optimize the experimental condition and data analysis process [32]. Sedimentation equilibrium experiments can take days or even weeks to complete. The method is most useful to study reversible protein aggregates. Unlike the sedimentation velocity analysis, the sedimentation equilibrium method usually is not sensitive enough to pick up the small amounts of protein aggregates typically observed in protein pharmaceuticals. The mathematical fitting of self-association models can be difficult and extremely time consuming due to the complexity of the protein aggregate distribution. Often the sample will be exposed to light and relatively high-pressure conditions caused by the centrifugal force; products that are sensitive to the high pressure or light exposure may not be adequately characterized by the AUC [33]. The data analysis of AUC greatly relies on the mathematical fitting and modeling, which may create artificial peaks for low levels of product-related impurities or reduce the accuracy of estimation for species that have very different conformation from the major species. Therefore, a careful evaluation of the data and understanding of the protein are essential for accurately interpreting the results [9].

Sedimentation velocity experiments are usually conducted in a double-sector centerpiece with sample and buffer on either side (Fig. 2.2). The experiment is carried out at relatively high rotor speed, and the speed can be optimized based on the size distribution of species. The sedimentation velocity experiment usually takes a few hours at a controlled temperature. Sedimentation equilibrium experiments are usually conducted using six-channel centerpieces (Fig. 2.2). Each centerpiece can hold up to three samples and three corresponding reference buffer solutions. The experiment is usually conducted at relatively low rotor speed and will take days to complete. Therefore, the stability of the protein should be carefully evaluated throughout the run.

The AUC measures protein concentration at a specific radial position and time point during the sedimentation process. The precision and accuracy of these measurements are essential for detection, particularly for measuring trace amounts of soluble aggregates. The precision and accuracy of AUC measurements very much rely on instrument and operating conditions. It has been previously shown that the wavelength drift, the signal-to-noise ratios, and variations in the rotor temperature can significantly impact the results [9]. Therefore, obtaining high precision requires careful maintenance of the instrumentation as well as additional steps to minimize both systematic and random noise. The wavelength and radial position accuracy as well as rotor temperature should be checked and calibrated regularly using reference or internal standards to ensure that the instrument is performing properly. The alignment of the AUC cell with the center of rotation can also be a factor [34]. An alignment tool can be used to improve the precision and accuracy of measurements. For the absorption system, it is important to avoid buffer or excipient components that have significant absorption at the wavelength of detection.

For accurate quantification, it is important to avoid the use of thermodynamically nonideal conditions, such as low-salt and high-protein concentration, since most analysis software and mathematical models are not designed to handle nonideal systems properly. The detection wavelength should be selected within a flat region of the absorbance peak so that the absorbance signal is not significantly impacted by a small wavelength drift. The numbers of scans within the specified time range are also important for quantitative analysis. In general, the more scans used for data analysis, the more reliable and reproducible the results will be. For the absorbance optical system, an increase in scan numbers can be achieved by lowering the temperature, using a larger radial step size or simply running a single cell in a run. For better quantitative analysis, it is also important to run the same sample multiple times, as this will provide statistical information on the results. Finally, as is true for any biophysical method, it is important to review the limitations and assumptions and verify the results from the AUC by using other orthogonal approaches.

The analysis of AUC data is a critical step and historically has been a time-consuming and difficult process. In a manner similar to SEC chromatograms analysis, the sedimentation coefficient distribution of each species can be plotted as a peak and easily integrated for quantitation. Several sedimentation velocity analysis methods have been developed over the years [23]. The c(s) method from SEDFIT is a more recent method that was developed by Peter Schuck. This method uses finite-element solutions of the Lamm equation by direct fitting of the velocity data [23]. The sedimentation coefficient distribution from this method has a much improved resolution and covers a broader size distribution, since it explicitly corrects for the broadening due to diffusion and all the scans can be used in the analysis. In addition, this method includes a sophisticated regularization routine to help in removing spurious peaks that are caused by the noise in the raw data. This method has been widely used in the biopharmaceutical industry for monitoring the size distribution of aggregates.

For sedimentation velocity data analysis using SEDFIT, it is important to assess whether the model fits well with the data in terms of the root mean square deviation (RMSD) and distribution of the residuals of the fit. The residuals bitmap plot from SEDFIT has been found to be very useful to identify the systematic deviations of the fitted curve from the raw data. The meniscus position in a sedimentation velocity experiment often occurs as an apparent absorbance peak using the absorbance optical system but is less noticeable using the interference optical system. The meniscus position corresponding to the starting position of sedimentation is a critical parameter for SEDFIT analysis. Although the meniscus position can be obtained by a least-square fitting, it does not always return to the correct position. As shown before, a slight shift of meniscus from the correct position can have a significant impact on the quantitative analysis of small amounts of protein aggregates [9].

In many cases, the assumption of a constant frictional ratio used in SEDFIT is valid, but this should be verified whether the aggregate can be separated and collected for further characterization [9]. For a system where there are significant differences in frictional ratio between two individual species, the c(s) analysis using a weight average value can produce significant errors on quantitation. This problem may be overcome by using a bimodal model where the frictional ratio for each individual species can be fitted separately [9].

2.3.3 Applications

The AUC is one of the most versatile tools to study protein aggregation. Sedimentation velocity has been used to analyze molecules with sizes from nanometer to micrometer [35]. It is an important orthogonal method to support SEC method development. Figure 2.3 shows examples of an mAb after storage at −70 and 40°C for six months. The sedimentation velocity data were analyzed using SEDFIT to yield a size distribution of protein degradation products. The major degradation products, including two fragments peaks and several major aggregate peaks, were resolved by both the SEC (Fig. 2.1a) and sedimentation velocity methods (Fig. 2.3). However, the sedimentation velocity method clearly shows better resolution of fragments and aggregates than those by the SEC method (Fig. 2.1a). In addition, more aggregate peaks were resolved by the sedimentation velocity method. Although the identities of those additional peaks are not fully understood and additional characterization work would be required to substantiate the presence of these peaks, the data clearly demonstrate the power of the sedimentation velocity method as an orthogonal method to monitor the size distribution of aggregates.

Recently with the introduction of the FDS, the sedimentation velocity method has shown a promising ability to analyze protein association in biologically relevant conditions [10]. To detect a protein sample with the fluorescence detector, the protein usually needs to be labeled with a fluorescent dye. Importantly, characterization studies were conducted to ensure that the labeling process did not significantly alter the protein structure and function. Figure 2.4 shows an example of omalizumab, a humanized anti-IgE mAb in human serum. The labeled mAb

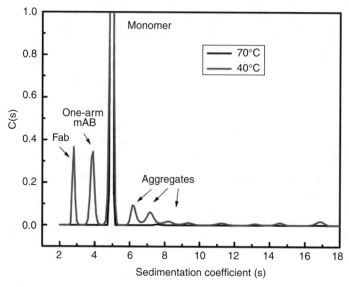

FIGURE 2.3 Sedimentation velocity analysis of an mAb in a liquid formulation after storage at −70 and 40°C for six months. The centrifuge experiments were conducted at 40,000 rpm and 10°C. The data were analyzed by SEDFIT using the continuous c(s) model. *(See insert for color representation of the figure.)*

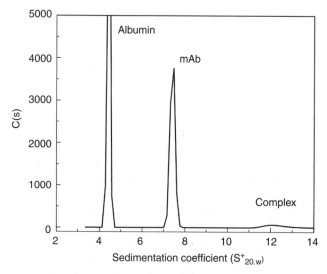

FIGURE 2.4 Sedimentation velocity analysis of fluorescently labeled omalizumab in human serum. The experiments were conducted at 40,000 rpm and 25°C. The data were collected using a fluorescence detector, and the size distribution of the sedimentation coefficient was determined by SEDFIT using a continuous c(s) model.

was mixed with human serum, and sedimentation was monitored with a fluorescence detector. Two major species were detected: the first peak at ~ 4.2 s was identified as human serum albumin, while the second peak at ~ 7.2 s is the monomer peak of the mAb. The fluorescence signal of albumin was not from intrinsic fluorescence, but from albumin-bound fluorescent molecules, such as flavins and hemoglobin oxidation products [10]. The sedimentation coefficient of the antibody in human serum, once corrected for serum density and viscosity, was very close to what is expected for an intact mAb in PBS. In addition to albumin and mAb, a trace amount of a large aggregate species at ~ 12s was also detected. This aggregate peak was not observed in PBS, but showed a similar size as intermediate complex formed by antibody and antigen, suggesting that it is likely due to the complex formed by omalizumab and the endogenous IgE.

Protein aggregates have also been detected by sedimentation equilibrium analysis. Although sedimentation equilibrium does not separate aggregates from monomer, the method can provide better estimates on the MW of aggregates. For a sample containing both monomer and HMS, sedimentation equilibrium will give a weight average MW. The data can be further fitted with a mathematical model to obtain the thermodynamic properties, such as binding affinity, stoichiometry, and virial coefficient [24]. Figure 2.5 shows a sedimentation equilibrium analysis of a self-associating mAb. The weight average MW determined by fitting the data as a single ideal species clearly demonstrates the concentration dependence of weight average MW, indicating the presence of protein self-association.

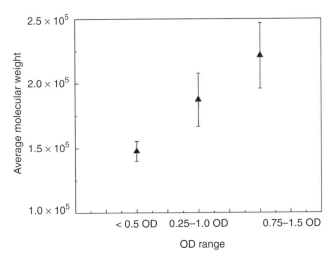

FIGURE 2.5 Sedimentation equilibrium analysis of an mAb as a function of protein concentrations. The experiments were conducted at 7000, 10,000, and 15,000 rpm at 20°C in PBS. The concentration was measured using a UV absorbance system. The data were analyzed using the Microsoft Windows-based software, Nonlin.

2.4   FIELD-FLOW FRACTIONATION

2.4.1   Theory, Instrumentation, and Background

The FFF refers to a family of flow-based separation techniques. The separation of protein molecules is achieved by applying an externally generated field that is perpendicular to a laminar flow in a channel. The field drives protein molecules toward an accumulation wall and differences in Brownian motion or diffusion create differences in the concentration distribution in the laminar flow, resulting in different elution times. The external vertical field can be gravitational, centrifugal, magnetic, electrical, temperature, or flow based [36]. The external field forms the basis of each FFF separation method. Among all these techniques, the flow FFF technique that uses a cross flow to create a vertical field has been widely used and is most suitable for the separation of protein aggregates [37]. For most protein molecules, the size of aggregates is well below ∼1 μm, and therefore, the separation purely relies on the diffusion coefficient of the protein species. This is also known as *normal mode FFF operation*. In contrast, for protein particles that are larger than ∼1 μm in size, the diffusion effect is essentially negligible [36]. The larger particles driven by the vertical field will accumulate at the wall and form a thicker layer as a result of their larger sizes. These particles will tend to distribute more close to the center of a laminar flow; therefore, the larger particles will be eluted earlier than the smaller particles. This is also known as *steric-hyperlayer mode* [38].

During the typical flow FFF operation under normal mode, protein samples are first injected into a thin and elongated channel. A semipermeable membrane, such as regenerated cellulose, that is permeable to the elution buffer but not to the protein samples serves as an accumulation wall, preventing larger protein molecules from exiting the channel via the cross flow. After injection, the protein samples will be focused and equilibrated into a narrow band by two opposite laminar flows and a vertical flow and then eluted with the channel flow into a detector. The smaller molecules have larger diffusion coefficients and tend to distribute closer to the center of laminar flow where the flow rate will be the fastest. This will result in an earlier elution of smaller molecules than larger molecules. In a normal elution mode, the retention time is related by a well-defined equation to the applied field and the translational diffusion of the proteins. The diffusion coefficient of different proteins, fragments, and aggregates can then be determined and MW can be calculated assuming spherical structure for all components.

Asymmetrical flow FFF is the most commonly used form of flow FFF technology in the industry. Unlike the symmetric flow FFF, where the channel is covered by two permeable walls with the cross flow passing through both walls, the asymmetric flow FFF channel is covered by one permeable wall and one solid transparent wall whereby the cross flow only passes through the permeable wall at a constant flow rate across its whole length (Fig. 2.6) [39]. The method has several advantages over the traditional symmetrical flow FFF system. It is widely available and has a simpler construction of the fractionation channel,

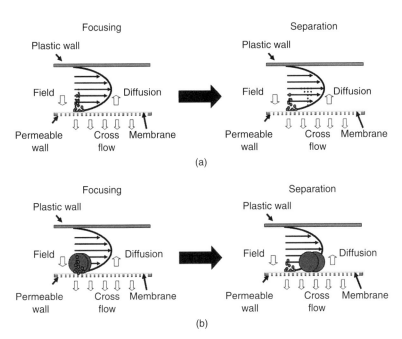

FIGURE 2.6   Schematic diagram of asymmetric flow FFF operation in (a) normal mode and (b) steric-hyperlayer mode.

and the channel can be visually monitored during the entire separation process through the transparent wall. In addition, it has much improved relaxation and focusing processes that may potentially improve the separation [40]. Like typical chromatography methods, flow FFF is usually connected with UV, RI, and LS detectors. The UV and RI detectors are mainly used to measure the concentration of proteins, and an online LS detector can be used for the characterization of protein and determination of the MW for each species. The mobile phase should be carefully filtered and degassed to avoid the interference with the detection signal and separation. The pH and components of buffers should be optimized for the protein samples and membrane. In addition, the buffer should contain appropriate excipients to minimize the nonspecific interaction of protein with the membrane [41].

2.4.2   Advantages, Challenges, and Key Consideration

Flow FFF has several advantages over SEC. Unlike conventional SEC, the flow FFF method does not use a stationary phase. Thus, all separations occur in a single phase, eliminating the potential problems caused by column fouling and matrix–protein interactions. Although membrane–protein interactions may compromise separation and recovery in a flow FFF channel, particularly at high cross flows, most of these problems can be mitigated by selecting low absorption membranes or lowering the cross-flow rate. For better separation, the membrane must be thin, smooth, flat, and free of creases.

The flow FFF method has a broad dynamic range and is capable of separating proteins over the entire colloidal size range (1–1000 nm) with a reasonable resolution [36]. The method can resolve protein fragments, soluble aggregates, and protein particles [9,39]. It has been successfully used for analyzing larger aggregates or particles that are filtered by an SEC column matrix or sediment instantaneously under a centrifugal field [38,41]. However, flow FFF also has several limitations. The separation of protein and aggregates is based on hydrodynamic properties, such as the diffusion coefficient, rather than the molecular mass. Therefore, an online LS detector is often connected to the flow FFF system to determine the molar mass of each species. The flow FFF system is also not suitable for the analysis of high-concentration protein solutions as the concentrated protein may form a viscous gel-like layer during the focusing and relaxation step and this would significantly compromise the resolution. For the best resolution, very often only small amounts of sample ($\sim$10 μg in the cases of mAbs) are loaded into the channel. This will create significant dilution of the protein during the elution process and is, therefore, not suitable to study aggregates that dissociate rapidly at lower concentrations. In addition, typical FFF instruments provide less resolution on some protein aggregates, particularly the aggregates formed by mAbs, than those by other commonly used methods, such as SEC and AUC [9].

The strength of the cross flow is the most important factor for the flow FFF operation. For a typical flow FFF instrument, the cross flow can be easily adjusted according to the size of the protein and aggregates. A cross-flow gradient can also be programmed for optimal separation. In the normal mode operation, an increase in the cross flow drives samples closer toward the accumulation wall and increases retention, selectivity, and fractionating power for sample components; however, the rate of cross flow is limited by either the pump or the channel pressure [42]. The high cross flow also results in an increase in separation time and sample dilution. An excessive cross flow may also lead to significant sample loss owing to increased interaction with the membrane [43]. For large particle separation, a lower cross flow is preferred as it minimizes the loss of protein due to nonspecific adsorption onto the membrane. The channel flow rate is another important experimental parameter in the flow FFF method; a decrease in the channel flow allows molecules to have more time to distribute into the localized laminar flow regions and, therefore, improves the fractionating power. However, the low channel flow will also result in longer separation times and increase of sample dilution [42].

Traditionally, flow FFF systems operate only at ambient temperature. With the recent introduction of a medium-temperature control apparatus with a temperature range from 5 to 80°C, it is now possible to analyze proteins by a flow FFF system at temperatures significantly different from ambient temperature. The increase in operating temperature can significantly increase the diffusion coefficients and potentially can reduce the separation time and enhance the resolution. In addition, the medium-temperature flow FFF system may potentially be used to separate the intermediate aggregates of thermally unfolded proteins during the temperature cycle.

2.4.3   Applications

Flow FFF has been successfully used to analyze protein aggregates [9,38,39]. Figure 2.7a shows an example of the asymmetrical flow FFF analysis of an mAb using a UV detector. The sample was stored at 30 and $-70°C$ for six months. When the cross flow was set at 6 mL/min, the main peak, corresponding to an mAb monomer, was resolved from two fragment peaks with molecular masses

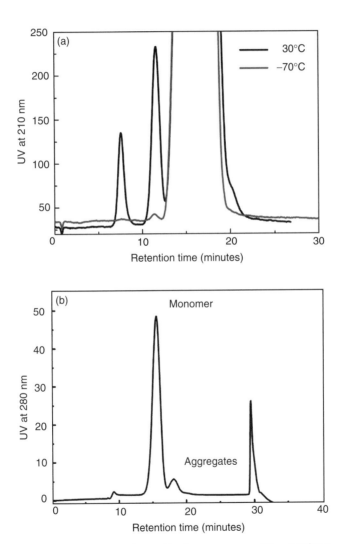

FIGURE 2.7   Flow FFF analysis of an mAb after storage at -70 and $30°C$ for six month. The eluted peaks were monitored using a UV absorption optical system at a wavelength of 210 or 280 nm. The flow FFF experiments were conducted using a regenerated cellulose membrane with a 10-kDa MW cutoff and a cross flow of PBS at (a) 6 mL/min and (b) 1 mL/min. *(See insert for color representation of part (a).)*

of 50 and 100 kDa as determined by an online LS detector, which is consistent with the size of a Fab and one-armed antibody, respectively. Both fragments have been identified as the major degradants for mAbs in liquid formulation on storage at elevated temperatures. The resolution of these fragments from the monomer at high cross flow is comparable to what is achieved by typical SEC chromatography. Although the high cross flow yields poor separation of protein aggregates, a much improved separation of protein aggregates was achieved with a low cross flow. As shown in Fig. 2.7b, at a low cross flow of 1 mL/min, the aggregates were clearly resolved from the monomer. Still, the low cross flow did not enable a separation of the fragments, and the aggregate peaks resolved in flow FFF appear to have a little broader distribution and lower resolution compared to what were observed using SEC and sedimentation velocity (Figs. 2.1a and 2.3). In spite of these drawbacks, flow FFF is still a useful method, particularly for monitoring large and insoluble aggregates [40].

Traditionally, the flow FFF operation is conducted at ambient temperature. With the recent introduction of a medium-temperature device, for the first time, the temperature effect on protein separation can be explored in flow FFF mode. Figure 2.8 shows the results of asymmetrical flow FFF experiments conducted at 20, 40, and 60°C. As the temperature increases, the diffusion coefficients also increase, resulting in an earlier elution of the peaks. The peak at 60°C is narrower and more homogeneous, suggesting that an increase in the temperature of operation can potentially improve the separation of protein aggregates.

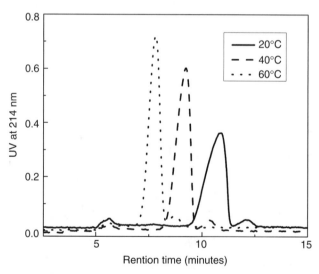

FIGURE 2.8 Asymmetrical flow FFF analysis of an mAb at temperatures of 20, 40, and 60°C. The flow FFF experiments were conducted using a regenerated cellulose membrane with 10-kD MW cutoff. The cross flow of PBS was set at 4 mL/min and the channel flow at 0.5 mL/min. The peak was monitored by a UV detector at 214 nm.

2.5 ELECTROPHORESIS

2.5.1 Theory and Background

Electrophoresis is a simple, rapid, and highly sensitive tool that has been widely used to analyze proteins [44]. The separation of proteins by gel electrophoresis is based on the fact that proteins will migrate through a gel matrix at a rate or distance as a function of the strength of the electric field as well as the protein charge, size, and conformation. Thus, gel electrophoresis can provide information about the size and charge distributions of proteins. Sodium dodecyl sulfate-polyacrylamide gel electrophoresis (SDS-PAGE) is the most commonly used gel electrophoresis technique for analyzing protein size distribution. SDS, an anionic detergent, denatures secondary and nondisulfide-linked tertiary and quaternary structures and binds to the polypeptide backbone with negative charges in proportion to the polypeptide mass. The larger proteins will move more slowly than the smaller proteins owing to the molecular sieving effect of the gel. The size of protein can be determined by directly comparing with MW standards.

Native or nondenaturing gel electrophoresis has also been used to analyze proteins, particularly for those molecules where the native structure or biological activity needs to be maintained. The electrophoresis is conducted in the absence of denaturant, such as SDS. Therefore, it is possible to recover active proteins in their native state after the separation. The native gel electrophoresis separates proteins based on their sizes, conformation, and surface charges. This makes them a great tool for detecting changes in charge, protein self-association, and unfolding. The separation of proteins using native gels usually is not as good as SDS-PAGE because of the complexity of the separation mechanism. Some of the limitations can be overcome by using two-dimensional gel electrophoresis where the second dimension electrophoresis such as SDS-PAGE or isoelectric focusing (IEF) allows for a better identification of each species [45].

With the introduction of capillary electrophoresis (CE) technology, the CE-SDS methods have evolved and rapidly become the methods of choice to replace the more traditional and labor-intensive SDS-PAGE [44]. The CE method provides high resolution, reproducibility, and rapid data analysis. The CE is a relatively simple system that uses a narrow capillary rather than a large gel slab and requires very small quantities of samples. The sample loading, separation, and detection process can be fully automated. The CE can also be incorporated into a microchip fluidic systems, which can largely increase the throughput of the analysis [46].

2.5.2 Advantages, Challenges, and Key Consideration for Method Development and Optimization

Gel electrophoresis has provided a rapid and reproducible method to study protein size distribution. The method is easy to use and has been employed in both QC and R&D environments for lot release, protein purity determination, and characterization. The CE-SDS is particularly useful as it largely increases the resolution and reproducibility of the protein separation when compared to the traditional gel electrophoresis. In addition, analysis of protein aggregates under reducing or nonreducing conditions can provide valuable information about the nature and mechanism of protein association, particularly for those aggregates linked through disulphide bonds [47]. However, the method also has several limitations. Proteins that contain an abundance of hydrophobic residues, such as membrane proteins, can load more than twofold of SDS than globular proteins, resulting in anomalous electrophoretic mobility compared to the usual globular protein standards [48]. The resolution for glycoproteins is poor as the sugar moieties do not bind well to SDS and the flexibility of the glycans may restrict the binding of SDS to the peptide backbone. In addition, some of the negatively charged glycans can impact the migration of proteins. The SDS is a strong denaturant and can disrupt noncovalent association; therefore, the method is most useful for the detection of covalently linked protein aggregates. Although native gel electrophoresis can overcome some of these limitations of SDS-PAGE, it usually has poorer resolution.

The CE-SDS and SDS-PAGE methods are quite easy to perform. The protein sample is first treated with SDS at elevated temperature to ensure that the protein is fully unfolded and covered by SDS. Gel electrophoresis under reducing conditions is achieved by incubating the samples at elevated temperatures with reducing agents such as dithiothreitol (DTT) or 2-mercaptoethanol (βME) to break the disulphide bonds. Following SDS-PAGE electrophoresis, proteins in the gel are usually visualized using Coomassie or silver staining methods. The Coomassie staining method provides a sensitive and robust staining for the proteins. Quantitation can be achieved using a scanning device to measure the relative density of the bands. Silver staining is a more sensitive method and it is capable of detecting low levels of protein in the nanogram range, but it is less useful for quantitation owing to the differential binding of silver stain to proteins as opposed to a more uniform staining by Coomassie [49]. The use of fluorescent dyes, such as 5-TAMRA (Tetramethylrhodamine), is a new type of protein staining method that offers both increased sensitivity and quantification for proteins [50]. For the CE-SDS method, the elution peak is usually measured using a UV or fluorescence detector. The UV detection is based on the intrinsic absorbance from the aromatic amino acids, such as Tyr and Trp, and it has good specificity. It can provide quantitative information about the size distribution of different protein species. Owing to the relatively poor sensitivity of UV detection and weak intrinsic fluorescence signal at low-protein concentrations, laser-induced fluorescence (LIF) methods have been developed to overcome these limits. Obviously, these methods require a more extensive sample preparation since the protein needs to be labeled with a fluorescent dye. The fluorophore usually is attached to the peptide or protein through primary amine groups on lysines or at the *N* terminus. The conditions of the labeling reactions often need to be optimized to ensure a reliable and consistent labeling of the protein.

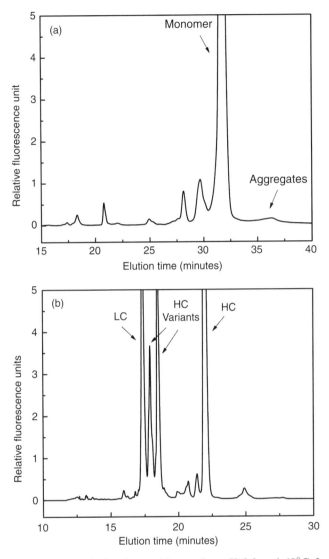

FIGURE 2.9 CE-SDS analysis of an mAb stored at pH 3.2 and 40°C for one week. Samples were prepared under nonreduced (a) and reduced (b) conditions. The reduced samples were treated with DTT and the nonreduced samples were alkylated by iodoacetamide and incubated at 75°C. The bands were detected using a fluorescence detector.

2.5.3 Applications

SDS gel electrophoresis has been successfully used for protein characterization. Figure 2.9 shows a typical profile of a degraded mAb after storage in acidic pH at 40°C for one week analyzed using nonreducing and reducing CE-SDS. Nonreducing CE-SDS separates the small amount of protein aggregates from the monomer peak. The amounts of protein aggregates are less than those observed by SEC, suggesting that some of the aggregates are noncovalent in nature and dissociated by SDS. There are a few minor fragment species that correspond to the variants containing combination of one to two heavy and light chains. Reducing CE-SDS resolves both heavy and light chains. In addition, two heavy chain variants, fragments, and nonreduced mAb were also detected. The aggregate peaks observed under the nonreducing condition are not visible under the reducing condition, suggesting that some of the soluble aggregates are linked by disulphide bonds.

SDS-PAGE has also been used to determine the mechanism of protein aggregation during formulation development. Andya et al. have previously shown that an mAb in a spray-dried formulation formed significant amounts of soluble protein aggregates while stored at 40°C for one year [51]. The sizes and levels of protein aggregates appeared to be impacted by the storage temperature. By using SDS-PAGE, it was shown that only part of the protein aggregates were dissociated by SDS, but all the aggregates were fully dissociated under a reducing and denaturing condition. This suggests that the soluble aggregates formed during storage are a mixture of both noncovalently and covalently linked aggregates.

2.6 OTHER POTENTIAL TECHNOLOGIES

In addition to these widely used separation methods described earlier, other chromatography methods such as ion exchange, reversed phase, and hydrophobic interaction chromatography have also been found to be useful for the detection of protein aggregates under certain conditions. Although these methods do not strictly separate aggregates based on their molecular size, the charge and hydrophobic distribution at the protein surface is modulated by its self-association and results in the separation of protein aggregates. The application of these methods has been demonstrated for a number of protein molecules, including antibodies, fibroblast growth factor, and peptides [52,53].

Electrospray differential mobility analysis (ES-DMA), also known as *gas-phase electrophoretic mobility molecular analysis*, is an emerging new technology to study protein aggregates [54]. The method is capable of resolving protein aggregates ranging from ∼3 to ∼250 nm. The separation of protein aggregates is based on charge to aerodynamic size ratio. Therefore, at a constant charge, the larger protein will take longer time owing to more increased aerodynamic drag. Pease et al. have recently shown that ES-DMA can effectively resolve protein aggregates from an IgG monomer [55]. This method can be potentially used as an orthogonal method for protein aggregate analysis and characterization.

2.7 SUMMARY

Protein aggregation is an important quality attribute and needs to be carefully monitored and controlled during manufacturing, shipping, handling, and long-term storage. Analytical methods based on separation mechanisms are very powerful and versatile tools. They have been the methods of choice and widely used in industry for protein aggregate analysis and characterization. With appropriate procedures and careful optimization, these methods can provide very useful quantitative information about the size and amounts of protein aggregates. This information is essential to have a better understanding of the potential impact of aggregates on the safety and quality of protein pharmaceuticals.

REFERENCES

1. Schellekens H. The immunogenicity of biopharmaceuticals. Neurology 2003;61: S11–S12.
2. Caughey B, Lansbury PT. Protofibrils, pores, fibrils, and neurodegeneration: separating the responsible protein aggregates from the innocent bystanders. Annu Rev Neurosci 2003;26:267–298.
3. Demeule B, Gurny R, Arvinte T. Where disease pathogenesis meets protein formulation: renal deposition of immunoglobulin aggregates. Eur J Pharm Biopharm 2006;62:121–130.
4. Ahern TJ, Manning MC, editors. Volume 2, Stability of protein pharmaceuticals. part A: chemical and physical pathways of protein degradation. New York: Plenum Press;1992.
5. Akers ML, Vasudevan V, Stickelmeyer M. Formulation development of protein dosage forms. In: Nail SL, Akers ML, editors. Development and manufacture of protein pharmaceuticals. New York: Springer; 2002. pp. 47–114.
6. Cromwell MEM, Hilario E, Jacobson F. Protein aggregation and bioprocessing. AAPS J 2006;8:E572–E579.
7. Watterson JG, Schaub MC, Waser PG. Shear-induced protein-protein interaction at the air-water interface. Biochimica et Biophysica Acta. 1974;356:133–143.
8. Cleland JL, Powell MF, Shire SJ. The development of stable protein formulations: a close look at protein aggregation, deamidation, and oxidation. Crit Rev Ther Drug Carrier Syst 1993;10:307–377. [erratum appears in Crit Rev Ther Drug Carrier Syst 1994;11(1):60].
9. Liu J, Andya JD, Shire SJ. A critical review of analytical ultracentrifugation and field-flow fractionation methods for measuring protein aggregation. AAPS J 2006;8:E580–E589.
10. Demeule B, Shire SJ, Liu J. A therapeutic antibody and its antigen form different complexes in serum than in phosphate-buffered saline: a study by analytical ultracentrifugation. Anal Biochem 2009;388:279–287.

11. Ahrer K, Buchacher A, Iberer G, Josic D, Jungbauer A. Analysis of aggregates of human immunoglobulin G using size-exclusion chromatography, static and dynamic light scattering. J Chromatogr A 2003;1009:89–96.

12. Shire SJ, Shahrokh Z, Liu J, Shire SJ, Shahrokh Z, Liu J. Challenges in the development of high protein concentration formulations. J Pharm Sci 2004;93:1390–1402.

13. Esue O, Kanai S, Liu J, Patapoff TW, Shire SJ. Carboxylate-dependent gelation of monoclonal antibodies. Pharm Res 2009;26:2478–2485.

14. Rosenberg AS. Effects of protein aggregates: an immunologic perspective. AAPS J 2006;8:E501–E507.

15. Hermeling S, Schellekens H, Maas C, Gebbink MFBG, Crommelin DJA, Jiskoot W. Antibody response to aggregated human interferon alpha2b in wild-type and transgenic immune tolerant mice depends on type and level of aggregation. J Pharm Sci 2006;95:1084–1096.

16. Berkowitz SA, Berkowitz SA. Role of analytical ultracentrifugation in assessing the aggregation of protein biopharmaceuticals. AAPS J 2006;8:E590–E605.

17. Irvine GB. High-performance size-exclusion chromatography of peptides. J Biochem Biophys Methods 2003;56:233–242.

18. Barth HG, Boyes BE, Jackson C, Barth HG, Boyes BE, Jackson C. Size exclusion chromatography. Anal Chem 1994;66:595R–620R.

19. Wen J, Arakawa T, Philo JS. Size-exclusion chromatography with on-line light-scattering, absorbance, and refractive index detectors for studying proteins and their interactions. Anal Biochem 1996;240:155–166.

20. Moore JM, Patapoff TW, Cromwell ME. Kinetics and thermodynamics of dimer formation and dissociation for a recombinant humanized monoclonal antibody to vascular endothelial growth factor. Biochemistry 1999;38:13960–13967.

21. Liu J, Nguyen MD, Andya JD, Shire SJ, Liu J, Nguyen MDH, Andya JD, Shire SJ. Reversible self-association increases the viscosity of a concentrated monoclonal antibody in aqueous solution. J Pharm Sci 2005;94:1928–1940.

22. Kanai S, Liu J, Patapoff T, Shire SJ. Reversible self-association of a concentrated monoclonal antibody solution mediated by Fab-Fab interaction that impacts solution viscosity. J Pharm Sciences 2008;97:4219–4227.

23. Schuck P, Perugini MA, Gonzales NR, Howlett GJ, Schubert D. Size-distribution analysis of proteins by analytical ultracentrifugation: strategies and application to model systems. Biophys J 2002;82:1096–1111.

24. Hansen JC, Lebowitz J, Demeler B. Analytical ultracentrifugation of complex macromolecular systems. Biochemistry 1994;33:13155–13163.

25. Laue TM, Stafford WF, 3rd. Modern applications of analytical ultracentrifugation. Annu Rev Biophys Biomol Struct 1999;28:75–100.

26. Cole JL, Lary JW, Moody TP, Laue TM. Analytical ultracentrifugation: sedimentation velocity and sedimentation equilibrium. Methods Cell Biol 2008;84:143–179.

27. Gonzalez JM, Rivas G, Minton AP. Effect of large refractive index gradients on the performance of absorption optics in the Beckman XL-A/I analytical ultracentrifuge: an experimental study. Anal Biochem 2003;313:133–136.

28. Minton AP. Analytical centrifugation with preparative ultracentrifuges. Anal Biochem 1989;176:209–216.

29. MacGregor IK, Anderson AL, Laue TM, MacGregor IK, Anderson AL, Laue TM. Fluorescence detection for the XLI analytical ultracentrifuge. Biophys Chem 2004; 108:165–185.

30. Kroe RR, Laue TM. NUTS and BOLTS: applications of fluorescence-detected sedimentation. Anal Biochem 2009;390:1–13.

31. Dam J, Schuck P. Sedimentation velocity analysis of heterogeneous protein-protein interactions: sedimentation coefficient distributions c(s) and asymptotic boundary profiles from Gilbert-Jenkins theory. Biophys J 2005;89:651–666.

32. Gabrielson JP, Arthur KK, Kendrick BS, Randolph TW, Stoner MR, Gabrielson JP, Arthur KK, Kendrick BS, Randolph TW, Stoner MR. Common excipients impair detection of protein aggregates during sedimentation velocity analytical ultracentrifugation. J Pharm Sci 2009;98:50–62.

33. Josephs R, Harrington WF, Josephs R, Harrington WF. On the stability of myosin filaments. Biochemistry 1968;7:2834–2847.

34. Arthur KK, Gabrielson JP, Kendrick BS, Stoner MR. Detection of protein aggregates by sedimentation velocity analytical ultracentrifugation (SV-AUC): sources of variability and their relative importance. J Pharm Sci 2009 Oct;98(10):3522–39.

35. Philo JS. A critical review of methods for size characterization of non-particulate protein aggregates. Curr Pharm Biotechnol 2009;10:359–372.

36. Giddings CJ. The field-flow fractionation family: underlying principles. In: Schimpf M, Caldwell K, Giddings J, editors. Field-flow fractionation handbook. New York: John Wiley & Sons; 2000.

37. Giddings JC. Field-flow fractionation: analysis of macromolecular, colloidal, and particulate materials. Science 1993;260:1456–1465.

38. Fraunhofer W, Winter G. The use of asymmetrical flow field-flow fractionation in pharmaceutics and biopharmaceutics. Eur J Pharm Biopharm 2004;58:369–383.

39. Ratanathanawongs Williams SK, Lee D. Field-flow fractionation of proteins, polysaccharides, synthetic polymers, and supramolecular assemblies. J Sep Sci 2006;29:1720–1732.

40. Schauer T. Symmetrical and asymmetrical flow field-flow fractionation for particle size determination. Part Part Syst Charact 2004;12:284–288.

41. Colfen H, Antonietti M. Field-flow fractionation techniques for polymer and colloid analysis. In: Advances in polymer science. Berlin/Heidelberg: Springer; 2000.

42. Schimpf ME. Optimization. In: Schimpf ME, Caldwell K, Giddings CJ, editors. Field-flow fractionation handbook. New York: John Wiley & Sons; 2000. pp. 95–102.

43. Ratanathanawongs Williams SK, Gidding CJ. Sample recovery. In: Schimpf ME, Caldwell K, Gidding CJ, editors. Field-flow fractionation handbook. New York: John Wiley & Sons; 2000. pp. 325–344.

44. Rustandi R, Washabaugh M, Wang Y. Applications of CE-SDS gel in development of biopharmaceutical antibody-based products. Electrophoresis 2008;29:8.

45. Stegemann J, Ventzki R, Schrodel A, de Marco A. Comparative analysis of protein aggregates by blue native electrophoresis and subsequent sodium dodecyl sulfate-polyacrylamide gel electrophoresis in a three-dimensional geometry gel. Proteomics 2005;5:2002–2009.

46. Dolnik V, Liu S. Applications of capillary electrophoresis on microchip. J Sep Sci 2005;28:1994–2009.

47. Andya JD, Hsu CC, Shire SJ. Mechanisms of aggregate formation and carbohydrate excipient stabilization of lyophilized humanized monoclonal antibody formulations. AAPS PharmSci 2003;5:E10.

48. Rath A, Glibowicka M, Nadeau VG, Chen G, Deber CM, Rath A, Glibowicka M, Nadeau VG, Chen G, Deber CM. Detergent binding explains anomalous SDS-PAGE migration of membrane proteins. Proc Natl Acad Sci U S A 2009;106:1760–1765.

49. Gromova I, Celis JE. Protein detection in gels by silver staining: a procedure compatible with mass-spectrometry. In:Celis JE, Carter N, Hunter T, Simons K, Small JV, Shotton D, editors. Cell biology: a laboratory handbook. 3rd ed. London, Elsevier, Academic Press; 2006.

50. Salas-Solano O, Tomlinson B, Du S, Parker M, Strahan A, Ma S, Salas-Solano O, Tomlinson B, Du S, Parker M, Strahan A, Ma S. Optimization and validation of a quantitative capillary electrophoresis sodium dodecyl sulfate method for quality control and stability monitoring of monoclonal antibodies. Anal Chem 2006;78:6583–6594.

51. Andya JD, Maa YF, Costantino HR, Nguyen PA, Dasovich N, Sweeney TD, Hsu CC, Shire SJ. The effect of formulation excipients on protein stability and aerosol performance of spray-dried powders of a recombinant humanized anti-IgE monoclonal antibody. Pharm Res 1999;16:350–358.

52. Shahrokh Z, Stratton PR, Eberlein GA, Wang YJ. Approaches to analysis of aggregates and demonstrating mass balance in pharmaceutical protein (basic fibroblast growth factor) formulations. J Pharm Sci 1994;83:1645–1650.

53. Sluzky V, Shahrokh Z, Stratton P, Eberlein G, Wang YJ. Chromatographic methods for quantitative analysis of native, denatured, and aggregated basic fibroblast growth factor in solution formulations. Pharm Res 1994;11:485–490.

54. Bacher G, Szymanski WW, Kaufman SL, Zollner P, Blaas D, Allmaier G. Charge-reduced nano electrospray ionization combined with differential mobility analysis of peptides, proteins, glycoproteins, noncovalent protein complexes and viruses. J Mass Spectrom 2001;36:1038–1052.

55. Pease LF 3rd, Elliott JT, Tsai D-H, Zachariah MR, Tarlov MJ. Determination of protein aggregation with differential mobility analysis: application to IgG antibody. Biotechnol Bioeng 2008;101:1214–1222.

3 Laser Light Scattering-Based Techniques Used for the Characterization of Protein Therapeutics

JOHN DEN ENGELSMAN

Analytical Development and Validation, Schering Plough Research Institute, Oss, The Netherlands

FABIAN KEBBEL and PATRICK GARIDEL

Pharmaceutical Development, Process Science/Biopharmaceuticals, Boehringer Ingelheim Pharma GmbH & Co. KG, Biberach an der Riss, Germany

3.1 INTRODUCTION

3.1.1 History of Light Scattering

Nowadays, techniques that use light scattering have been extensively applied in the food, chemical, and pharmaceutical industries to characterize particles in solution. These techniques are widely used because of the speed, nondestructive (the original sample can be recovered), and noninvasive nature (the direct measuring system is not in direct contact with the sample; there is no impact of the laser beam on the properties of the sample) of such methods. Especially in the biopharmaceutical industry, the use of light scattering methods has taken a flight to determine the presence of unwanted protein aggregates. Light scattering techniques are noninvasive and are very well suited for determining the molecular weight, hydrodynamic size, and quaternary structure of biomolecules and aggregates thereof. However, proper interpretation of the data requires extensive knowledge of the fundamentals of light scattering. This chapter explains the theory of the two mainly used light scattering detection techniques, static light scattering (SLS) and dynamic light scattering (DLS), for the investigation of protein pharmaceuticals. After a brief summary of the important events that have led to the concepts of light scattering, the theories of SLS and DLS are explained.

Analysis of Aggregates and Particles in Protein Pharmaceuticals, First Edition.
Edited by Hanns-Christian Mahler, Wim Jiskoot.
© 2012 John Wiley & Sons, Inc., Published 2012 by John Wiley & Sons, Inc.

Light scattering is a natural phenomenon of light deviating from its main trajectory in the presence of nonuniformities. It takes place when a light beam, in its free propagation through an initially homogeneous medium, encounters heterogeneities. When the light impinges on matter such as protein molecules, the electric field of the light induces an oscillating polarization of electrons in the molecules, resulting in scattering of the light.

The scientists, Michael Faraday (1792–1867), James Clerk Maxwell (1831–1879), and Lord Rayleigh (John William Strutt 1842–1919), are mainly accountable for the basic research that gave an explanation for the scattering of light by particles. Many other scientists have also made significant contributions to this phenomenon including Einstein, Tyndall, Debye, Gans, etc. (for a thorough historical overview, see [1]).

Faraday, a pioneer in the study of light scattering, was interested in the scattering of light passing through a gold dispersion. A narrow beam of (laser) light passing through a gold dispersion (colloidal system) will form a visible cone of scattered light. This is the so-called Faraday–Tyndall effect, which can also be observed for protein solutions, especially for highly concentrated ones. Maxwell later continued Faraday's work and developed the classical electromagnetic theory unifying previous unrelated observations, experiments, and equations of electricity, magnetism, and optics into one consistent theory. The set of equations (Maxwell's equations) demonstrated that electricity, magnetism, and light are all manifestations of the same phenomenon: the electromagnetic field.

In the nineteenth century, Lord Rayleigh (John William Strutt) described the wavelength-dependent scattering of light from particles in air, with a diameter much smaller than the diameter of the wavelength (1/20th) of the incident light. This theory explained why the sky is blue on a clear day. Small particles in the air scatter light with shorter wavelengths more effectively (intensity $\sim 1/\lambda^4$); therefore, the (scattered) light we see is blue shifted. Furthermore, he observed that the intensity of the scattered light is proportional to the power of six to the diameter of the scattering particle. This is the reason larger particles scatter much stronger than the smaller ones. Rayleigh's theories are the basis of more sophisticated theories and experimental techniques for obtaining information about molecules by analyzing the way they scatter light.

In 1906, Gustav Mie developed a mathematical–physical theory [2] of the scattering of electromagnetic radiation by spherical particles, which is called the *Mie theory* (also called *Lorenz–Mie theory* or *Lorenz–Mie–Debye theory*). This is a complete analytical solution of Maxwell's equations for the scattering of electromagnetic radiation by spherical particles (also called *Mie scattering*). This solution takes the particle shape and the difference in refractive index (RI) between the particles and the supporting medium into account. The Mie theory predicts the scattering intensity as a function of the angle at which light is scattered at the point of interaction with a spherical particle. The Mie theory is applicable to a wide size range.

Rayleigh's theory was later extended to describe larger macromolecules in solution, which was called the *Rayleigh–Gans–Debye (RGD) approximation* to recognize all scientists who made a considerable contribution. In the 1940s, Bruno Zimm laid the foundations to condense the RGD equations into a "simple" equation (Eq. 3.1) [3,4]. This development made it possible to accurately determine the molecular weight, root mean square (rms) radius, and second virial coefficient of particles in solution using ultrasensitive detectors and sophisticated software [3,5].

In summary, different scattering regions are generally considered on the basis of the relationship between the particle size (d is the particle diameter) and the wavelength (λ).

1. *Rayleigh scattering, valid for $d < \lambda/20$*: The scattered light is independent of the scattering center and the phase of the wave is only marginally altered with regard to the dimension of the scattering center [6–8]. The scattering center is polarized by the electromagnetic wave and as a result a scattering field with dipole characteristics is observed. The scattering intensity is independent of the scattering angle and proportional to d^6.

2. *RGD scattering, valid between $\lambda/20$ and $\lambda/6$*: This model assumes that there is no homogeneous polarization over the scattering center, but infinitely small volume elements with different dipole moments. The overall scattering field is, therefore, the sum of the single scattering contributions.

3. *Mie scattering, valid between $\lambda/6$ and 4λ*: This scattering theory allows an exact mathematical solution for spherical particles having refractive indices being not constant over the scattering center volume [2].

4. *Fraunhofer scattering, valid between 4λ up to a few micrometers:* This scattering is, however, beyond the scope of this chapter.

3.2 STATIC LIGHT SCATTERING

3.2.1 Introduction to the Theory of SLS

When light hits a particle in a solution, this particle scatters the light in multiple directions. The Rayleigh theory predicts the scattering properties of a beam of light that hits such a particle. A prerequisite for the Rayleigh theory to apply is that the particles do not absorb the incident light, and scattering from the solvent is relatively low.

The scattering of the particles depends on the size of the particles and the wavelength of the incident light. Small particles ($d < \lambda/20$) that are hit by a laser beam scatter light uniformly in all directions (isotropic scattering), where larger particles scatter most light in the forward direction (anisotropic scattering). The theory of light scattering is based on the detection of those scattered signals. The RGD theory expression is formulated into a simple form, which is commonly used these days for SLS measurements; see Equation 3.1 (for further theoretical considerations beyond the scope of this chapter, see Refs 3–5,9–11):

$$\frac{K_c}{R_\theta} = \frac{P(\theta)^{-1}}{M_w} + 2A_2c, \tag{3.1}$$

where K is an optical constant (also called *contrast constant*; see Eq. 3.2), c the particle concentration, M_w the molecular weight, A_2 the (osmotic) second virial coefficient, $P(\theta)$ the light scattering function, and R_θ the excess Rayleigh scattering (Eq. 3.3):

$$K = \frac{4\pi^2 n_0^2}{\lambda^4 N_A} \left(\frac{dn}{dc}\right)^2, \tag{3.2}$$

where λ is the wavelength of light in a vacuum, n_0 the RI of the solvent, N_A Avogadro's number, and dn/dc the RI increment of the scattering species in the solvent used. The value is approximated by the measurement of the incremental change in the RI of a solution with the concentration of the solute.

The molecular weight (M_w) and osmotic second virial coefficient (A_2) of particles in solution can be determined using the above-mentioned equations. However, for proper interpretation of the equations, several items need to be further clarified.

The excess Rayleigh scattering (R_θ) is the difference between the Rayleigh scattering of the sample and a pure solvent (usually toluene). It is difficult to measure the magnitude of the incident light interacting with the particle. Therefore, excess Rayleigh scattering is used R_θ is defined by Equation 3.3.

$$R_\theta = \frac{I_A n_0^2}{I_T n_T^2} R_T, \tag{3.3}$$

where I_A is the intensity of the analyte (sample$_1$–solvent$_1$); n_0 the solvent RI; I_T the intensity of a standard (usually toluene); n_T the RI of the standard (usually toluene); and R_T the known Rayleigh ratio of the standard, which is a quantity used to characterize the scattered intensity as a function of the scattering angle.

The osmotic second virial coefficient is a property describing the interaction strength between the particles and solvent. For samples where the osmotic second virial coefficient > 0, the particles have more interaction with the solvent than with themselves [12,13]. When the osmotic second virial coefficient < 0, the particles have more interaction with themselves (self-interaction) than with the solvent and might, therefore, interact and form associates and/or aggregates. The knowledge of the osmotic second virial coefficient is very helpful when working with proteins to understand solution properties because interactions between proteins are common and might be indicative for protein aggregation. Note that this is only true in cases where the interaction between native proteins is the rate-limiting step for colloidal stability. This is not the case when, for example, protein adsorption or conformational changes are the rate-limiting step for aggregation (i.e., colloidal instability); A_2 will not be predictive at all [12,13,29].

The RI increment (dn/dc) is strongly dependent on the properties of both the solute (or the particle) and the solvent. The RI increment is an indication of the contrast and describes to what extent the RI changes with sample concentration.

$P(\theta)$, the light scattering function (shape or form factor), is the ratio between the actual light scattering and the scattering that would occur by isotropic scattering, thus from a small particle. This ratio gives information about the shape and size of the particle (r_g) and describes the angular dependence of the intensity of the scattered light (Eq. 3.4):

$$P(\theta)^{-1} = 1 + \frac{16\pi^2}{3\lambda^2} r_g^2 \sin^2(\theta/2),\qquad(3.4)$$

where r_g is the radius of gyration.

The $P(\theta)$ function can be calculated more precisely by increasing the number of detection angles. The radius of gyration is the rms distance of the particle from its center of gravity.

For spherical particles that exceed 1/20th of the wavelength, anisotropic scattering occurs. A characteristic of this anisotropic scattering is a strong angular dependence of the scattered intensity, which is represented by the function $P(\theta)$ (Eq. 3.1). This angular dependence arises from constructive and destructive interference of light scattered from different positions of the same particle. When particles are very small compared to the wavelength of the light $(d < \lambda/20)$, particles can be regarded as point scatterers and will scatter the light in an isotropic manner (Fig. 3.1). Under these conditions, according to Rayleigh scattering, the angular dependence of the scattering intensity is lost; therefore, $P(\theta)$ is equal to 1 and Equation 3.1 is reduced to Equation 3.5:

$$\frac{K_c}{R_\theta} = \frac{1}{M_w} + 2A_2c.\qquad(3.5)$$

This simplified version of the general light scattering equation can be written as a linear function $(y = A + Bx)$. Hence, for small particles, an experiment can be performed at a single detection angle. The lower the detection angle, the lesser the interference of multiple scattering to the scattering signals. In such a case, the measured intensity of the scattered light is related to the concentration and molecular weight of the molecule (Eqs. 3.1 and 3.5). Therefore, M_w and A_2 can be directly determined from a simple plot where the concentration is plotted against K_c/R_θ. This is known as the *Debye plot* (Figs. 3.6 and 3.7). From the intercept with the y-axis, the inverse of the molar mass is determined

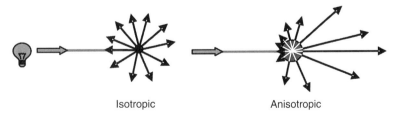

Isotropic   Anisotropic

FIGURE 3.1   Isotropic and anisotropic scattering of particles.

and the slope of the calibration line represents the second virial coefficient (A_2) multiplied by 2.

Protein pharmaceuticals are often analyzed by multiangle laser light scattering (MALLS) equipment (combined with, e.g., size-exclusion chromatography (SEC)) to obtain an accurate M_w. In a MALLS instrument, the signal is collected at multiple detectors; therefore, MALLS is less sensitive to particle contamination (e.g., dust). Extracting the molecular weight, second virial coefficient, and radius of gyration from data obtained with MALLS is more tedious compared to that obtained with, for instance, low-angle laser light scattering (LALLS), where the angle at which is measured is close to $0°$ of the incident light. In this case, a method known as the *Zimm plot* is often applied [3,10,14,15]. To extract the required data from the MALLS experiment, some mathematical approximations have to be applied.

Equation 3.6 shows that the term in brackets goes to unity (1) when θ, the scattering angle, is equal to 0 (this is, however, physically impossible). To achieve this experimentally, data points need to be plotted for a variety of scattering angles (θ) at a constant concentration (c) after which extrapolation to a zero scattering angle can be done:

$$\frac{K_c}{R_\theta} = \frac{1}{M_w}\left[1 + \frac{16\pi^2}{3\lambda^2}r_g^2\sin^2\left(\frac{\theta}{2}\right)\right] + 2A_2c. \tag{3.6}$$

Now that the expression between brackets is forced to unity, that is, $\theta \to 0$; we are left with Equation 3.5. This equation is identical to the one used in the earlier mentioned Debye plot. Solving this part of the equation experimentally implies that data points for a constant scattering angle (θ) at varying concentrations (c) need to be plotted, and thereafter extrapolation to zero concentration can occur (Eqs 3.5 and 3.7):

$$c = 0 \to \frac{K_c}{R_\theta} = \frac{1}{M_w}\left[1 + \frac{16\pi^2}{3\lambda^2}r_g^2\sin^2\left(\frac{\theta}{2}\right)\right]. \tag{3.7}$$

In summary, an experiment should be performed at various angles and several different concentrations. From the resulting Zimm plot, A_2 (the slope of the $\theta = 0$ line), r_g (the slope of the $c = 0$ line), and M_w (the intercept with the y-axis of both lines is the inverse of M_w) can be derived. In this Zimm plot, Equation 3.5 is adjusted with a stretch factor, k, for the readability of the plot and leads to Equation 3.8. $\frac{K_c}{R_\theta}$ is plotted against $\sin^2\left(\frac{\theta}{2}\right) + kc$ (Fig. 3.2):

$$\theta = 0 \to \frac{K_c}{R_\theta} = \frac{1}{M_w} + \frac{2A_2}{k}c. \tag{3.8}$$

The above-mentioned equations clearly show that to obtain information about the molecular weight, radius of gyration, and second virial coefficient of the sample, data regarding the RI of the solvent, precise concentration of the solutions, and the RI increment of the scattering species in the solvent are required.

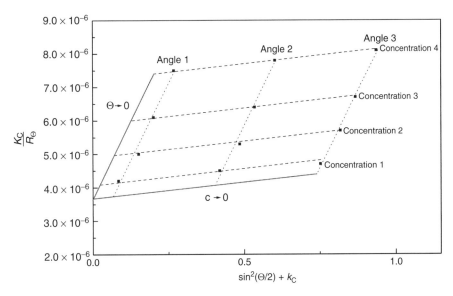

FIGURE 3.2   Example of a Zimm plot.

3.3 DYNAMIC LIGHT SCATTERING

3.3.1 Introduction

DLS is also known as *photon correlation spectroscopy* (*PCS*), *quasielastic light scattering* (*QELS*), or *intensity fluctuation spectroscopy* (*IFS*). It is a noninvasive technique capable of measuring particle size in colloidal systems. It is based on the measurement of the Brownian motion of (spherical) particles in the solution. During a DLS experiment, intensity fluctuations of the scattered light, which arise from particles moving relative to each other, are monitored. Note that in a typical SLS experiment, the light scattering intensity is recorded by sensitive detectors [3,5,14] over a period of time ranging from 10 s to 1 min. This time averaging "removes" the inherent fluctuations in the signal and, hence, the term *static light scattering*. The intensity fluctuations measured in DLS are related to the diffusion coefficient of the particles in solution and, hence, by the hydrodynamic diameter of the particles. Therefore, it is possible to compute the particle size distribution from the intensity fluctuations. For further reading on DLS instrumentation, see Ref. 16.

3.3.2 The Speckle Pattern

The measurement of particles by DLS is based on (i) the fact that particles undergo Brownian motion, also called *random walk*, and (ii) the assumption that particles are analyzed as though they were spherical. As a result of Brownian motion, particles move randomly in time, dependent on their hydrodynamic size (the smaller the particles, the faster they will move). In DLS, size measurements of particles present in a defined measurement field (scattering volume) are performed using a "speckle pattern." The speckle pattern is mainly generated by constructive and destructive light interference. This means that two beams of scattered light interfere and can cancel out each other or enhance each other [16,17]. The intensity of the scattered light changes in time because of the continuously changing position of particles relative to each other. Information on the particle size and species distribution can be obtained by correlating the intensity fluctuations in time through the autocorrelation function (see Section 3.3.5).

3.3.3 Size Calculation

Since the scattering intensity of a particle strongly increases with an increasing particle diameter, even extremely low concentrations of large particles or aggregates can be detected by DLS. The detectable size range usually varies between less than a nanometer to several microns. However, the method is not specific to certain particles, that is, particles are detected independent of their chemical nature and origin.

The velocity of the Brownian motion is defined by the translational diffusion coefficient (D), obtained through the autocorrelation function (see Section 3.3.5). This value is used to calculate the particle diameter or radius using the Stokes–Einstein equation (Eq. 3.9):

$$D = \frac{k_b T}{6\pi\eta r} \tag{3.9}$$

where η is the dynamic viscosity of the sample (mPa·s), T the temperature (K), D the diffusion coefficient (m^2/s), k_b the Boltzmann constant (1.3807×10^{-23} J/K), and r the hydrodynamic sphere radius (m).

3.3.4 Nonspherical Particles

A main assumption is that all particles are spherical. This is often not the case. However, in a DLS experiment, this is compensated as follows: because of the Brownian motion, a particle randomly moves around. For instance, an elongated particle moves rapidly in elongated directions and slowly in the other directions. The detector gets an image over time, which is an average of the rapid and slow movements of the particle. Therefore, in DLS experiments, an equivalent sphere is calculated. However, the molecular weight derived from the particle diameter based on the equivalent sphere will not always give an accurate value in the case of complex-shaped particles.

It should be noted that in a DLS experiment, not the real radius but the hydrodynamic radius of particles is measured (cf. Eq. 3.9). This value is influenced by ionic strength and the presence of surface coatings. By the addition of appropriate amount of salt to the sample, the hydrodynamic radius will be close to the actual particle radius.

3.3.5   The Autocorrelation Function

The particle size (or better, the translational diffusion coefficient, D) is obtained from the speckle pattern using an autocorrelation function. With time, particles randomly move (away) from their original place (the Brownian motion). Therefore, the correlation of a measurement field in time decreases in comparison to the situation at $t = 0$.

The time passed since $t = 0$ is called the *sample time* (τ) and $I(t)$ is the intensity of the scattered light. The value of the correlation varies between 1 and 0, where 1 is the perfect correlation and 0 no correlation. At $t = 0$, the correlation is 1 because no particles have moved yet. When the sample time increases slightly, the correlation slightly decreases until no correlation is present anymore. Because larger particles move slower than the smaller ones, the correlation for larger particles decreases less rapidly when compared to that of the smaller ones.

As described earlier, the autocorrelation function measures the correlation to $t = 0$ in a time-dependent manner. For a sample consisting of same sized particles, a monodisperse sample (described as a single exponential decay), the autocorrelation function is described by Equation 3.10. For a sample consisting of different sized particles, a polydisperse sample (described as a sum of exponentials), the autocorrelation function is described by Equation 3.11:

$$G(\tau) = A[1 + B\exp(-2\Gamma\tau)] \tag{3.10}$$

$$G(\tau) = A[1 + Bg_1(\tau)^2] \tag{3.11}$$

where A is the baseline of the autocorrelation function, the average intensity of the scattered light; B the intercept of the autocorrelation function, the efficiency factor. This depends on the size of the scattered volume and the fixed angle at which the scattered signal is collected; $g_1(\tau)$ the sum of all exponential decays contained in the correlation function; $\Gamma = Dq^2$, where q is the scattering vector, a constant related to the frequency of the scattering light; and D the translational diffusion coefficient.

3.3.6   Processing the Autocorrelation Function by Cumulants Analysis

The measured autocorrelation function is used to calculate different parameters, which are used for the interpretation of DLS data. Applying a monoexponential fit (a good fit is obtained only in the case of a perfectly monodisperse system) to the measured autocorrelation function in the form of Equation 3.10 (cumulants analysis) enables to calculate the intensity-weighted mean diameter (z-average) and polydispersity index (PDI) (determined by the deviation from the monoexponential fit) of a sample [18–20]. Both are powerful parameters for the determination of changes in the colloidal composition of a solution caused by the formation of aggregates or fragments, for example, during stresslike heating, stirring, or shaking.

Figure 3.3a shows the z-average in dependence of the molar ratio of two particle sizes (30 and 80 nm). In the case of pure 80-nm latex particles, the

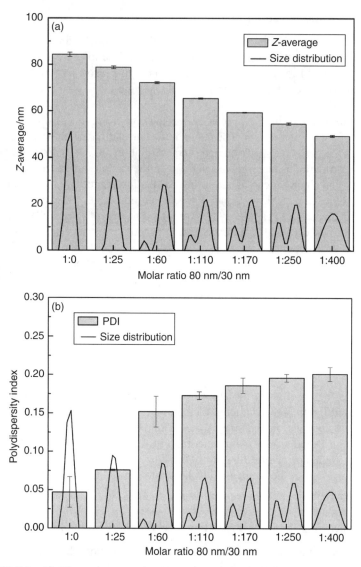

FIGURE 3.3   (a) The z-average of a blend composed of 80/30 nm latex particles in molar ratios from 1:0 to 1:400 in WFI (water for injection, 20°C) analyzed with multiple narrow algorithm. (b) The polydispersity index (PDI) of a blend composed of 80/30 nm latex particles in molar ratios from 1:0 to 1:400 in WFI (water for injection, 20°C) analyzed with multiple narrow algorithm.

z-average is about 80 nm. Hence, if a sample consists of only one population (monomodal), the z-average is equivalent to the hydrodynamic diameter d_H. The presence of smaller particles in the solution (30 nm in the present case) leads to a decrease in z-average. The higher the content of 30 nm particles, the lower the

z-average (50 nm at a molar ratio of 1:400). Similarly, the higher the content of aggregates in a protein solution, the higher will be the measured z-average.

Furthermore, the example in Fig. 3.3a illustrates a case with a mixture of two particle populations. As can be seen from this figure, particles with diameters of 30 and 80 nm can be resolved as single populations at certain molar ratios. However, at a large numerical excess of the 30 nm particles, the overall particle distribution is dominated by a single particle population corresponding to the 30-nm particles.

The PDI describes the deviation of the single-exponential-fitted autocorrelation function (for perfectly monodisperse particles) to the measured one. This parameter can be used to obtain an indication of the presence of more than one population in a sample [18–20]. Figure 3.3b shows the PDI in dependence of the molar ratio of two particle sizes (30 and 80 nm). If the sample is unimodal (only one population of 80 nm), the PDI is < 0.1. At a molar (80 nm/30 nm particles) ratio of 1:60, two populations at 30 and 80 nm are observed and the PDI increases to 0.15 in this case.

3.3.7 Processing the Autocorrelation Function by NNLS

In addition to the described cumulants analysis used to calculate the z-average and PDI, data from DLS can be used to calculate distributions by intensity, volume, and number with the intensity distribution being the most common. Intensity distributions are calculated by applying a multiexponential fit to the autocorrelation function using nonnegatively least square (NNLS) algorithms (Eq. 3.11) [18–20]. Most manufacturers of DLS equipment have developed their own specific algorithms [29]. They differ among others in the grade of "smoothing" the autocorrelation function before the analysis, which leads to a loss of information and with it differences in the calculated distributions [1,21]. The grade of smoothing is defined in the so-called regularizer, α-parameter, or smoothing parameter. For instance, the "smoothing-parameter" Malvern instruments used for the algorithms "Contin", "general purpose," and "multiple narrow" are listed in Table 3.1. A higher smoothing parameter leads to a stronger smoothing [1,9,22].

Figure 3.4 shows the size distributions for a blend of latex standards (30/80/1000 nm in a molar ratio of 180,000:4000:1) calculated with the above-mentioned three different algorithms. Because of the smoothing of the autocorrelation function, Contin and general purpose calculate only one and two populations, respectively. Using "multiple narrow mode" as an algorithm

TABLE 3.1 Smoothing Parameter of Three Different PCS Algorithms

Algorithm	Smoothing Parameter
Contin	Variable, standard = 0.1
General purpose	0.01
Multiple narrow	0.001

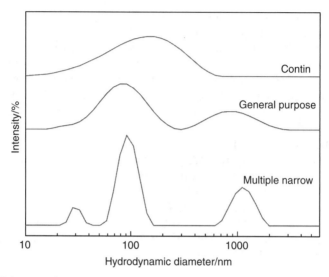

FIGURE 3.4   Intensity-weighted size distributions of a blend composed of 30/80/1000 nm latex particles at 20°C in water in a molar ratio of 180,000:4000:1 calculated with the Contin, general purpose, and multiple narrow algorithms.

with a low smoothing degree, three populations of 30, 80, and 1000 nm are resolved. Because of the high-resolution power of this algorithm, it seems to be most suitable for the characterization of protein solutions. However, a drawback of this algorithm is that in the case of samples with a broad distribution of species (e.g., during thermal protein denaturation) erroneously only a few discrete populations might be observed. Moreover, processing unsmoothed autocorrelation functions can lead to the creation of nonexistent "ghost peaks." Especially at longer delay times, noise in the autocorrelation often occurs. If left unsmoothed, this might introduce ghost peaks (for more details, see Refs [1,9,29]).

The intensity-weighted size distributions can subsequently be converted into volume or number distributions. Figure 3.5 shows these distributions for a blend composed of 30-, 80-, and 1000-nm latex particles in molar ratios from 180,000:4000:1 calculated with the algorithm multiple narrow mode and Mie theory. Small particles contribute relatively little to the scattering intensity ($\sim d^6$) and volume ($\sim d^3$). On the other hand, a negligible number of large particles (1 μm) lead to high scattering intensities and volumes. This behavior is based on the scattering physics, with the scattering intensity being proportional to d^6 (Section 3.1.1) [18]. These results demonstrate why DLS (as well as SLS) is so sensitive to small amounts of large aggregates and much less to small species (e.g., protein monomers).

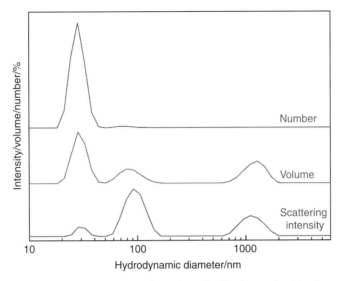

FIGURE 3.5 Intensity-, volume-, and number distributions of a blend composed of 30/80/1000 nm latex particles in a molar ratio of 180,000:4000:1 calculated with the multiple narrow algorithm and Mie theory.

3.4 CASE STUDIES AND DRAWBACKS OF LIGHT SCATTERING-BASED METHODS

As mentioned earlier, large particles have a strong contribution to the scattering property of a sample. The presence of such large particles can mask the existence of smaller particles. Therefore, it can be helpful to carefully prepare different fractions of the sample of interest by filtration or centrifugation of the sample. Although such handling can affect the sample, it allows narrowing the potential particle population in the sample, allowing a more accurate determination of the size of individual particle populations by light scattering. Various filters can be used, starting with filters in the range of 3–4 μm, to 1 μm, down to 0.4, 0.2, or 0.1 μm. Using centrifugation, such filters are not required; however, centrifugation may be quite time consuming and may require optimization to obtain good fractionation efficiency.

3.4.1 Static Light Scattering

3.4.1.1 Aggregate Analysis Using SLS   SLS can be used to assess whether aggregation has taken place in a protein sample. Figure 3.6 shows an example of how SLS can be used for this purpose. In this experiment, bovine serum albumin (BSA) in PBS (at pH 7.0) was freshly prepared and not treated, stressed

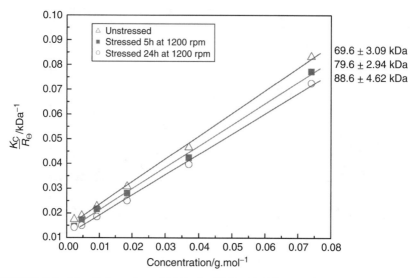

FIGURE 3.6 The Debye plot of BSA (in PBS, pH 7.0) as a fresh sample and after stirring for 5 and 24 h at 1200 rpm at 22°C.

by stirring for 5 h or stressed for 24 h at 1200 rpm. A concentration range was prepared from these samples, and a Debye plot was generated (Section 3.2.1). The BSA in the unstressed sample had an average M_w of 69.6 kDa, which is fairly close to the expected M_w of 66 kDa. The slightly higher value is caused by the unavoidable presence of low abundance oligomers (dimers, trimers, etc.) in the sample. The BSA in stressed samples showed average M_ws of 79.6 and 88.6 kDa for the 5- and 24-h stirred samples, respectively. This increase in M_w on stirring indicates the formation of aggregate species. The presence of these aggregate species was confirmed by DLS experiments (data not shown). Even a slight increase in the quantity of aggregate species will significantly contribute to the determination of the average M_w; note that $I \sim d^6$. However, it is impossible to determine the quantity of the formed aggregates by SLS (or DLS).

3.4.1.2 Using the Second Virial Coefficient A_2 for the Prediction of Colloidal Protein Stability SLS can be used to determine the second virial coefficient, A_2, as explained in Section 3.2.1. To illustrate this, hen egg white lysozyme was dissolved at pH 2 and 7 and analyzed using SLS. In Fig. 3.7, two linear plots can be seen. The slightly positive slope observed at pH 2 indicates that the protein molecules tend to have more interaction with the surrounding solvent, while the negative slope of the curve observed at pH 7 indicates that the particles tend to have more interaction among themselves. This is in accordance to recently presented studies [13]. Potentially, the hen egg white lysozyme dissolved at pH 7 would be more susceptible to aggregation.

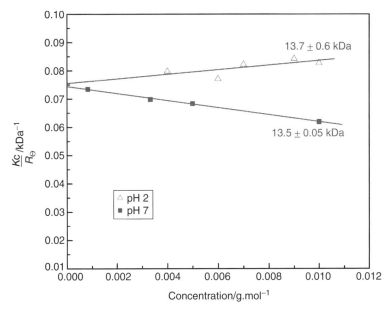

FIGURE 3.7   The Debye plot of hen egg white lysozyme at pH 2 and 7.

3.4.1.3 Drawbacks of SLS   If performed appropriately, SLS will give the absolute molecular weight of the protein being analyzed and will give information whether the protein might be prone to aggregation. However, if the sample is not monodisperse, the determination of the molecular weight will be skewed. This can be of use to assess whether aggregation occurs. Trace amounts of large particles of nonproteinaceous nature, for example, dust particles or particles coming from the used excipients or container, will also skew the determination of the molecular weight. Therefore, it is recommended to perform a DLS analysis before the SLS experiment to assure monodispersity.

Often proteins display some sort of self-associative behavior. In this case, obtaining a linear Debye plot with SLS is impossible and the determination of the molecular weight is difficult if not impossible.

3.4.2 Dynamic Light Scattering

3.4.2.1 Discrimination of Different Proteins Using DLS   To illustrate the different hydrodynamic diameters of several proteins, Fig. 3.8 shows the size distributions of BSA (2 mg/mL in water for injection (WFI), pH 6.0, 0.2 μm filtered), lysozyme (10 mg/mL in WFI, pH 2), and an antibody (1 mg/mL in WFI, pH 6) at 20°C, each of them calculated with the multiple narrow algorithm. These monomeric proteins (based on high-performance SEC) show hydrodynamic diameters of 3.8 nm (lysozyme), 7.5 nm (BSA), and 11 nm (antibody).

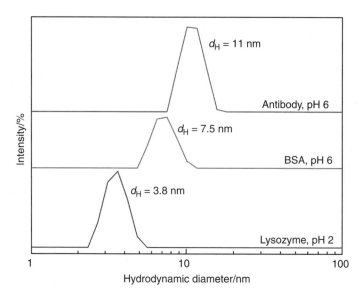

FIGURE 3.8   Size distributions of BSA (2 mg/mL in WFI, pH 6.0, 0.2 μm filtered), lysozyme (10 mg/mL in WFI, pH 2), and an antibody (1 mg/mL in WFI, pH 6) at 20°C calculated with the multiple narrow algorithm.

3.4.2.2 Characterization of the Colloidal Stability of Protein Solutions Using DLS

Figure 3.9 shows the size distributions of a solution of BSA (0.2 mg/mL in WFI, pH 6.0) as fresh solution (not filtered) as well as after stirring for 1 h at 5000 rpm and 20°C. The native, monomeric protein shows a hydrodynamic diameter of 7.5 nm. Even without the applied stress, the protein tends to form larger aggregates. Stirring the solution leads to the formation of aggregates with a diameter of about 700 nm, while the other populations change in relative intensity. Simultaneously, the aggregation leads to an increasing z-average (52–251 nm) and PDI (0.25–0.55). The aggregation during stirring is caused by the unfolding of the protein at the hydrophobic solvent–air interface [23–25]. This example illustrates the power of DLS for investigations of protein aggregation during physical stress.

The colloidal and thermal stability of proteins can be influenced by several parameters, for example, pH, buffer, protein concentration, and excipients [24,26]. Figure 3.10 shows the influence of the pH on the size distribution of lysozyme (10 mg/mL in WFI, pH 2 and 10). Under acidic conditions (pH 2), there is only a monomeric population with $d_H \approx 4$ nm detected. Increasing the pH to 10 is followed by the formation of aggregates with $d_H \approx 1$ μm. This aggregation kinetics is fast, and the formation of protein aggregates is observed within minutes. The isoelectric point of lysozyme is pH 10.8. Here, the net charge of the protein at pH 10 is close to 0, and the electrostatic repulsion between the molecules is negligible—protein aggregation can easily occur.

As mentioned earlier, the choice of the buffer conditions can have great influence on the colloidal stability of an antibody. As an example, Fig. 3.11 shows

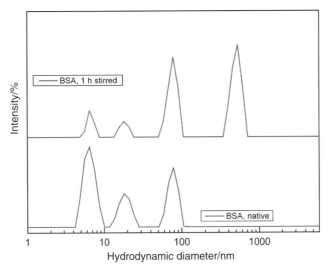

FIGURE 3.9   Size distributions of BSA (0.2 mg/mL in WFI, pH 6.0) as a fresh sample and after stirring for 120 min at 5000 rpm at 20°C using the multiple narrow algorithm.

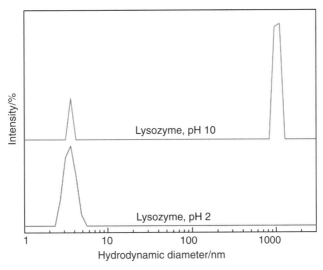

FIGURE 3.10   Size distributions of lysozyme (10 mg/mL in WFI, pH 2 and 10) at 20°C using the multiple narrow algorithm.

the size distribution of an immunoglobulin after shaking for one week at 20°C in two different buffers (25 mM phosphate or citrate, each pH 6.1). The antibody in phosphate buffer did not show any aggregates after shaking. In contrast, using 25-mM citrate as a formulation leads to antibody aggregation.

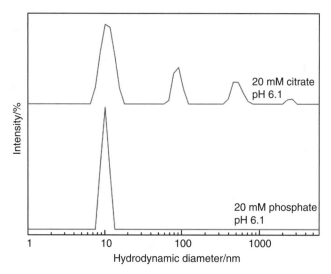

FIGURE 3.11   Size distributions of an antibody solution (2.5 mg/mL) after shaking for one week at 20°C under different buffer conditions (25 mM phosphate or 25 mM citrate, each pH 6.1) using the multiple narrow algorithm.

These examples show that DLS can potentially be used as a screening tool to identify the best formulation conditions for a specific protein. However, the detection of protein aggregates is limited by different reasons. First, DLS can only measure in a size range from ~ 1 nm to 5–7 μm. Larger particles cannot be detected owing to directed movements and because larger particles tend to sediment, making them undetectable.

3.4.2.3   Characterization of Thermally Induced Protein Aggregation Kinetics Using DLS

Figure 3.12 shows the size distributions of an antibody (1.2 mg/mL in 20 mM citrate, pH 6.1) during a temperature scan from 40 to 67°C. At low temperatures ($T \leq 40°C$), the antibody solution consists of only one population with $d_H = 11$ nm, reflecting the native, monomeric antibody. The populations with sizes from 20 to 100 nm at 64 and 65°C indicate the formation of antibody aggregates. Increasing the temperature to 67°C leads to the formation of larger aggregates with diameters of about 50 and 1000 nm. After cooling down the sample to room temperature, DLS indicated that the formed aggregates were not reversible (data not shown).

In general, studying thermally induced antibody aggregation by DLS can be helpful, for example, to identify suitable formulation conditions for protein pharmaceuticals and support other studies of the thermodynamic behavior such as differential scanning calorimetry or intrinsic fluorescence spectroscopy [27].

3.4.2.4   DLS as an In-Process-Control Assay

The processing of biopharmaceuticals includes several steps, for example, filtration, purification, and

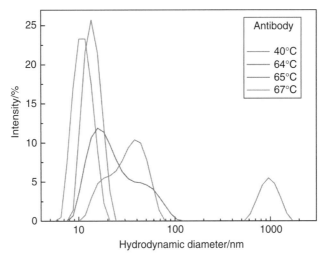

FIGURE 3.12   Size distributions of an antibody (1.2 mg/mL in 20 mM citrate, pH 6.1) at elevating temperatures from 40 to 67°C using the multiple narrow algorithm. *(See insert for color representation of the figure.)*

filling [28]. All these processes can cause undesirable protein aggregation and need to be monitored carefully [29]. DLS can be used as such as an "in-process-control" technology. Figure 3.13 shows the size distribution of an antibody before and after sterile filtration using a filter with 0.2-μm pores. The unfiltered solution shows the monomeric antibody population at 10 nm and

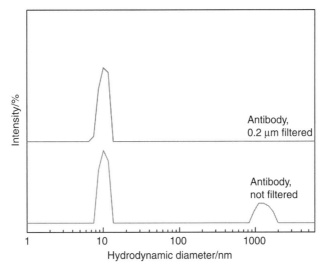

FIGURE 3.13   Size distributions of an antibody (1.2 mg/mL, pH 6.1) before and after sterile filtration at 20°C calculated using the general purpose algorithm.

a small population of large aggregates at ~1300 nm. After one appropriate filtration step, the large particles are completely removed from the sample.

3.4.2.5 Drawbacks of DLS

For "absolute" size measurements with DLS, several sample specific parameters have to be known. As part of the Stokes–Einstein relation (Eq. 3.9), the dynamic viscosity of the solvent has a direct influence on calculating sizes from DLS data. Figure 3.14 shows the influence of the dynamic viscosity on the size measurement of a 275-nm latex standard. Using the correct viscosity of the solvent, the calculated size is nearly constant. Using the viscosity of water at 20°C (1.033 mPa·s), the measured sizes are very high. Hence, absolute measurements require the knowledge of the dynamic viscosity of the solvent. Temperature is also a parameter that has to be controlled, as it affects the viscosity, and temperature differences may lead to convection.

Another important parameter influencing DLS results is the choice of the algorithm for the calculation of size distributions (Section 3.3.7). For the measurement of an unknown protein solution, the use of general purpose seems to be appropriate. However, the DLS application dictates the algorithm to be used. It is very useful to first analyze the autocorrelation function that may help to choose the correct algorithm.

The RI of the solution as part of the scattering vector q (Eqs. 3.10 and 3.11) is another sample parameter, which should be known for absolute DLS

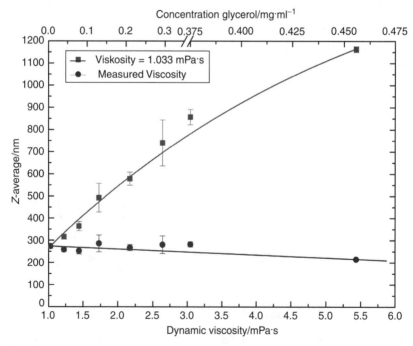

FIGURE 3.14 Influence of the dynamic viscosity on DLS measurements of a latex standard (275 nm).

measurements. Even the choice of the cuvettes can influence the result of a DLS measurement. Cuvettes made of quartz glass lead to a better quality of the scattered light, while plastics can cause multiple scattering.

3.5   CONCLUSIONS AND DISCUSSION

SLS and DLS are powerful methods for the determination of particle size. Because of the fact that the intensity of the scattered light is proportional to the sixth power of the size of the protein/particle (i.e., a particle that is 10 times larger in size will scatter a million times more light), light scattering-based techniques are very sensitive to small amounts of particles including aggregates. This shows a drawback of these techniques, that is, dust particles or other larger size impurities can drastically disturb measurements and may lead to faulty conclusions. Therefore, particular attention should be given to proper sample preparation. This means that the sample preparation should preferably be carried out in laminar air-flow cabinets and all solutions needed for dilution of the samples should be filtrated. Furthermore, the use of equipment with large scattering angles (e.g., the back scattering detector ($173°$) used in the Malvern Zetasizer) reduces the sensitivity to large (contaminating) particles (see anisotropic scattering). On the other hand, some new DLS devices provide a software-based dust filter [30], which excludes bad data from the analysis. In addition, the use of very concentrated samples might be problematic because multiple scattering can occur, that is, the probability of a scattered light beam hitting a second particle (secondary scattering) is high. This causes the hydrodynamic radius to be underestimated. Furthermore, highly concentrated samples can overload the photomultiplier in the DLS equipment owing to excessive light intensity, which influences the determination of the size. This phenomenon can be minimized by measuring at low protein concentrations (e.g., 1 mg/mL). However, various approaches, such as photon cross-correlation spectroscopy (PCCS), are now available, enabling the investigation of highly concentrated protein solutions up to protein concentrations of ~ 200 mg/mL, which would not be possible with other techniques [16,31,32]. With these new applications, DLS allows the measurement of highly concentrated protein formulations in its original protein concentration.

Excipients used in pharmaceutical preparations to stabilize the proteins more than occasionally interfere with data analysis. For instance, nonionic detergents are often used to prevent protein aggregation. When added above their critical micelle concentration (CMC), they form micelles with sizes in the nanometer range, which can be in the size range of native and aggregated species.

In the case of SLS (MALLS and LALLS), the time-averaged light intensity scattered by the particles in solution is measured. This will give the mean molecular weight of the particles in solution. However, when a sample is polydisperse (more than one species present in the solution or dust), accurate determination of the molecular weight of the main species is impossible. In this case, DLS is a good technique for determining the PDI of a sample. A way to overcome this problem is the separation of the protein sample into its individual species (a sample containing protein aggregates is by definition polydisperse). This can be achieved by SEC or asymmetrical flow field-flow fractionation (aFFFF) before light scattering analysis (Chapters 2, 4, and 5). Using DLS as an additional online detector would be greatly beneficial as size analysis is not based on concentration, and, thus, no concentration detector is required.

When used in batch mode, DLS is not capable of separating species that differ <2.6-fold in size. This means that protein dimers and trimers cannot be separated from the monomer protein peak. An indication whether dimers and/or trimers are present can be obtained from an increase in the PDI. Furthermore, the presence of dimers or trimers can be detected (but not quantified) by an increasing half-power width of the intensity-weighted size distribution.

The use of light scattering techniques for the analysis of the association states of proteins in solution, such as MALLS and DLS, provides an advantage in that they are relatively fast and noninvasive methods [33]. Thus, the sample can be reused for other investigations. On the other hand, scattering techniques are not specific for proteins, that is, nonproteinaceous particles that scatter light are also detected.

For drawing proper conclusions, a basic level of understanding the phenomenon of light scattering is necessary. Furthermore, data analysis with both SLS and DLS techniques is tedious. For instance, extracting the molecular weight from MALLS experiments requires the knowledge of complicated mathematical transformations. Fortunately, advanced software packages ease this progress. However, still the results need to be carefully scrutinized. In the case of DLS, not only the size distributions should be examined but also other "underlying" data, such as the correlation plot, need to be carefully investigated.

REFERENCES

1. Berne BJ, Pecora P. Dynamic light scattering, with applications to chemistry, biology and physics. New York: Wiley Interscience; 1976.

2. Mie G. Beiträge zur Optik trüber Medien, speziell kolloidaler Metallösungen. Ann Phys 1908;25(3):377–445.

3. Zimm BH. Apparatus and methods for measurement and interpretation of the angular variation of light scattering; preliminary results on polystyrene solutions. J Chem Phys 1948;16(12):1099–1117.

4. Zimm BH. Molecular theory of the scattering of light in fluids. J Chem Phys 1945;13:141–146.

5. Wyatt PJ. Light scattering and the absolute characterization of macromolecules. Anal Chim Acta 1993;272:1–40.

6. Rayleigh L, Strutt JW. On the light from the sky, its polarisation and colour. Philos Mag 1871a;41(271):107–120.

7. Rayleigh L, Strutt JW. On the light from the sky, its polarisation and colour. Philos Mag 1871b;41(273):274–279.

8. Rayleigh L, Strutt JW. On the scattering of light by small particles. Philos Mag 1871c;41(275):447–454.

9. Harding SE, Sattelle DB, Bloomfield VA. Laser light scattering in biochemistry. Cambridge: Royal Society of Chemistry; 1992.

10. Andersson M, Wittgren B, Wahlund K-G. Accuracy in multiangle light scattering measurements for molar mass and radius estimations. Model calculations and experiments. Anal Chem 2003;75(16):4279–4291.

11. Slotboom DJ, Duurkens RH, Olieman K, Erkens GB. Static light scattering to characterize membrane proteins in detergent solution. Methods 2008;46:73–82.

12. LeBrun V, Friess W, Schultz-Fademrecht T, Muehlau S, Garidel P. Insights in lysozyme - lysozyme self-interactions as assessed by the osmotic second virial coefficient: impact for physical protein stabilisation. Biotechnol J 2009;4(9):1305–1319.

13. LeBrun V, Friess W, Bassarab S, Garidel P. Correlation of protein-protein interactions as assessed by affinity chromatography with colloidal protein stability: a case study with lysozyme. Pharm Dev Technol 2010.. DOI: 10.1080/10837450903262074.

14. Zimm BH. The scattering of light and the radial distribution function of high polymer solutions. J Chem Phys 1948;16:1093–1100.

15. Berry GC. Thermodynamic and conformational properties of polystyrene. I. Light-scattering studies on dilute solutions of linear polystyrenes. J Chem Phys 1966;44:4550–4565.

16. Xu R. Photon Correlation Spectroscopy, Chapter 5. Particle Characterization: light scattering methods. Dordrecht, The Netherlands: Kluwer Academic Publishers; 2000. pp 223–283.

17. Rabal HJ, Braga RA Jr. Dynamic laser speckle and applications. USA: Taylor & Francis Group, LLC; 2009.

18. Wehr LR. Untersuchungen zu Proteinaggregationsprozessen mittels dynamischer und elektrophoretischer Lichtstreuung [PhD thesis]. Berlin, Germany: Freie Universitaet. 2002.

19. Gun'ko MV, Klyueva AV, Levchuk YN, Leboda R. Photon correlation spectroscopy investigations of proteins. Adv Colloid Interface Sci 2003;105:201–328.

20. Finsy R. Particle sizing by quasi-elastic light-scattering. Adv Colloid Interface Sci 1994;52:79–143.

21. Provencher SW. CONTIN: a general purpose constrained regularization program for inverting noisy linear algebraic and integral equations. Comput Phys Commun 1982;27:229–242.

22. Malvern Instruments. FAQs, Zetasizer Nano ZS. What's the best DLS algorithm?. Worcestershire, UK: Malvern Instruments. 2009.

23. Garidel P, Bassarab S. Impact of formulation design on stability and quality. In: Lyscon N, editor. Quality for biologics: critical quality attributes, process and change control, product variation, characterisation, impurities and regulatory concerns. Hampshire: Biopharm Knowledge Publishing; 2009. pp. 94–113. Chapter 7.

24. Wang W. Instability, stabilization, and formulation of liquid protein pharmaceuticals. Int J Pharm 1999;185:129–188.

25. Chi EY, Krishnan S, Randolpf TW, Carpenter JF. Physical stability of proteins in aqueous solution: mechanism and driving forces in nonnative protein aggregation. Pharm Res 2003;20(9):1325–1336.

26. Zheng JY, Janis LJ. Influence of pH, buffer species, and storage temperature on physicochemical stability of a humanized monoclonal antibody LA298. Int J Pharm 2006;308:46–51.

27. Garidel P. Steady-state intrinsic tryptophan protein fluorescence spectroscopy in pharmaceutical biotechnology. Spectrosc Eur 2008;20(4):7–11.

28. Bowen WR, Hall NJ, Pan L-C, Sharif AO, Williams PM. The relevance of particle size and zeta-potential in protein processing. Nat Biotechnol 1998;16:785–787.

29. Garidel P, Kebbel F. Protein therapeutics and protein aggregates characterised by photon correlation spectroscopy: an application for high concentration liquid formulations. Int Bioprocess 2010;8(3):38–46.

30. Malvern Instruments Ltd.Handbook Zetasizer NanoZS. Worcestershire, UK: Malvern Instruments Ltd. 2009.

31. Lämmle W. Particle size and stability analysis in turbid suspensions and emulsions with photon cross correlation spectroscopy. VDI Ber 2008;2027:97–103.

32. Minton AP. Static light scattering from concentrated protein solutions, I: general theory for protein mixtures and application to self-associating proteins. Biophys J 2007;93(4):1321–1328.

33. Fernández C, Minton AP. Static light scattering from concentrated protein solutions II: experimental test of theory for protein mixtures and weakly self-associating proteins. Biophys J 2009;96(5):1992–1998.

4 Online Detection Methods and Emerging Techniques for Soluble Aggregates in Protein Pharmaceuticals

TAPAN K. DAS

BioTherapeutics Pharmaceutical Sciences, Pfizer, St. Louis, Missouri, USA

4.1 INTRODUCTION

In contrast to pharmaceutical development of small molecules, biotherapeutic candidates exhibit much higher degree of instability owing to their structural complexity. Hence, studying biologics molecules requires a comprehensive set of biochemical as well as biophysical tools applied to either a heterogeneous mix of species (e.g., isoforms, degradation products such as aggregates) in solution or to the separated components from a heterogeneous mixture. Some of the tools such as UV–vis spectroscopy, refractive index (RI) measurement, and fluorescence spectroscopy measure bulk properties (ensemble average of mixture of species) in solution. These tools, in most cases, can also be coupled with separation techniques such as high performance liquid chromatography (HPLC) to study physicochemical properties of the fractionated species from a drug substance or drug product solution. Separation of fractions can also be achieved by other techniques such as asymmetrical flow field-flow fractionation (AF4) and centrifugal methods (e.g., analytical ultracentrifugation (AUC)) described in Chapter 2. Dynamic light scattering, on the other hand, can provide size information of constituent species in an unfractionated sample, albeit with limited size resolution as discussed in Chapter 3.

The principle of online detection techniques is that as the constituent species in a formulation of a protein pharmaceutical are being separated, one or more detectors are used either simultaneously or sequentially to study the desired physicochemical properties of the separated species. Traditional absorbance, RI, and fluorescence detectors are most often used online with size-, charge-, or

Analysis of Aggregates and Particles in Protein Pharmaceuticals, First Edition.
Edited by Hanns-Christian Mahler, Wim Jiskoot.
© 2012 John Wiley & Sons, Inc., Published 2012 by John Wiley & Sons, Inc.

hydrophobicity-based separation techniques for quantitation of fractionated species. For characterization of separated species, such as to determine molecular mass, online static light scattering (SLS) [1,2] is one of the most reliable methods. Online fluorescence detectors can also provide information on protein conformation especially when data is collected in spectral mode. Protein solutions containing aggregates can also be studied using batch mode assays (i.e., not online); however, the batch mode analysis obviously does not provide resolution of various soluble aggregates forms such as dimer and trimer from the monomer.

It should be noted that the term *online* detection used in this chapter as well as elsewhere in protein pharmaceuticals characterization literature refer to throughput detection during sample fractionation achieved via an integrated system. For process monitoring in manufacturing, however, online refers to ability to detect/monitor certain parameter(s) without having to take a sample out of process stream. Therefore, the type of online applications referred here (e.g., size-exclusion (SE-)HPLC with UV detection) would generally be termed as *at-line* in process monitoring in which a sample aliquot may have to be taken out to inject in the SE-HPLC system.

The following sections discuss online detection and characterization techniques for soluble aggregates. Additionally, some of the emerging techniques and novel methods for soluble aggregate detection are highlighted along with a brief description of the technical principles, sample requirements, and their applications in aggregate detection, as well as their advantages and limitations.

In the context of this chapter, soluble aggregates are defined as the *aggregate species* that are small enough to enter the column of a chromatographic separation. However, it should be noted that much larger size aggregates such as a 1000-mer of IgG2 can remain in solution (i.e., soluble) without much change in appearance (i.e., visibility). In principle, the online detection systems are able to detect larger aggregate species if fractionation is achieved, and the quantity of the fractionated species is above the limit of detection of the online detector.

4.2 ONLINE METHODS FOR SOLUBLE AGGREGATE DETECTION

An important prerequisite for a method to be suitable as an online detection method is its rapid response, thus enabling fast data acquisition. The commonly used online detection methods, including various UV–vis absorbance, light scattering methods, RI, fluorescence, circular dichroism (CD), and intrinsic viscosity (IV), fulfill this requirement. For example, when various aggregated species are being fractionated by HPLC, these detectors are able to collect data as they are passing through the channel. Table 4.1 provides a listing of the commonly available online techniques including their attributes, strengths, and limitations. In contrast to these rapid response techniques, some of the biochemical methods (e.g., sodium dodecyl sulfate–polyacrylamide gel electrophoresis (SDS–PAGE)) are not readily suitable for online application. On the other hand,

TABLE 4.1 Online Methods for Soluble Aggregate Detection in Protein Pharmaceutical Development

Online Method	Attribute(s) Monitored	Strengths	Limitations	Area(s) of Application
UV–vis detector	Concentration, %aggregate	High precision, accurate quantitation, robust, high throughput, QC compatible, low cost, easy to use, compatible with various separation methods (SE-HPLC, AF4, AUC)	May not work well for nonamino acid part of protein molecules such as PEG, carbohydrates; mostly insensitive to protein conformational changes	Release, stability, comparability, development
Fluorescence detector	Conformational change in protein, concentration possible with calibration curve	High sensitivity, excellent limit of detection (nanograms of protein), choice of intrinsic fluorescence and external dye, high throughput, low cost, easy to use, compatible with various separation methods (SE-HPLC, AF4, AUC)	Various quenching pathways can complicate data interpretation; Trp fluorescence intensity value not absolute; broad Trp fluorescence emission band—uncertainty in accurate emission maximum determination	Development
Refractive index detector	Concentration, % aggregate, concentration of nonamino acid content (e.g., PEG, carbohydrate)	Modest precision (less than UV–vis), accurate quantitation, robust, high throughput, low cost, easy to use, compatible with various separation methods (SE-HPLC, AF4, AUC); does not depend on the presence of UV or fluorescence chromophores. Works with higher protein concentration than UV.	Need isocratic mobile phase, need steady flow rate of mobile phase, difficulty detecting low %aggregates	Development
Viscosity detector	Intrinsic viscosity, hydrodynamic size (when coupled to SLS detector)	Sensitive to aggregation, protein unfolding, high throughput, low cost, compatible with SE-HPLC	Must be coupled to mass determination detector (SLS), hydrodynamic size data may not be reliable for low %aggregates	Development

(continued)

TABLE 4.1 (*Continued*)

Online Method	Attribute(s) Monitored	Strengths	Limitations	Area(s) of Application
Multiangle light-scattering and low-angle light-scattering detectors	Molecular mass, radius of gyration	Very reliable method for mass determination can handle broad size range (dynamic range of SE-HPLC), works in both MALS and LALS modes, compatible with various separation methods (SE-HPLC, AF4), integrated systems (with RI, UV) available	Must be coupled with concentration detector (UV–vis, RI), no radius of gyration data for smaller than 10 nm protein species, difficulty in mass determination of low %aggregates	Development
Dynamic light-scattering detector	Hydrodynamic radius	Can handle broad size range (dynamic range of SE-HPLC), compatible with SE-HPLC, can also provide shape information (when coupled with MALS, from radius of gyration and hydrodynamic radius)	Optimization of flow rate, injected mass, and collection time needed, very sensitive to beads leaching from SE-HPLC column	Development
Circular dichroism detector	Structural change (secondary, tertiary)	Choice of wavelengths to monitor various CD bands (helical, Trp, Tyr, etc.), direct information on assignable secondary structure changes	Much less sensitive than fluorescence and UV–vis detectors, limited access to far-UV wavelengths (>220 nm)	Development

capillary electrophoresis (CE) methods can be used for throughput separation of protein monomer and aggregates under nondenaturing and denaturing (with urea or SDS) conditions [3–6]. SDS typically dissociates noncovalent aggregates; therefore, CE with SDS can yield an estimate of the aggregate populations that are covalent in nature [3].

The following sections briefly describe the principles, mode of online operation, sample requirements, and relevance to aggregate detection of selected online detectors. Some of these are used more regularly (such as SLS) compared to others (such as evaporative light scattering, CD). Strengths and drawbacks of these online detectors are also discussed.

4.2.1 UV–vis Detector

The most commonly used online detector with SE-HPLC and other separation methods is UV and visible absorbance. UV–vis spectrophotometric techniques are described in greater detail in Chapter 8. Absorbance detection is very useful in quantifying percentage of fractionated species such as monomer and aggregates. Fast sampling rate, typically in the range of 20–160 Hz, enables high speed absorbance detection compatible with HPLC applications. Most UV–vis detectors cover a wavelength range of 190–600 nm, but additional coverage up to 950 nm is also available. For quantification of fractionated protein species, typically absorbance is monitored either at 280 nm or at a wavelength in the 214–220 nm range. Using programmable slits, these detectors can cover a wide range of absorbance values, approximately three orders of magnitude, thereby facilitating the detection of species in both low concentration and high concentration protein samples. Additionally, a variety of flow cells are available with micro- to nanoliter sample volume, various pathlengths, and compatibility with a range of pressures, thereby offering flexibility with types of samples and amount of sample injected. For example, antibody formulations in a wide range of strengths from less than 1 mg/mL to higher than 100 mg/mL can be handled with reproducible aggregate detection of approximately 0.5% as the limit of quantitation.

Absorbance can be monitored at one or more preset wavelengths, or full spectra can be collected using a diode-array detector. UV–vis detectors provide very high quality and robust data, which make it a reliable quantification method suitable for quality control (QC) applications [7]. However, absorbance value (or RI) by itself cannot determine the molecular size of the separated species; hence, most commonly online UV–vis detectors are used in conjunction with other detectors such as SLS to determine mass of monomer and aggregates as discussed later.

It should be noted that the online UV–vis detector (as well as the other online detectors discussed below) may not be able to distinguish between chemical natures of the aggregates (such as covalent vs noncovalent) without additional biochemical treatment. Solubilizing chemicals can be used (such as SDS) in the mobile phase in SE-HPLC to distinguish between covalent versus noncovalent aggregates; however, cleaning of SDS from the HPLC system can be quite difficult. Alternatively, off-line methods such as SDS–PAGE can conveniently distinguish between covalent and noncovalent aggregates.

4.2.2   Fluorescence Detector

Fluorescence techniques are described in detail in Chapter 9. The fluorescence detector is another commonly used online detector used with SE-HPLC. Fluorescence detection typically includes excitation at a chosen wavelength suitable for the available chromophores (e.g., 280 nm for Trp) and detection of emission at or near the emission maxima (typically between ~330 and 345 nm for folded proteins). Additionally, the emission spectrum can be recorded to determine a shift in emission maximum indicative of conformational differences between native protein (monomer) and variants including aggregates. The fluorescence detectors can help achieving sensitivity of an order of magnitude better than UV depending on the type of fluorescence reporter group used [8]. Both intrinsic (such as tryptophan and tyrosine) and extrinsic (dye) fluorescent reporters [9] can be used with SE-HPLC systems to characterize aggregates. Tryptophan is present in most proteins and is a natural choice as fluorescence probe without need to label. Tryptophan fluorescence of proteins is known to be sensitive to its local environment [10,11]. Therefore, it offers an excellent method of aggregate characterization for conformational changes. Tryptophan fluorescence can exhibit intensity change, emission maximum shift, alteration in spectral band width, and sometimes a change in the number of bands depending on the type of denaturation and/or aggregation. Therefore, instead of collecting fluorescence intensity at a preset wavelength, collection of fluorescence emission spectra during elution (of the separated species) may be useful in aggregate characterization such as finding any conformational change and/or intensity quenching. Online fluorescence spectra can be collected by rapid scan techniques (e.g., at the rate of 28 ms per data point) without interrupting chromatographic elution, where the fluorescence detector is equipped with excitation and emission monochromators utilizing holographic concave grating.

4.2.3   Refractive Index Detector

Refraction of light occurs when incident light traverses from one medium to an optically denser (or lighter) second medium. The RI is a measure for the extent to which light is retarded by a medium (e.g., a solvent) or substance (e.g., a protein). A differential refractometer is commonly used as an RI detector and can be coupled with various separation techniques such as SE-HPLC. Differential RI between the reference (e.g., mobile phase) and protein sample is measured as analytes such as protein monomers and aggregates are being separated. The RI signal can be used to measure concentration of fractionated species irrespective of any absorbance or fluorescence emanating from the analytes. This attribute makes an RI detector a more universal detector than absorbance or fluorescence for measuring concentration.

In practical applications of protein aggregate measurements, one does not need to determine optical properties (absorbance maxima, fluorescence excitation/emission) of unknown aggregates if using RI to measure concentration. Concentration can be calculated from the RI signal (proportional to concentration) if the *dn/dc* (RI increment by solute concentration) value is known. For proteins without nonamino acid content, the *dn/dc* value is nearly constant (0.186 mL/g) [12]. The same *dn/dc* value can be used for protein monomer and its aggregates. When an SLS detector is coupled with RI detection in a SE-HPLC or AF4 separation, relative percentage (by RI) of monomer and aggregates as well as their molecular mass (by SLS) can be conveniently determined.

Although the mobile phase used in RI detection does not need to be UV transparent, significant drift in baseline is a frequent issue especially if (i) the mobile phase composition changes (such as in nonisocratic conditions), (ii) flow rate needs to be varied, and (iii) quality of flow is poor (may be the case in slow elution AF4 experiments). Another issue with RI detection is its low sensitivity (compared to UV absorbance and fluorescence) rendering concentration measurements for low amounts of aggregates practically impossible. Depending on the UV wavelength (at or near 280 nm) and the extinction coefficient, the UV absorbance signal of a protein can be approximately 2- to 10-fold stronger than the RI signal. On the other hand, if the UV signal is saturated with high protein load, the RI signal can be used instead.

Another important application of RI detection is the determination of relative ratio of protein-based (amino acids) species and nonprotein portion such as in carbohydrate-containing proteins and PEG–protein conjugates [13]. The extent of pegylation in each of the SE-HPLC fractions can be determined from the RI/UV absorbance ratio to establish heterogeneity of pegylation in a drug product. Additionally, the presence of any depegylated species as well as aggregates formed by depegylated protein can be differentiated from aggregates formed by pegylated protein as long as these species can be separated by SE-HPLC or other separation techniques. It is important to note that the *dn/dc* values of the protein and nonprotein components need to be determined (or known) in such measurements.

4.2.4 Viscosity Detector

Coupled with light scattering, UV, and RI detectors, a viscometer can be added to SE-HPLC-based separations to determine the IV, which relates to hydrodynamic size. The IV of proteins in solution increases when proteins aggregate or change shape [14,15], resulting in increased hydrodynamic radius. The IV is part of the solution viscosity contributed by the solutes, and it is defined as the *ratio of specific viscosity* (η_{sp}) to concentration in infinitely dilute solution. The SLS detector can determine the mass; hence, the change in size calculated from viscometry can be attributed to a change in either mass (e.g., because of aggregation) or shape (e.g., because of denaturation).

The design of an online viscometer is a differential viscometer that uses a four-capillary bridge shown in Fig. 4.1 [16]. The four capillaries (denoted as

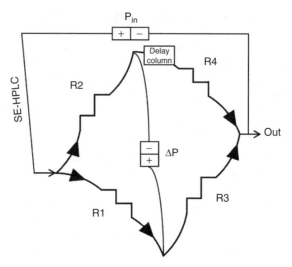

FIGURE 4.1   Schematics of a differential viscometer with a four-capillary bridge.

R1, R2, R3, and R4) of same resistance are configured in a way so that R1 and R3 are parallel to R2 and R4. A delay column is installed between the R2 and R4 capillaries. The differential pressure, ΔP, would be zero when the reference solvent (with viscosity η_0) flows through all four capillaries. In the next step, when the protein fractions (monomer, aggregates, etc.) flow through the bridge, the resistance in the capillaries R1, R2, and R3 increase in proportion to the IV of the fractionated species, while the reference solvent continues to flow through R4 because of the holdup volume in the delay column. Hence, the differential pressure increases proportionally to the specific viscosity of the protein fractions, and these are no longer zero. Differential pressure transducers are used to measure the pressure difference, ΔP, across the midpoint of the bridge. The relationship of specific viscosity (η_{sp}) to recorded parameters differential pressure (ΔP) and inlet pressure (P_{in}) is expressed as

$$\eta_{sp} = \frac{\eta - \eta_0}{\eta_0} = \frac{4\Delta P}{P_{in} - 2\Delta P}$$

Under the dilute solution assumption, that is, at low concentration of the protein fractions, the IV can be approximated as the ratio of specific viscosity to concentration. It should be noted that the IV does not have the units of viscosity; instead, it is in inverse density unit. With molecular weight (M_w) determined using the SLS detector, the IV value can yield an estimate of hydrodynamic radius (R_h) from the following equation, with N_A being the Avogadro number:

$$IV \cdot \frac{M_w}{N_A} = \frac{10}{3}\pi R_h^3$$

Therefore, an integrated system with SLS, RI, and viscosity detectors coupled to the SE-HPLC can provide an estimate of the hydrodynamic radius along with the molecular weight of protein monomer and aggregates from a single measurement [17]. One potential disadvantage of estimating hydrodynamic size from the IV is that the viscosity change is also caused by protein unfolding (denaturation), protein conformational changes, and changes in protein hydration; hence, for a complex system undergoing aggregation and the above mentioned events, reliability of size data will mainly depend on the ability to separate (SE-HPLC) and to determine molecular weight (SLS) of the individual species from the mixture.

4.2.5   Multiangle Light Scattering Detection

Light scattering techniques are described in detail in Chapter 3. Various modes of SLS are available for molecular mass measurement with protein solutions that may or may not contain aggregated forms. Determination of molecular mass of a macromolecule from scattered light is governed by the fundamental equation known as the *Zimm equation* [1,2], which includes angular dependence of scattered light and molecular mass (see Chapter 3). For most protein monomers and their aggregates that are fractionated by separation techniques such as SE-HPLC, size is typically $\lesssim 50$ nm and most often in the range of few nanometers to ~ 20 nm, depending on protein size. This size group falls in the category of $\lesssim 1/10$th (more strictly $< 1/20$th) of the incident laser wavelength in the visible range (~ 400–750 nm); hence, they are considered point masses with respect to the incident beam and can be treated as Rayleigh scatterers [18]. Larger size protein aggregates, with diameters closer to the incident beam wavelength, cause interference (reduction in intensity) of the scattered light emanating from different parts of the molecules. Mie scattering principles [19] can be applied for size ranges $\gtrsim 1/10$th of the laser wavelength. It should be noted that protein pharmaceuticals can form larger size species including subvisible and visible aggregates, but these are beyond the scope of this chapter.

SLS studies can be performed using light scattering detectors that are commercially available in various configurations such as low angle light scattering (LALS), right-angle light scattering (RALS), and multiangle light scattering (MALS). These LS detectors will have to be coupled with a concentration measurement detector (absorbance, RI, or both) to extract molecular mass of the fractionated species. A LALS detector employs light scattering measurements at low angle [17] where the reduction of scattered intensity due to intramolecular interference is negligible for molecules of sizes up to ~ 150 nm. Scattered light from molecules $\lesssim 10$ nm have negligible angular dependence; hence, both RALS and LALS will show similar intensity. For molecules $\gtrsim 10$ nm (up to ~ 150 nm), the Rayleigh ratio at low angle (calculated from LALS data) can be approximated to the value at zero angle. This approach simplifies data processing as the data is obtained from a single low angle detector and still provides reliable data on molecular mass. One of the commercially available detectors uses a low angle of 7° and determines molecular mass of a range of protein monomer and aggregates without need for extrapolation.

MALS measurements are also frequently used in the development of protein pharmaceuticals, in which a series of detectors are placed around the flow cell at various angles to collect angular dependence information, to aid the determination of molecular weight of different species separated via SE-HPLC or other techniques. When the angle increases, intramolecular interference results in a reduction of light scattering intensity for molecules larger than ~10 nm (and more prominently for molecule sizes of >1/20th of the incident beam wavelength). In addition to deriving molecular mass using a MALS detector, the angular dependence of the scattering intensity can provide size (the radius of gyration) information of the separated aggregate species. MALS detectors are commercially available, and an array of detectors can be placed in a range of angles (approximately from low (20°) to high (160°)). Size information is obtained in the form of root mean square radius, also referred to as *radius of gyration*. However, if the shape of the separated aggregates is not known, it is difficult to accurately estimate the dimension or radius. Angular dependence is diminished when the size (diameter) of protein monomer or aggregate is ≲10 nm (with incident laser light wavelength in the visible range), and consequently size can no longer be determined accurately. Range of molecular mass determined by online SLS is from several hundred Daltons to millions of Daltons and higher. However, practically when a mixture of species is fractionated using separation techniques (such as SE-HPLC, AF4, etc.), some of the components can be present in small quantity and determining their molecular mass (and size) by MALS can be very challenging due to a low signal-to-noise ratio.

In either MALS or LALS mode, an integrated unit of several detectors (e.g., absorbance, RI, LS, etc.) is commercially available that provides a convenient option to researchers to get a wealth of data from a single sample injection.

4.2.6 Dynamic Light Scattering Detection

DLS (also known as *quasielastic light scattering*) is most frequently used in batch mode (see Chapter 3) with unfractionated samples placed either in a sample cell or in well plates. More recently, online DLS has been made available coupled to SE-HPLC separation. DLS measures hydrodynamic radius using spherical approximation of a protein species according to the Stokes–Einstein equation [20]. Quality of online DLS data of the fractioned aggregates and monomer depends on the concentration of fractionated species, flow rate, and size of the aggregates/monomer. Unlike in batch mode, data collection over longer time is not practical in online mode. Therefore, some optimization between flow rate, injected protein mass, and data collection time will be necessary to get a reasonable quality of data. Additionally, the detection of a few percentage of aggregates may be challenging in online DLS mode and requires higher sample load than that in SLS to detect such species. Advantage of online DLS is that it collects autocorrelation function data of individual species; hence, ambiguity of data analysis and interpretation is less compared to that in batch mode, provided that the data of the individual (diluted) fractions are good enough. DLS of unfractionated samples (batch mode) yields only average hydrodynamic radius unless the two species (e.g., monomer and aggregate) are widely apart in molecular weight (such as monomer vs >10-mer). However, the capability of a DLS detector coupled with SE-HPLC is obviously limited to the separable size range by SE-HPLC; hence, any large protein aggregates (e.g., 100-mer and 1000-mer) present along with monomer will not be individually detected. Batch mode DLS is able to detect such large aggregates (up to few micrometers depending on detection angle) along with the monomers.

4.2.7   Circular Dichroism Detector

The use of online CD detectors in online separation techniques for aggregate characterization has been very limited. The far-UV region (~180–250 nm) is used to monitor secondary structural changes, while the near-UV range (~250–320 nm) can be probed for tertiary structural changes. Far-UV CD spectrum of proteins displays a signature of secondary structural contents (helical, β-sheet, etc.) [21]. Therefore, in principle, CD detectors can be helpful in identifying any structural differences between monomer and aggregates separated by SE-HPLC. However, the online CD detectors have nearly two orders of magnitude lower sensitivity (limit of detection) than that of a fluorescence detector [8]. The lower sensitivity of the CD detector is due to the fact that CD detection is based on very small absorption differences between right- and left-circularly polarized light [8]. Additionally, the CD signal intensity will also depend on the protein type (e.g., helical vs β-sheet structure) and wavelength of detection. Although CD signals in the near-UV region are more sensitive to conformational changes, due to the very weak CD signals in the near-UV region, it is very challenging to collect good quality data in online mode (with SE-HPLC). On the other hand, much stronger protein CD bands are seen in the far-UV CD region, but these bands are less sensitive to subtle structural/conformational changes. Extensive structural changes, for example, in aggregates formed by unfolded monomers, can be detected. Finally, because most proteins contain a mix of secondary structure types, comparison of spectra (as opposed to intensity at a single wavelength) is often essential for the assessment of protein structural changes. However, the online CD detectors are not capable of recording full spectra in the far-UV range. Because of several limitations of the online CD detector as discussed above, off-line CD analysis is a more popular practice.

4.2.8   Application of Online Detection Methods in the Development of Protein Pharmaceuticals

The use of various online detection methods for aggregation-related phenomena may depend on stages of development as well as type of information sought during development. There is an increasing need of minimizing investment in pre-proof-of-concept stages; therefore, detailed formulation and analytical characterization may not be available in early stages. Application of online aggregation detection systems may be helpful in early stages as these are amenable for high throughput operation. However, only few of the detection systems discussed above, such as light scattering detectors along with UV and/or RI, provide optimum benefit for most molecule types in characterizing aggregates in formulation development studies. The less commonly used detectors (e.g., CD) may be essential for certain molecule types and for specialized applications. One example of specialized application is when a protein is suspected of undergoing significant unfolding before forming aggregates, detectors that provide direct information on secondary (CD) or tertiary structure (CD, fluorescence) are quite beneficial.

During late-stage developments (e.g., fine tuning of formulations for phase 3 and commercial dosage forms), it may be necessary to identify and characterize more subtle structural changes associated with aggregate formation. Additionally, a detailed structural analysis of protein pharmaceuticals, their degradation profile, and stability is needed to be included in a CMC (chemistry, manufacturing and controls) package. While SE-HPLC with a UV detector is most commonly used for quantifying soluble aggregates for release and in stability studies, the online detectors as discussed above may provide additional structural characterization data.

4.3   EMERGING TECHNIQUES AND NOVEL METHODS FOR SOLUBLE AGGREGATE DETECTION

Many of the physical degradation events including aggregation, particulate formation, and related structural alterations associated with adsorption, misfolding, denaturation (by heat, chemicals, chaotrophs, etc.), partial misfolding, nucleating species, and sometimes chemical degradation will require the use of specialized techniques for comprehensive characterization. This section highlights some of the emerging techniques that may provide valuable supporting data in aggregation-related studies during formulation and process development, especially at later stages of development.

In the past several years, there has been much focus on emerging techniques and novel methods to study aggregation and particulates in biotherapeutics. Emerging techniques for studying visible and subvisible particulates are discussed in Chapter 7. The following sections discuss some of the emerging techniques as well as novel methods using traditional techniques applied to studying smaller size aggregates. The techniques discussed below encompass a number of applications for either detection of aggregates (such as mass spectrometry (MS)) or measuring physical properties that are sensitive to or potentially predictive of aggregate formation (such as quartz crystal microbalance (QCM) with dissipation monitoring, ultrasonic resonator technology (URT), and second virial coefficient determination).

4.3.1   Quartz Crystal Microbalance with Dissipation Monitoring (QCM-D)

QCM technology is known for several decades and has been used to study small changes in mass adsorbed on rigid surfaces. Quartz crystal microbalance with dissipation (QCM-D) is a relatively new technique for applications in biotechnology. QCM relies on a voltage being applied to a quartz crystal, causing it to oscillate at a specific frequency. When protein mass is adsorbed onto the crystal surface, the corresponding changes (damping) in frequency are measured. Additionally, when the oscillation is made to stop by disconnecting power, dissipation of energy can be monitored over time. Dissipation rate depends on the mass of the adsorbed biomolecule and its structural properties such as its viscoelastic behavior. The formation of a soft protein layer on the crystal surface increases the rate of damping (dissipation).

In recent years, a number of publications describe the use of QCM-D in various fields including adsorption studies of protein [22–25], DNA [26], nanoparticles [27], and lipid vesicles [28]. Although QCM-D principally analyzes the adsorption layer(s), the central hypothesis for its application to soluble protein aggregates is that the major components in a protein solution reversibly adsorb to the crystal surface. Therefore, it has been proposed that the state of self-association and its dissociation kinetics on dilution can be monitored at nanometer resolution using QCM-D (Das and Ho, unpublished data). It is to be recognized that utility and applications of QCM-D in solution aggregation studies are not established at present. From a practical point of view, it is important that the sensor crystals are regenerated by UV/ozone treatment to ensure a clean surface when reused.

Recent applications of this technology include studying dissipation behavior with liquid-phase samples. Herewith, the method becomes potentially applicable to studying the dimension of an adsorbed layer of protein monomer or aggregates in equilibrium with bulk protein solution. With protein solutions, adsorbed protein layers are often soft (i.e., not rigid), especially when large macromolecules and reversible/loose aggregates are studied. In addition, for cases of significant protein–protein interactions, viscoelastic behavior of any adsorbed layer will be highly different from that of a rigid adsorbed layer. For these types of applications, dissipation of crystal's oscillation data at the fundamental frequency (viz. 5 MHz) as well as overtones (e.g., 15, 25 and 35 MHz) can be collected that enable applying the Voigt model [26] for viscoelastic behavior to extract thickness, viscosity, and elasticity of soft layers.

Commercially available QCM-D equipment can detect adsorbed mass on the crystal surface as low as 0.5 ng/cm^2 in equilibrium with bulk liquid, thus offering high sensitivity of mass detection. Additionally, the adsorbed protein layer thickness of as low as a few nanometers can be detected, which opens the possibility of distinguishing a protein monomer versus a protein aggregate. However, it remains to be seen if it is able to detect and distinguish a fraction of soluble aggregates in a protein formulation in the presence of excess monomer. One of the potentially major applications of QCM-D is to detect concentration-dependent self-association behavior. The assumption is that the adsorbed layer on the quartz surface represents the state of protein in bulk solution. Additionally, it is possible that interaction with surface may induce aggregation.

QCM-D has been used in studying protein in solution such as high concentration monoclonal antibody to determine solution pH conditions at which the antibody formulation exhibits greatest liquidlike (i.e., least protein–protein interactions) behavior [23]. Knowles et al. [22] showed that precise determination of the growth rates of ordered protein aggregates such as amyloid fibrils can be achieved through real-time monitoring of the changes in the numbers of molecules in the fibrils from variations in their masses. Hovgaard et al. [24] used QCM-D to monitor the changes in layer thickness and viscoelastic properties accompanying multilayer amyloid deposition in situ for glucagon fibrillation.

Using a custom-built ultrasonic shear rheometer capable of operating at megahertz frequencies, Kalonia et al. studied the nature of protein–protein interactions in high protein concentration solutions [29,30].

In summary, the QCM-D technique is far from being proven as a mature technology for studying protein aggregation, but it holds potential for unique applications in the areas of protein self-association and high concentration formulations.

4.3.2   Ultrasonic Resonator Technology (URT)

URT measures ultrasonic velocity as well as absorption of ultrasonic waves when passed through a medium [31]. The discussion here focuses on ultrasonic velocity, as it is more relevant to measuring protein structural changes. Compressibility of a solute (e.g., protein) can modulate the propagation of ultrasound in solution. Therefore, a change in ultrasonic velocity indicates a change in compressibility, which, in turn, is linked to structure and level of hydration of the solute [32,33]. Ultrasonic velocity is lower in medium containing high compressibility solutes than one containing "hard" solutes. The ultrasonic resonator method has been used to study protein hydration by measuring relative specific sound velocity increment in solution [32]. The relative specific sound velocity increments in conjunction with the apparent specific volume data yield apparent specific adiabatic compressibility of a protein. Compressibility data has also been used in protein unfolding studies to assess heat-induced structural changes, and such structural changes were verified by orthogonal techniques such as CD spectroscopy [34,35].

Researchers have attempted to apply URT for studying protein stability, phase separation, and aggregation [36–38]. The underlying hypothesis is that such structural events cause a detectable change in ultrasonic velocity. Liu et al. measured the hydration differences between two phases of a high concentration antibody formulation and proposed that the protein molecules in the bottom phase may be more hydrated and, therefore, less likely to interact with each other to form aggregates [36]. Mathis et al. [38] suggested that a high concentration of protein aggregates results in a decrease in ultrasonic velocity, related to an overall decrease in hydration water due to the reduced surface-to-volume ratio of protein aggregates compared to monomers.

One inherent problem of applying URT technology in protein formulation studies is that it is sensitive to many factors, including hydration of all the components present in a formulation and their temperature dependence. Hence, the dependence of any observed changes in ultrasonic velocity to formulation variables (e.g., a change in salt/excipient concentration, a change in protein concentration) must be carefully segregated. It is often very difficult to assign the change in velocity measured by URT to a particular phenomenon. Such an assignment requires identification of the structural event using a biophysical method such as CD or fluorescence spectroscopy. It remains to be seen if URT holds any promise becoming an important aggregation characterization technique in formulation development of protein pharmaceuticals.

4.3.3 Taylor Dispersion (TD)

When a solution is flown slowly through a capillary, the solutes spread out under the combined action of molecular diffusion and the variation of velocity over the cross section [39]. This phenomenon known as *Taylor dispersion (TD)* is named after Sir Geoffrey Taylor. The distribution of solute concentration, however, remains symmetrical and moves with the mean speed of the flow in spite of flow asymmetry. The dispersion along the capillary is governed by a virtual coefficient of diffusivity that can be calculated from the measured distribution of solute concentration [39]. The concentration distribution data (band broadening) can be analyzed to determine the diffusion coefficient, thereby providing an alternative method of estimation of a protein's hydrodynamic radius. The hydrodynamic radius can be used to make an assessment if the protein solution contains only monomers or a mixture with aggregates [40]. Several applications of TD for measuring the diffusion coefficient of protein molecules have been reported [40–44].

The TD method allows proteins to be analyzed in their native form, without any labeling or denaturation. A plug of protein solution is injected into a capillary, driven by applied pressure, and detected using UV area imaging before and after the solution is looped through the capillary. The radius of the protein is determined by analysis of band broadening due to TD using the following equation:

$$R_h = \frac{4k_B T (\tau_2^2 - \tau_1^2)}{\pi \eta r^2 (t_2 - t_1)} \quad \text{and} \quad \tau^2 = \frac{r^2 t}{24D}$$

where R_h is the hydrodynamic radius, T the temperature in Kelvin, k_B the Boltzmann constant, η the viscosity, τ the variance (of peaks 1 and 2), t the center point of peaks, and D the diffusion coefficient. Using two windows (for UV imaging) helps eliminate sources of variance other than TD.

The advantages of the TD method are that it may provide an alternative (to DLS) measurement of R_h. This method has the potential for high throughput operations when coupled to a commercially available CE system. The method is applicable over a wide concentration range ($\sim$0.1–100 mg/mL) and uses small volume (tens of nanoliters to 1 μL) of sample.

In the currently available configurations of TD equipment, the R_h data of a solution containing a mixture of protein monomer and small aggregates (dimer, trimer, etc.) will be derived as weight average radius. The method is not able to sensitively detect the presence of a few percent of aggregates. When multiple aggregate species of different sizes are present, it may be possible to extract individual R_h values using a multicomponent fit. Currently available systems can be used to precisely measure R_h from 0.3 to approximately >20 nm.

In summary, the TD method appears to be much less versatile compared to DLS with respect to measurable size range and the type of applications but may offer certain advantages such as low sample volume requirements and coverage of a wide range of concentrations.

4.3.4   Second Virial Coefficient Estimation Using High Throughput Methods

The second osmotic virial coefficient (often denoted as B_{22}) is a qualitative measure of nonideal solution behavior arising from two-body interactions. B_{22} has been studied extensively by physical chemists and protein chemists applied to predict crystallization [45,46] and aggregation (or reduced solubility) [47,48] propensities. In protein formulation, B_{22} is defined as a two-state interaction between protein monomers. A positive B_{22} value reflects net repulsive forces between monomers, while a negative value indicates net attractive forces, suggesting propensity to attraction or aggregation. While B_{22} is considered to be useful providing guidance on self-association in a qualitative manner, there has been no success for consistent prediction of aggregation propensity, across a range of protein pharmaceuticals that can be applied to storage stability.

Some of the popular methods for measuring B_{22} are SLS [49,50], sedimentation equilibrium (AUC-SE) [51,52], and self-interaction chromatography (SIC) [53,54]. Winzor et al. recently noted that using SLS as the method, the measured B_{22} values reflect not only protein–protein interactions but also protein–cosolute interactions contributing to protein nonideality, whereas B_{22} values measured by sedimentation equilibrium provide an unequivocal measure of the osmotic virial coefficient for protein self-interaction [52,54]. Advancements in analytical and biophysical methods enable B_{22} determination in high throughput manner as demonstrated by SLS measurements [55,56], SIC [53,54], and SE-HPLC [57]. This section focuses on recent developments using light scattering and chromatography to measure B_{22} in a high throughput manner relevant to protein formulation and aggregation.

A concentration gradient SLS method was employed by Attri and Minton [55,58] for continuous measurement of scattered light and UV absorbance. This method is based on simultaneous measurement of the Rayleigh light scattering and UV absorbance of a solution whose composition is varied with time, thus allowing the determination of association behavior of proteins. A second approach uses a custom-designed dual-detector cell, which simultaneously measures protein concentration and the corresponding scattered light intensity at $90°$, after the protein elutes from a size-exclusion column for the measurement of the B_{22} value of proteins in aqueous solutions in flow mode [56]. The dual-detector cell eliminates the issues of interdetector band broadening and delay volume when two separate detectors are used.

Using the methods as described above, Minton et al. and Kalonia et al. demonstrated high throughput determination of the B_{22} values of a number of proteins including lysozyme, chymotrypsinogen, chymotrypsin, β-lactoglobulin, and hemoglobin under various solution conditions [55,56,58]. The method developed by Attri and Minton [55,58] also has been commercialized for potential use in formulation development studies.

Various chromatography-based techniques may be amenable to higher throughput applications to measure B_{22}. An HPLC approach that has gained more attention from researchers is SIC [53,54]. The magnitude of B_{22} is calculated from the elution volume of the protein in zonal chromatography on an affinity column with the same protein as immobilized ligand. This assumes that the immobilized protein retains its conformation and that its self-interaction sites are not selectively blocked during immobilization. Le Brun et al. conducted a detailed investigation with lysozyme in various solution conditions including ionic strength and showed that B_{22} values determined using HIC correlates with protein solubility as well as physical protein stability [53]. It remains to be seen whether such correlation is universal for other types of proteins with different surface charge and hydrophobicity.

The quality of B_{22} data collected using various methods as well as their respective interpretations depend on how they are measured, and the methods are still evolving. The use of the high throughput methods enables rapid collection of data under various solution conditions; therefore, it is hoped that a comprehensive evaluation of the predictive power of B_{22} for various aggregation pathways will become available in the near future.

4.3.5 Mass Spectrometry

MS is a powerful tool in the development of protein pharmaceuticals and provides key data on drug substance characterization including the identification of post-translational modifications. The major applications of MS are beyond the scope of this section. Instead some of the recent developments on the use of MS on aggregate characterization are highlighted here. An advantage of aggregate detection by MS is that the mass determination is a label-free analysis, and one does not need to separate the monomer and aggregate components before analysis [59]. An important limitation is the maximum size limit that can be reached by MS, discussed later. Moreover, sample preparation protocols as well as MS detection methods must be carefully selected to ensure that noncovalent aggregates remain integral. Electrospray ionization (ESI) MS has been successfully used to detect native heterotetrameric (noncovalent) hemoglobin as well as aggregated (hexameric and octameric) forms of hemoglobin [60,61]. Ahrman et al. [62] reported successful detection of a dodecameric form (252.7 kDa) of Hsp21 protein using nano-ESI (nano-ESI) MS by careful manipulation of gas pressures to preserve noncovalent interactions. This approach demonstrates that large protein oligomers can be transported intact (assuming that sample handling does not generate any new aggregates) through the mass spectrometer so that the oligomeric mass can be determined and, thereby, the oligomer stoichiometry can be established. Robinson and coworkers used nano-ESI MS for reliable mass determination of the 800 kDa complex of chaperone GroEL [59]. Pinkse et al. identified a dodecameric form of assembly of urease α-/β-subunits ($\sim$1064 kDa) using nano-ESI MS [63].

Although ESI may be gentle enough to keep aggregate structures undissociated, finding the right conditions to keep multimeric forms intact can be challenging. Additionally, the impact of sample preparation methods including the use of aqueous volatile buffers and need for desalting is a serious limitation, because it can affect the aggregation state already before analysis.

Another ionization method, matrix-assisted laser desorption ionization (MALDI), may be suitable to study protein formulations without need for desalting. Holmberg et al. [64] studied stability and aggregation of albumin and IgG using MALDI MS. The authors reported that significant heterogeneity was present in albumin, with visible peaks of monomer, dimer, trimer, and tetramer ($\sim$272 kDa). For the IgG, monomer, dimer ($\sim$303 kDa), and higher order aggregates up to tetramer were detected. Furthermore, iodine labeling of the protein was shown not to affect its aggregation behavior.

A difficulty with MALDI, however, is the need for detection of very high m/z ions that result when $z = 1$ (as is usually the case with MALDI); in addition, high laser powers are needed to produce gas-phase ions from high mass analytes [65]. Recent developments in detector technology, such as the development of an ion conversion dynode (ICD) detector allows for the sensitive detection of ions with m/z above 100 kDa [65].

The impact of significantly intense laser power used in MALDI to produce gas-phase ions and its potential of dissociating an aggregated structure was investigated by Michel et al. [66]. They studied a stable and functional complex of the wild-type full-length integrase and the cellular cofactor LEDGF/p75 in the absence and the presence of a chemical cross-linker (cross-linking performed to preserve the integrity of the functional complex). High mass MALDI time-of-flight (ToF) MS analysis in the absence of cross-linker identified the mass of the two components of integrase and LEDGF, showing that the MS method induced disruption of the complex. However, the cross-linked complex exhibited a series of protein complexes with various stoichiometries, with molecular mass ranging from 99.8 to 267.4 kDa. The high mass MALDI ToF MS applied in this study is a relatively new technique to push the mass limit detection to nearly 1200 kDa by adding an ICD detector [65–68]. High mass MALDI ToF MS was applied by Pimenova et al. [65] to characterize the multimeric state of the human plasma protein haptoglobin (mass range of 150–300 kDa) as well as higher order structures of hemoglobin-based oxygen carriers and their interactions with human haptoglobin.

Modern mass spectrometers are capable of providing mass accuracy of better than 100 ppm (0.01%) for intact proteins, depending on the instrumentation used and the molecular mass being measured. This translates to 3 Da accuracy of a 30-kDa protein at 100 ppm. However, for the detection of high molecular weights using the high mass MALDI ToF MS (upper detection limit of 1.2 MDa), the resolution is much lower [69] ($\sim$0.1% for 200 kDa to $\sim$0.45% for higher mass), but still adequate for identifying the valency of a protein aggregate.

In summary, advancements in MS detection enable the identification of aggregated proteins and functional complexes without the need to separate or isolate them. However, application of MS to characterizing noncovalent and reversible aggregates that might be present in formulations of protein pharmaceuticals has been very limited due to concerns of altering formulation conditions and disruption of aggregates.

4.4 SUMMARY

This chapter discussed online detection and characterization techniques for soluble aggregates. Additionally, some of the emerging techniques and novel methods for soluble aggregate detection by direct or indirect methods were discussed along with a brief description of the technical principles and their applications in the development of protein pharmaceuticals, in relevance to the detection of aggregates. Although SE-HPLC with UV detection is the most commonly used method for quantifying soluble aggregates for release and in stability studies (development as well as QC applications), the other online detectors described here can be useful during development and in characterization. Some prior knowledge of the identity of the aggregates is required to use SE-HPLC as an appropriate stability-indicating assay.

Many of the physical degradation events including aggregation, particulate formation, and related structural alterations associated with adsorption, misfolding, heat denaturation, partial misfolding, nucleating species, and chemical reactions degradation require the use of specialized and emerging techniques for comprehensive characterization. The section on emerging techniques highlighted some of the techniques that can be employed in aggregation-related studies during formulation and process development, especially at later stages of development. These techniques and methods are primarily intended for aggregate characterization and investigational purposes, for example, when a critical stability issue arises during product development. A good understanding of the commonly observed factors causing aggregation and the forced degradation profile using orthogonal techniques is important to develop stable, safe, and efficacious protein pharmaceuticals and such data are part of the key information submitted with biologics license applications to regulatory agencies.

Acknowledgments

The author thanks Drs. Kevin King, Satish Singh, and David Steinmeyer of Pfizer, and the editors, Drs. Wim Jiskoot and Hanns-Christian Mahler, for reviewing this article.

REFERENCES

1. Zimm BH. Molecular theory of the scattering of light in fluids. J Chem Phys 1945;13:141–145.
2. Wyatt PJ. Light scattering and the absolute characterization of macromolecules. Anal Chim Acta 1993;272:1–40.
3. Rustandi RR, Washabaugh MW, Wang Y. Applications of CE SDS gel in development of biopharmaceutical antibody-based products. Electrophoresis 2008;29:3612–3620.
4. Dolnik V. Capillary zone electrophoresis of proteins. Electrophoresis 1997;18: 2353–2361.
5. Bermudez O, Forciniti D. Aggregation and denaturation of antibodies: a capillary electrophoresis, dynamic light scattering, and aqueous two-phase partitioning study. J Chromatogr B Analyt Technol Biomed Life Sci 2004;807:17–24.
6. Gates AT, Lowry M, Fletcher KA, Murugeshu A, Rusin O, Robinson JW, Strongin RM, Warner IM. Capillary electrophoretic screening for the inhibition of homocysteine thiolactone-induced protein oligomerization. Anal Chem 2007;79:8249–8256.
7. Krishnamurthy R, Sukumar M, Das TK, Lacher NA. Emerging analytical technologies for biotherapeutics development. Bioprocess Int 2008;6:32–42.
8. Luykx DM, Goerdayal SS, Dingemanse PJ, Jiskoot W, Jongen PM. HPLC and tandem detection to monitor conformational properties of biopharmaceuticals. J Chromatogr B Analyt Technol Biomed Life Sci 2005;821:45–52.
9. Hawe A, Friess W, Sutter M, Jiskoot W. Online fluorescent dye detection method for the characterization of immunoglobulin G aggregation by size exclusion chromatography and asymmetrical flow field flow fractionation. Anal Biochem 2008;378:115–122.
10. Lakowicz RJ Principles of fluorescence spectroscopy. 2nd ed. New York: Kluwer Academic Publishers and Plenum Press; 1999.
11. Das TK, Mazumdar S. Conformational substates of apoprotein of horseradish peroxidase in aqueous solution: a fluorescence dynamics study. J Phys Chem 1995;99:13283–13290.
12. Wen J, Arakawa T, Philo JS. Size-exclusion chromatography with on-line light-scattering, absorbance, and refractive index detectors for studying proteins and their interactions. Anal Biochem 1996;240:155–166.
13. Kendrick BS, Kerwin BA, Chang BS, Philo JS. Online size-exclusion high-performance liquid chromatography light scattering and differential refractometry methods to determine degree of polymer conjugation to proteins and protein-protein or protein-ligand association states. Anal Biochem 2001;299:136–146.
14. Dutta PK, Hammons K, Willibey B, Haney MA. Analysis of protein denaturation by high-performance continuous differential viscometry. J Chromatogr 1991;536:113–121.

15. Hess EL, Cobure A. The intrinsic viscosity of mixed protein systems, including studies of plasma and serum. J Gen Physiol 1950;33:511–523.

16. Haney MA. The differential viscometer. I. A new approach to the measurement of specific viscosities of polymer solutions. J Appl Polym Sci 1985;30:3023–3036.

17. Qian RL, Mhatre R, Krull IS. Characterization of antigen-antibody complexes by size-exclusion chromatography coupled with low-angle light-scattering photometry and viscometry. J Chromatogr A 1997;787:101–109.

18. Yguerabide J, Yguerabide EE. Light-scattering submicroscopic particles as highly fluorescent analogs and their use as tracer labels in clinical and biological applications. Anal Biochem 1998;262:137–156.

19. Mie G. Beiträge zur Optik trüber Medien, speziell kolloidaler Metallösungen. Ann Phys 1908;25:377–445.

20. Burchard W, Schmidt M, Stockmayer WH. Information on polydispersity and branching from combined quasi-elastic and integrated scattering. Macromolecules 1980;13:1265–1272.

21. Martin SR, Schilstra MJ. Circular dichroism and its application to the study of biomolecules. Methods Cell Biol 2008;84:263–293.

22. Knowles TP, Shu W, Devlin GL, Meehan S, Auer S, Dobson CM, Welland ME. Kinetics and thermodynamics of amyloid formation from direct measurements of fluctuations in fibril mass. Proc Natl Acad Sci U S A 2007;104:10016–10021.

23. Patel AR, Kerwin BA, Kanapuram SR. Viscoelastic characterization of high concentration antibody formulations using quartz crystal microbalance with dissipation monitoring. J Pharm Sci 2009;98:3108–3116.

24. Hovgaard MB, Dong M, Otzen DE, Besenbacher F. Quartz crystal microbalance studies of multilayer glucagon fibrillation at the solid-liquid interface. Biophys J 2007;93:2162–2169.

25. Kao P, Patwardhan A, Allara D, Tadigadapa S. Human serum albumin adsorption study on 62-MHz miniaturized quartz gravimetric sensors. Anal Chem 2008;80:5930–5936.

26. Tsortos A, Papadakisa G, Gizeli E. Shear acoustic wave biosensor for detecting DNA intrinsic viscosity and conformation: a study with QCM-D. Biosens Bioelectron 2008;24:836–841.

27. Tretiakov KV, Bishop KJ, Kowalczyk B, Jaiswal A, Poggi MA, Grzybowski BA. Mechanism of the cooperative adsorption of oppositely charged nanoparticles. J Phys Chem A 2009;113:3799–3803.

28. Pfeiffer I, Hook F. Quantification of oligonucleotide modifications of small unilamellar lipid vesicles. Anal Chem 2006;78:7493–7498.

29. Saluja A, Badkar AV, Zeng DL, Nema S, Kalonia DS. Ultrasonic storage modulus as a novel parameter for analyzing protein-protein interactions in high protein concentration solutions: correlation with static and dynamic light scattering measurements. Biophys J 2007;92:234–244.

30. Saluja A, Kalonia DS. Nature and consequences of protein-protein interactions in high protein concentration solutions. Int J Pharm 2008;358:1–15.

31. Eggers F, Funck T. Ultrasonic measurements with milliliter liquid samples in the 0.5-100MHz range. Rev Sci Instrum 1973;44:969–977.

32. Chalikian TV, Totrov M, Abagyan R, Breslauer KJ. The hydration of globular proteins as derived from volume and compressibility measurements: cross correlating thermodynamic and structural data. J Mol Biol 1996;260:588–603.

33. Kaatze U, Eggers F, Lautscham K. Ultrasonic velocity measurements in liquids with high resolution—techniques, selected applications and perspectives. Meas Sci Technol 2008;19:1–21.

34. Ulrih NP, Anderluh G, Macek P, Chalikian TV. Salt-induced oligomerization of partially folded intermediates of equinatoxin II. Biochemistry 2004;43:9536–9545.

35. El Kadi N, Taulier N, Le Huerou JY, Gindre M, Urbach W, Nwigwe I, Kahn PC, Waks M. Unfolding and refolding of bovine serum albumin at acid pH: ultrasound and structural studies. Biophys J 2006;91:3397–3404.

36. Liu L, Luo Y. Compressibility study of protein-therapeutics at high concentration using ultrasonic resonator technology. 2007 National Biotechnology Conference. San Diego (CA): AAPS; 2007.

37. Stromer T, Lange A, Bierbaum H, Funck T, Gau D. Ultrasonic resonator technology: a sensitive new tool to study thermal stability of proteins from low to high concentrations. 2006 National Biotechnology Conference. Boston (MA): AAPS; 2006.

38. Mathis K, Gruber F, Parlitz R, Gau D, winter G. Use of alternative analytical methods to detect small amounts of protein aggregates. 2006 Annual Meeting. San Antonio (TX): AAPS; 2006.

39. Taylor G. Dispersion of soluble matter in solvent flowing slowly through a tube. Proc R Soc Lond A 1953;219:186–203.

40. Ostergaard J, Jensen H. Simultaneous evaluation of ligand binding properties and protein size by electrophoresis and Taylor dispersion in capillaries. Anal Chem 2009;81:8644–8648.

41. Bello MS, Rezzonico R, Righetti PG. Use of Taylor-aris dispersion for measurement of a solute diffusion coefficient in thin capillaries. Science 1994;266:773–776.

42. Clark SM, Leaist DG, Konermann L. Taylor dispersion monitored by electrospray mass spectrometry: a novel approach for studying diffusion in solution. Rapid Commun Mass Spectrom 2002;16:1454–1462.

43. Clark SM, Konermann L. Diffusion measurements by electrospray mass spectrometry for studying solution-phase noncovalent interactions. J Am Soc Mass Spectrom 2003;14:430–441.

44. Wakeham WA, Salpadoru NH, Caro CG. Diffusion coefficients for protein molecules in blood serum. Atherosclerosis 1976;25:225–235.

45. George A, Chiang Y, Guo B, Arabshahi A, Cai Z, Wilson WW. Second virial coefficient as predictor in protein crystal growth. Methods Enzymol 1997;276:100–110.

46. Tessier PM, Lenhoff AM. Measurements of protein self-association as a guide to crystallization. Curr Opin Biotechnol 2003;14:512–516.

47. Ho JG, Middelberg AP, Ramage P, Kocher HP. The likelihood of aggregation during protein renaturation can be assessed using the second virial coefficient. Protein Sci 2003;12:708–716.

48. Chi EY, Krishnan S, Kendrick BS, Chang BS, Carpenter JF, Randolph TW. Roles of conformational stability and colloidal stability in the aggregation of recombinant human granulocyte colony-stimulating factor. Protein Sci 2003;12:903–913.

49. Bajaj H, Sharma VK, Badkar A, Zeng D, Nema S, Kalonia DS. Protein structural conformation and not second virial coefficient relates to long-term irreversible aggregation of a monoclonal antibody and ovalbumin in solution. Pharm Res 2006;23:1382–1394.

50. Liu W, Cellmer T, Keerl D, Prausnitz JM, Blanch HW. Interactions of lysozyme in guanidinium chloride solutions from static and dynamic light-scattering measurements. Biotechnol Bioeng 2005;90:482–490.

51. Alford JR, Kendrick BS, Carpenter JF, Randolph TW. Measurement of the second osmotic virial coefficient for protein solutions exhibiting monomer-dimer equilibrium. Anal Biochem 2008;377:128–133.

52. Winzor DJ, Deszczynski M, Harding SE, Wills PR. Nonequivalence of second virial coefficients from sedimentation equilibrium and static light scattering studies of protein solutions. Biophys Chem 2007;128:46–55.

53. Le Brun V, Friess W, Schultz-Fademrecht T, Muehlau S, Garidel P. Lysozyme-lysozyme self-interactions as assessed by the osmotic second virial coefficient: impact for physical protein stabilization. Biotechnol J 2009;4:1305–1319.

54. Winzor DJ, Scott DJ, Wills PR. A simpler analysis for the measurement of second virial coefficients by self-interaction chromatography. Anal Biochem 2007;371:21–25.

55. Attri AK, Minton AP. New methods for measuring macromolecular interactions in solution via static light scattering: basic methodology and application to nonassociating and self-associating proteins. Anal Biochem 2005;337:103–110.

56. Bajaj H, Sharma VK, Kalonia DS. Determination of second virial coefficient of proteins using a dual-detector cell for simultaneous measurement of scattered light intensity and concentration in SEC-HPLC. Biophys J 2004;87:4048–4055.

57. Bloustine J, Berejnov V, Fraden S. Measurements of protein-protein interactions by size exclusion chromatography. Biophys J 2003;85:2619–2623.

58. Attri AK, Minton AP. Composition gradient static light scattering: a new technique for rapid detection and quantitative characterization of reversible macromolecular hetero-associations in solution. Anal Biochem 2005;346:132–138.

59. Benesch JL, Ruotolo BT, Simmons DA, Robinson CV. Protein complexes in the gas phase: technology for structural genomics and proteomics. Chem Rev 2007;107:3544–3567.

60. Griffith WP, Kaltashov IA. Highly asymmetric interactions between globin chains during hemoglobin assembly revealed by electrospray ionization mass spectrometry. Biochemistry 2003;42:10024–10033.

61. Simmons DA, Wilson DJ, Lajoie GA, Doherty-Kirby A, Konermann L. Subunit disassembly and unfolding kinetics of hemoglobin studied by time-resolved electrospray mass spectrometry. Biochemistry 2004;43:14792–14801.

62. Ahrman E, Lambert W, Aquilina JA, Robinson CV, Emanuelsson CS. Chemical cross-linking of the chloroplast localized small heat-shock protein, Hsp21, and the model substrate citrate synthase. Protein Sci 2007;16:1464–1478.

63. Pinkse MW, Maier CS, Kim JI, Oh BH, Heck AJ. Macromolecular assembly of Helicobacter pylori urease investigated by mass spectrometry. J Mass Spectrom 2003;38:315–320.

64. Holmberg M, Stibius KB, Ndoni S, Larsen NB, Kingshott P, Hou XL. Protein aggregation and degradation during iodine labeling and its consequences for protein adsorption to biomaterials. Anal Biochem 2007;361:120–125.

65. Pimenova T, Pereira CP, Schaer DJ, Zenobi R. Characterization of high molecular weight multimeric states of human haptoglobin and hemoglobin-based oxygen carriers by high-mass MALDI MS. J Sep Sci 2009;32:1224–1230.

66. Michel F, Crucifix C, Granger F, Eiler S, Mouscadet JF, Korolev S, Agapkina J, Ziganshin R, Gottikh M, Nazabal A, Emiliani S, Benarous R, Moras D, Schultz P, Ruff M. Structural basis for HIV-1 DNA integration in the human genome, role of the LEDGF/P75 cofactor. EMBO J 2009;28:980–991.

67. Nazabal A, Wenzel RJ, Zenobi R. Immunoassays with direct mass spectrometric detection. Anal Chem 2006;78:3562–3570.

68. Bich C, Scott M, Panagiotidis A, Wenzel RJ, Nazabal A, Zenobi R. Characterization of antibody-antigen interactions: comparison between surface plasmon resonance measurements and high-mass matrix-assisted laser desorption/ionization mass spectrometry. Anal Biochem 2008;375:35–45.

69. Bovet C, Ruff M, Eiler S, Granger F, Wenzel R, Nazabal A, Moras D, Zenobi R. Monitoring ligand modulation of protein-protein interactions by mass spectrometry: estrogen receptor alpha-SRC1. Anal Chem 2008;80:7833–7839.

5 Analytical Methods to Measure Subvisible Particulates

SHAWN CAO, LINDA NARHI, YIJIA JIANG, and RAHUL S. RAJAN

Process and Product Development, Amgen Inc., Thousand Oaks, California, USA

5.1 INTRODUCTION

Protein aggregation refers to the undesired self-association of a protein and can result in species of any size, from dimers to visible particles. As described in Chapter 1, there are many different pathways by which protein aggregates can form, and this has been the focus of numerous articles and reviews [1–5]. Unfolding or partial unfolding of a monomer can expose hydrophobic regions in the interior of the folded protein that are prone to self-association when not protected, while colloidal instability can favor the association of even the native protein depending on the solvent conditions. Heteronucleation, where small foreign particles, such as stainless steel shed from pumps during the manufacturing process, act as nucleation sites and catalyze the formation of larger protein particles, has also been reported [6]. In addition to the large size range, the aggregates can also have conformations ranging from native, through near native and partially unfolded intermediates, to fully unfolded species. Because of this complexity, dissecting the underlying mechanism of aggregation of a specific protein can be very difficult, and this is an area of active research. With the advent of biotechnology, understanding how to maintain a protein in its native state has become even more important, as a protein pharmaceutical ideally consists of a homogeneous preparation of folded, native protein. Many of the stresses that can unfold proteins are encountered during the manufacturing process for protein pharmaceuticals, including processes where heteronuclei are shed, exposure to extremes of pH and other solution conditions, surface interfaces during process and storage that can induce aggregation, etc. [1–5]. Thus, the ability to analyze and control aggregate formation is critical in the development and production of protein pharmaceuticals.

Analysis of Aggregates and Particles in Protein Pharmaceuticals, First Edition.
Edited by Hanns-Christian Mahler, Wim Jiskoot.
© 2012 John Wiley & Sons, Inc., Published 2012 by John Wiley & Sons, Inc.

One of the difficulties in discussing analytical methods for aggregation characterization is the lack of consistent terminology used. Aggregate can be used to mean all self-associated species but is also sometimes applied to specific species (often the oligomers). Aggregates can also be defined by size, chemical nature of the interactions (covalent vs noncovalent), and conformation of the protein in the aggregate, etc. The terms insoluble and soluble are also occasionally used to differentiate between visible precipitate and aggregate that is not visible but can still often be irreversible. There are several reviews of the analytical methods for assessing aggregates of different sizes, especially in the micrometer and visible range [3,7]. For the purposes of this chapter, the aggregates are classified solely based on size: oligomer refers to aggregates that are on the order of nanometers, subvisible particles span the range of submicrometer to about 150 μm, and visible particles are defined as anything larger than 150 μm, the size that can be seen by the majority of trained inspectors [8].

The analytical methods most commonly used to quantitate the smallest aggregates, or oligomers, were described in Chapter 4. These methods (such as field-flow fractionation (FFF), analytical ultracentrifugation (AUC), size-exclusion chromatography (SEC), etc.) quantify protein aggregates in terms of mass concentration or weight percent, with limits of detection of the order of 0.1–1%. For particles above about 50 nm, the quantitation is reported in terms of numbers of particles, the sensitivity is typically a few particles per container or per milliliter for above micrometer particles, and they are categorized by size (e.g., diameter), rather than by molecular weight or degree of aggregation (e.g., dimer). This difference in sensitivity presents difficulties when trying to connect the formation of oligomers to the formation of subvisible and, finally, visible particles.

This chapter describes methods that can be used to address the analytical challenges presented by the subvisible particles. Currently, there are no consistent, quantitative methods for measuring the submicrometer particles (e.g., 0.05–1 μm), though dynamic light scattering and related techniques can be used to qualitatively characterize these particles. This is an area of ever-evolving technical development, with some of the techniques discussed below showing the most promise. However, the recent regulatory concerns have focused on the subvisible particles in the micrometer range. Therefore, this is the primary focus of this chapter as well.

The amount of visible and subvisible particles allowed in therapeutics is governed by the pharmacopeia of the individual countries in which the drug is marketed. In the United States, it is governed by United States Pharmacopoeia (USP) <788> ([9]). The current USP <788> has been harmonized with the European Pharmacopoeia (EP 2.9.19) and Japanese Pharmacopoeia (JP). The compendial method for the quantitation of subvisible particles based on USP <788> was written to control contamination by foreign particles, with preventing theoretical adverse effects such as capillary occlusion from foreign particles more than 10 μm that might be found in traditional small-molecule therapeutics delivered intravenously as one of the chief goals. To this end, it lays out specifications for subvisible particles at ≥10 and 25 μm; for small-volume parenterals, the amounts of subvisible particles should not exceed 6000 particles at ≥ 10 μm and 600 particles at ≥ 25 μm per container. The primary method described uses light obscuration, with isolation and microscopic analysis as a secondary screen.

The number of protein pharmaceuticals on the market has exponentially grown in the last two decades. These products are often formulated at high concentration and have a tendency to self-associate. The subvisible and visible particles that can occur in these products are thus often inherent properties of the specific protein pharmaceutical. The compendial subvisible particle requirements and testing procedures have increasingly been applied to these protein pharmaceuticals. The proteinaceous subvisible and visible particles that might be present at a low level in protein pharmaceuticals have received ever-increasing attention from the regulatory agencies as a potential safety issue. A recent commentary coauthored by academic scientists and members of the Food and Drug Administration (FDA) laid out the case for more careful analysis of these particles [10]. At the same time, the guidance around whether products can contain any visible particles that are intrinsic to the product (differentiated from the presence of foreign particles) has been inconsistent, with the EP requiring labels that claim "... without visible particles" (for monoclonal antibodies) or "... and practically free from particles" (for any other parenteral preparations), the USP requiring parenterals to be "... essentially free from visible particulates" and the JP stating "... free from readily detectable foreign insoluble matters." While these issues are about visible particulates, it is likely that subvisible particles may be closely related to the formation of product-containing visible particles (as opposed to foreign particles). Analytical methods with adequate performance are, therefore, needed to address these questions and to study the mechanism of particle formation. Ideally, these methods should be applied throughout the development cycle, from process characterization and formulation development through lot release and stability testing. In addition to qualification parameters, the methods should also include appropriate sample handling to minimize false-positive results from contaminants and microbubbles introduced during sample preparation, handling, or measurement, utilize a small enough volume that performing the analysis is not prohibitive during early development, and include a statistically relevant sampling plan for stability [11]. The method or methods should be able to determine both the size distribution of the particles and population distribution based on shape, morphology, optical properties, chemical composition, etc. The latter is necessary to be able to determine what percent of the total particles consist of protein and what percent can be attributed to other materials, such as silicone oil droplets that, for example, may originate from the container surface itself. In the absence of a single method that can determine all these properties, a combination of techniques may be desired. During the early phases of development, the amount of material available for testing can be very limited, and obtaining reliable and "fit-for-purpose" results with a small amount of material is the key, while during lot release the method must be capable of producing robust and precise results to satisfy release and stability requirements. The subvisible analytical methods available, their strengths and weaknesses, and some case studies showing how these techniques can be applied to address particle characterization during the product lifecycle are discussed in this chapter, with a focus on the USP<788>-based compendial methods.

5.2   USP <788>-BASED COMPENDIAL TESTING OF SUBVISIBLE PARTICLES

5.2.1   Introduction

The compendial method USP <788>, "Particulate Matter in Injections," defines particulate matter in injections and parenteral infusions as "mobile undissolved particles, other than gas bubbles, unintentionally present in the solutions," and specifies two procedures for the determination of these particles. Method 1, light-obscuration particle count test, is the preferred method, while method 2, microscopic particle count test, is the method to use when method 1 is not applicable and can also be used concurrently with method 1 to confirm its results. The compendial methods for quantifying subvisible particles have been harmonized: although the discussion below is specific for the USP, the EP and JP methods are very similar.

To perform a single test with either method per the USP specification, a minimum sample volume of 25 mL is required. For parenterals having a volume of 25 mL or more, single units are tested individually. For parenterals <25 mL in volume, the contents of 10 or more units are combined to obtain a volume of not <25 mL; where justified and authorized, the test solution may be prepared by mixing the contents of a suitable number of units and diluting to 25 mL with an appropriate solvent. The USP specifies that the results obtained in examining a discrete unit or group of units cannot be extrapolated with certainty to the other untested units in a large group, and a statistically sound sampling plan must be developed and used to draw valid inferences.

The compendial method sets acceptance criteria for greater than ($\geq$) 10 μm and $\geq$25 μm. For preparations supplied in containers with a nominal content of 100 mL or less, the limits are 6000 and 600 particles per unit for the $\geq$10 and $\geq$25 μm particles, respectively, as determined by the light-obscuration particle count test, and 3000 and 300, respectively, as determined by the microscopic particle count test, reflecting inherent differences between the two methods. For preparations supplied in containers with a nominal content of more than 100 mL in volume, the limits are 25 and 3 per mL, respectively, for the $\geq$10 and $\geq$25 μm particles as determined by the light-obscuration particle count test, and 12 and 2 particles per mL, respectively, as determined by the microscopic particle count test.

One exception to the above classification is that for preparations supplied in containers with a nominal content of 100 mL, the JP is not harmonized with the USP or EP criteria and applies the "more than 100 mL" acceptance criteria of 25 and 3 particles by light obscuration, and 12 and 2 by microscope for $\geq$10 and $\geq$25 μm particles, respectively, to this volume.

5.2.2 Light-Obscuration-Based Measurements

5.2.2.1 Principle   The typical light-obscuration test apparatus is an electronic particle-counting system consisting of a syringe-type sample-feeding device, commonly known as the *sampler*, connected to a particle counter commonly known as the *sensor*. Different volume syringes and flow rates are available to enable drawing and testing of liquid of specific volume at an appropriate flow rate. During normal operation, the sampler syringe drive first draws the sample liquid from its container through the sensor (via a sensor probe) into the syringe and then pushes the plunger up, sending the liquid from the syringe to a waste container. The aforementioned process is repeated until the testing task is complete. Particle determination takes place when the liquid sample passes the sensor.

The working principle of the sensor, light obscuration (also known as *light blockage* or *light extinction*), is depicted in Fig. 5.1. As a liquid sample is taken by the syringe sampler and passes through the sensor flow cell, the particles obscure (or block/diminish) the light falling on the light-sensitive detector. When the concentration of particles lies within the normal range of the sensor, these particles pass through the detection zone discretely and are detected one by one. The passage of each particle through the detection zone reduces the incident light on the detector, and the voltage output of the detector is momentarily reduced. The changes in the voltage register as electronic pulses that are used to quantitate the number of particles. The cross section of the particle producing a pulse is used to determine its size. A calibration curve can be generated for a sensor by passing monosized polystyrene latex (PSL) spheres through the sensor and plotting the voltage responses to the diameters of the PSL spheres used, as shown in Fig. 5.2. The sizes of particles in the test sample are calculated by the interpolation of the measured voltages onto the calibration curve. Thus, the determination of the size of the particles (sizing) and the number of particles (counting) is achieved.

5.2.2.2 Measurement   To ensure that particles are reproducibly sized and counted, and the results obtained truly reflect the particles present in the sample as defined by the USP, special attention must be paid to instrument preparation, test environment control, sample preparation and handling, appropriate testing methods and techniques, and data analysis and interpretation.

Instrument Preparation.   The instrument used must have a suitable particle concentration and the size ranges appropriate for the purpose of the test. Typically, light-obscuration sensors have an upper concentration limit of 10,000–20,000 particles/mL, at which coincidence counts due to simultaneous presence of two or more particles in the sensor view volume are no more than 10%. Coincidence particles will be counted as a single particle larger than the individual particles, resulting in undercounting but oversizing. The lower sizing limit is typically 1–2 µm, below which measurements become less robust owing to decreasing signal-to-noise ratio and limits of the extinction efficiency. The upper sizing limit is 100–400 µm and is dependent on the dimension of the sensor flow cell used.

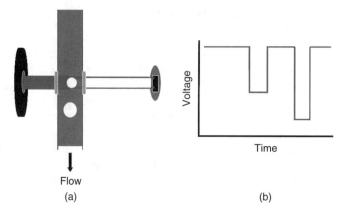

Flow
(a)   (b)

FIGURE 5.1   The light-obscuration principle. When particles pass through the detection zone of the flow cell, they obscure some of the light falling onto the photosensitive detector (a). This decrease in detected light intensity is converted into discrete electronic pulses (b). Particle sizing and quantitation are achieved by the analyzed number and amplitudes of the pulses. The polarity of the pulses is depicted arbitrarily only for illustration purpose.

Procedures need to be conducted periodically to ensure that critical instrument performance parameters such as the sample volume accuracy, sample flow rate, calibration curve, sensor resolution, and count accuracy are appropriate. Figure 5.2 and Table 5.1 show representative calibration curves and count accuracy results, conducted over two preventative maintenance sessions at six months apart for two different systems, and demonstrate that the performances changed little during that period of time. Together with routine performance verification checks such as the negative (particle-free water) and positive (PSL particle-counting standards) controls conducted as part of each test session, these procedures provide assurance that an instrument performs as expected.

Test Environment Control. To ensure that the particles being measured were not environmental particles introduced during testing, the amount of extraneous particles in the testing environment, including the atmosphere of the room, the glassware, container closure systems, reagents used, etc., must be minimized. In general, rinsing glassware and equipment with filtered deionized (DI) water is effective, and mild detergents and organic solvents such as 30% isopropyl alcohol (IPA) may also be used to facilitate the cleaning and long-term storage of the instrument. The test is preferably carried out in a laminar-flow hood, although best laboratory practices are generally adequate and the blank control requirement can be met.

Sample Preparation and Handling. Like test environment control, sample preparation should be carried out in a manner that minimizes false-positive and false-negative contributions, including extraneous/environmental contamination, air bubbles, and sample inhomogeneity. Most of these false contributions can be kept at a minimum with good laboratory practice. Solutions containing detergents may have a lower level of microbubbles.

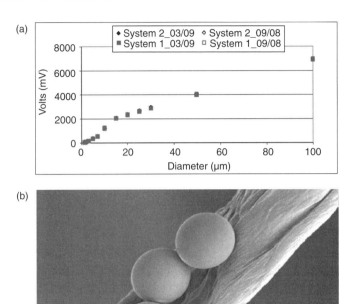

FIGURE 5.2   The overlay of four calibration curves for two different light-obscuration systems, each calibrated at six months apart (a). The calibration curves can vary from instrument to instrument. For the same instrument, the calibration curve changed little after six months. The calibration is done with monodisperse PSL spheres with certified sizes. (b) An image of 5-μm PSL spheres showing their spherical nature and homogeneity.

When preparing protein therapeutic samples, some additional precautions are needed. Protein samples often attract and trap air bubbles easily, fill volumes are small (e.g., 1 ml) and so content pooling is necessary. Protein particles are often fragile and unstable on agitation; the pooling steps such as pipetting and mixing with magnetic stir bars can either break up the particle or generate new particles. Special attention and techniques are often needed and should be used to minimize the impact of sample preparation on the product's native particle profile including concentration and concentration versus size distribution. Gentle pipetting and mixing by hand swirling are often necessary. Proper and consistent analyst training is crucial in minimizing inter- and intra-analyst variation. For particles that are stable toward dilution, this may also be a viable choice to produce the required sample volume for testing. Eliminating gas bubbles by allowing to stand or sonicating can be either not effective or not appropriate. Degassing

TABLE 5.1   Particle-Counting Accuracy Tests on Two Light-Obscuration Systems Each at Six Months Apart, Using the USP Particle Count Reference Standards

		USP Results (System 1)			
Size (μm)	Particles/mL	Spec	Ratio (10/15)	Spec	Date
10	4489	2860–4617			
15	2959		1.52	1.102–3.149	March 2009
10	3813	3381–4298			
15	1933		1.97	1.294–3.242	September 2008
		USP Results (System 2)			
Size (μm)	Particles/mL	Spec	Ratio (10/15)	Spec	Date
10	3951	2860–4617			
15	2431		1.63	1.102–3.149	March 2009
10	4304	2860–4617			
15	2235		1.93	1.102–3.149	September 2008

An instrument passes if the ≥ 10 μm and the ratio of the counts obtained at ≥ 10 μm to those obtained at ≥ 15 μm conform to the values that accompany the USP particle count reference standards.

with a gentle vacuum (e.g., ~10% of ambient pressure for 1 h) has been found to be effective and appropriate for protein pharmaceuticals [11].

Test Methods.   For each test session, negative and positive controls need to be tested before the samples to ensure the appropriateness of the environment, instrument, and test procedure. Negative control is typically done with filtered distilled water to ensure the cleanness of the environment and setup. For the positive control, PSL particle-counting standards with certified size and concentration (e.g., 15.0 ± 0.1 μm PSL spheres at 2000 ± 200 particles/mL) are typically used. Once the control tests pass their respective preset acceptance criteria, the appropriately prepared and homogenized product samples can be tested. The instrument needs to be cleaned appropriately before testing each sample to avoid cross contamination.

The test is conducted by introducing the liquid sample into the sampler. A test consists of consecutively removing a preset number of aliquots (also known as *runs* or *draws*) of a specified sample volume, averaging the results of a subset of these runs (typically four runs per test, the first run is discarded and the last three averaged), and reporting this average as the test result.

The compendial test consists of four (or more) 5-mL runs, with the results obtained from the first run discarded, and the mean number of ≥ 10 and ≥ 25 μm particles per container calculated by averaging the results from the last three runs. A single such test requires a minimum of 25 mL of the sample.

5.2.2.3   Strengths and Weaknesses

Strengths.   Some of the strengths of the light-obscuration particle count test are the simplicity of its operating principle and the robustness of its hardware. The instrument is fairly easy to operate, and data analysis is straightforward.

Weaknesses. The numbers of particles of different sizes are determined based on the equivalent circular diameter as compared against the PSL calibration spheres. The optical and morphological properties of the actual protein particles and high protein concentration formulations could differ considerably from those of the PSL particle standards and water, affecting both the size and number of particles reported. It does not provide any information on particle shape, morphology or composition, which are important clues often necessary to identify particle type or origin. This is potentially one of the biggest shortcomings of this technique. Most of the operational steps are manual and require the analyst's undivided attention; as a result, it is labor intensive and the throughput is not high.

5.2.2.4 *How Best to Apply to Protein Pharmaceuticals*   The light-obscuration particle count test has been applied to protein pharmaceuticals for both product development and release.

For product release and potentially for stability, the current practice is to quantitate the amounts of the ≥ 10 and ≥ 25 µm particles and compare this against the USP acceptance criteria, thus determining whether a product complies with the compendial requirement and can be released for patient administration. In some cases, the results can also be useful for stability trending. Abnormal results, even within the compendial limits, can be indicative of problems with either the test itself or the product lot tested and can be used to trigger additional monitoring and investigational activities to identify the source of the problem and corresponding corrective actions.

However, the current safety concerns for protein particles arise from the potential immunogenicity of these particles, rather than ones such as capillary occlusion [10]. The smaller particles (e.g., < 10 µm) that are present in greater abundance may be as much if not more of an immunogenic concern. Therefore, testing and monitoring these smaller particles in addition to the ≥ 10 and ≥ 25 µm may be helpful in better understanding potential correlations between subvisible protein particles and immunogenicity.

The compendial light-obscuration particle count test as written (i.e., 25 mL per test to quantitate ≥ 10 and ≥ 25 µm particles) is difficult to use routinely during product development owing to volume and sensitivity limits. During development, particularly in early development, where the need for particle testing is great, sample availability is often very limited, and the 25-mL sample volume required for a single test is prohibitive. In addition, the ≥ 10 and ≥ 25 µm results are often not sensitive or precise enough to be useful in determining the effect of the conditions under examination. However, methods that are modified versions of the compendial method, with reduced sample volumes (e.g., 0.7 mL tare + four 0.2 mL runs per test) and extended size range (e.g., ≥ 2 µm), have been found to generate reproducible and indicative results, as listed in Table 5.2. Such methods can be routinely used throughout a product's lifecycle including development.

TABLE 5.2   Particle Concentrations of Different Sizes Measured for a Set of In-Process Samples with Different Filtration Steps

Sample	Particles/mL at >2 μm	Particles/mL at >5 μm	Particles/mL at ≥10 μm	Particles/mL at ≥25 μm
Control (unfilt, lot 1)	339 ± 78	29 ± 2	Below LOQ	Below LOQ
1× Filtration lot 1	29 ± 6	11 ± 5	Below LOQ	Below LOQ
2× Filtration lot 1	19 ± 9	14 ± 9	Below LOQ	Below LOQ
5× Filtration lot 1	50 ± 14	12 ± 9	Below LOQ	Below LOQ
Control (unfilt, lot 2)	680 ± 51	36 ± 4	Below LOQ	Below LOQ
1× Filtration lot 2	20 ± 3	5 ± 2	Below LOQ	Below LOQ

The results demonstrate that the filtration is effective at removing subvisible particles, and 1× filtration is sufficient. Measuring only the ≥10 and ≥25 μm particles was not indicative of this effect since the concentrations of those large particles are below the limit of quantitation.

For high protein concentration formulations, it is often necessary to dilute the samples to reduce the optical interference from the protein solution itself.

5.2.3   Microscopic Particle Count Test

5.2.3.1 Principle   The microscopic particle count test consists of first collecting the particles via a filtration step, examining the particles retained on the filter membrane under an optical microscope, and then reporting size and quantity.

To collect the liquid-borne particles, the liquid sample is filtered through a microporous membrane. The filter membrane used is of suitable size (e.g., 25 mm) and porosity (e.g., ≤1 μm), black or dark gray in color, and often gridded to retain the particles of interest, to facilitate differentiation of the particle from the background, and to optimize particle counting. A gentle vacuum is often applied to facilitate the filtration process. The filter membrane is then air dried and placed under a suitable microscope to count the particles retained on the membrane.

The binocular microscope used for this test is equipped with an ocular micrometer, a circular diameter graticule consisting of a large circle divided by crosshairs into quadrants with 10- and 25-μm reference circles to facilitate particle sizing (as shown in Fig. 5.3). An internal illuminator provides episcopic illumination, and an adjustable external auxiliary illuminator provides reflected oblique illumination at an angle of 10–20°. Projecting the images onto a monitor screen can help with the microscopic system setup and calibration process. The magnification is set at 100 ± 10. The relative error of the graticule is measured by comparing a certified stage micrometer with the internal built-in linear scale of the graticule.

The membrane filter is scanned under the microscope, and the ≥10 and ≥25 μm particles are counted with the aid of the circular diameter graticule. The particle-sizing process is carried out by estimating the equivalent diameter of a particle in comparison with the 10- and 25-μm reference circles on the graticule. Either a total count procedure with which the entire membrane is examined or a partial count procedure in which a known representative fraction of the membrane is examined can be used, whichever is more appropriate.

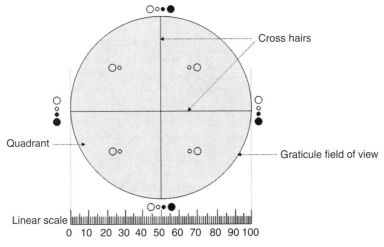

O 25 micrometer reference circle (transparent)
o 10 micrometer reference circle (transparent)
● 25 micrometer reference circle (opaque)
• 10 micrometer reference circle (opaque)

FIGURE 5.3   The microscope's circular diameter graticule. The linear scale is used together with a certified external micrometer to determine the relative error of the graticule. The 10- and 25-μm reference circles are used to facilitate the sizing of spotted particles.

5.2.3.2 USP Description   To perform a USP microscopic particle count test, preferably in a laminar-flow hood, a minimum sample volume of 25 mL is needed. Large- or small-volume parenterals having a content volume of 25 mL or more may be tested individually. For small-volume parenterals <25 mL in volume, the contents of 10 or more units are combined and tested; where justified and authorized, the test solution may be prepared by mixing the contents of a suitable number of units and diluting to 25 mL with an appropriate solvent. The number of units to be tested must be based on an appropriate sampling plan to ensure that the test results provide a statistically sound assessment of the level of particulate matter in a large group of units.

The solution is filtered through the filter assembly, fitted with a membrane with 1.0 μm or finer nominal pore size. The ≥ 10 and ≥ 25 μm particles are counted with the aid of a microscope, and the average number of particles thus determined to be present in the units tested are compared to the microscopic particle count test criteria: no more than 3000 per container for the ≥ 10 μm particle and 300 per container for the ≥ 25 μm particles for products with ≤ 100 mL content volume, and no more than 12 and 2 per mL for the ≥ 10 and ≥ 25 μm particles, respectively, for products with >100 mL content volume.

5.2.3.3 Strengths and Weaknesses   While the light-obscuration particle count test relies on calibration with PSL spheres, the microscopic particle count test is a direct measurement based on first principle: particles are collected on a filter membrane, placed under a microscope, and sized and counted directly by a trained operator.

The actual experimental procedure, however, is very labor intensive since all the steps are manual operations that need to be executed with great care. A single test could take as long as 1 h or more. Examining the particles under the microscope is very taxing on the analyst. The process of seeing the particle and sizing it could be subjective. Not all particles are retained on the filter; depending on the orientation during the isolation step, it is possible for some of the irregular particles to filter through the pores. As a result, the microscopic particle count test is often regarded to be of very low throughput and poor reproducibility.

5.2.3.4 Challenges in Applying to Protein Pharmaceuticals   Particles in protein pharmaceuticals, such as protein particles, are often fragile, amorphous, and translucent. Some of these particles do not survive the filtration process well: they break apart during filtration and are lost instead of being retained. For the ones that do get retained on the membrane, as previously mentioned protein particles are often amorphous and translucent in nature, and these particles might not all be counted since it is very difficult and subjective to distinguish them from the stains and discoloration normally present on the membrane filter. As a result, the discrepancy between the results from the microscopic and light-obscuration tests for protein products is often on the order of $10\times$ or more, with the light-obscuration method being more sensitive, which is much larger than the $2\times$ discrepancy as expected for conventional injectables. In addition, the method is limited to analysis of the ≥ 10 and ≥ 25 μm particles but cannot be used to quantify the subvisible particle in the $1-10$ μm range.

Because of the low throughput, labor-intensive procedure, the subjectivity of the analysis, under counting concerns, and the limited information it generates, the microscopic particle count test has not found wide usage in biotech laboratories: its applications are limited to quality control (QC) laboratories as a secondary test for product release and stability and are used only when a product fails the light-obscuration test or is not suitable to be tested by it.

5.3 OTHER TECHNIQUES FOR SUBVISIBLE PARTICLE MEASUREMENTS

In addition to the light-obscuration and microscopic techniques as described in Section 5.2, a number of other techniques can also be used to measure subvisible particles. This section provides a discussion on three such techniques that have been used to characterize subvisible particles in protein pharmaceuticals: electrical-sensing zone (ESZ)-based methods, flow-imaging-based methods, and light-scattering-based methods. ESZ-based methods are described in detail. Since flow-imaging and light scattering methods are described elsewhere in this book (Chapters 3 and 7, respectively), these topics are summarized briefly in the context of the other methods described in this chapter.

5.3.1 Electrical-Sensing-Zone-Based Methods

Using the ESZ principle, also known as the *Coulter principle* or *electrozone sensing*, this technique was originally developed by Wallace Coulter in the late 1940s to early 1950s for rapidly counting blood cells [12]. It has since found many applications in characterizing particles of a wide range of material types in addition to blood and other cells. The current ESZ technology can putatively be applied over a size range of approximately 0.5 to more than 1000 μm, making it a viable candidate for measuring subvisible particles in parenterals, including protein pharmaceuticals, depending on the product solution.

ESZ Principle   In an ESZ measurement, particles of interest are suspended in a weak electrolyte solution, typically 1–2% NaCl and phosphate salt. Two electrodes are immersed in the electrolyte solution, separated by a small aperture (or an orifice). A constant current flows through the electrodes, resulting in a conductivity-dependent voltage across the aperture. This voltage creates a "sensing zone" near the aperture; the volume of this sensing zone is about 2.5× the volume of the aperture. When a particle traverses the sensing zone, it displaces a volume of electrolyte equal to its own volume, causing a momentary change in the impedance or resistance across the aperture, which results in a voltage pulse. The Coulter principle, which has been theoretically derived and experimentally proven [13,14], states that the amplitude of this pulse is directly proportional to the volume of the particle that produced it. The proportionality, or calibration constant, between the pulse height and volume of the particle can be determined by calibrating the instrument with particles of known volume, such as the monosized PSL spheres used to calibrate the light-obscuration instruments. The particle concentration is kept sufficiently low so that the particles traverse the sensing zone individually, and discrete positive pulses are produced, slightly analogous to the picture depicted in Fig. 5.1. The heights of the individual pulses can then be converted into the equivalent spherical (or volume) diameters of the particles using the calibration constant, while the number of pulses represents the number of particles. By drawing a specified volume (e.g., 2 mL) of the sample solution through the aperture and counting and analyzing the resulting pulses, particle sizing and quantitation can be achieved.

ESZ Measurement   To ensure a successful ESZ measurement, special attention must be paid to sample preparation, electrolyte selection, and instrument preparation.

  Sample Preparation.   In general, all the precautions required in preparing samples for the light-obscuration measurement as discussed in the above section also apply here. Efforts must be made to minimize or eliminate false-positive and false-negative contributions. For example, eliminating air bubbles as discussed for the light-obscuration method is also important for ESZ, since air bubbles impede the conductivity across the aperture and, therefore, are "sensed" and counted as particles.

Electrolyte Selection.   The electrolyte used in an ESZ measurement serves two functions: to provide a stable suspension for the particles and to provide suitable conductivity for the measurement. A commonly used aqueous electrolyte that provides adequate conductivity is phosphate-buffered saline (PBS) (e.g., 150 mM sodium chloride, 20 mM sodium phosphate, pH 7.4) that many protein formulation laboratories routinely stock and use. PBS can be used as the electrolyte to suspend the particles and conduct the experiment provided that diluting in PBS does not change the particle profile of the product, as assessed by any other method. However, in many cases, the particle profile of a product is sensitive to the ionic strength and composition of the diluent. For instance, diluting a protein sample in PBS may cause rapid particulation. In such cases, a more suitable electrolyte needs to be used. Determining the effect of the electrolyte solution on the product being analyzed must be part of method development; in some cases, it might not be possible to find a buffer that is compatible with both the product and the technique.

Instrument Preparation.   Modern ESZ instruments are fairly easy and robust to operate. Some of the key instrument setup and preparation steps are aperture selection and instrument calibration.

Aperture Selection.   The dynamic size range of an aperture, which is the effective particle size range over which an aperture can be used, is typically about 2–60% of the nominal diameter of the aperture. For example, for a 100-µm aperture, the upper size limit is about 60 µm and the lower size limit is about 2 µm. The 2-µm lower size limit is essentially determined by the electrical noise: the voltage pulses generated by particles smaller than 2 µm are comparable to the background instrumental noise. The 60-µm upper size limit is determined by concerns of aperture blockage by particles (particularly nonspherical particles) with sizes comparable to the aperture diameter and the increasing nonlinearity of the size-to-voltage relationship when the particle size approaches the aperture diameter.

For testing subvisible particles in protein pharmaceuticals, a common aperture choice is the 100-µm aperture tube with a standard dynamic size range of 2–60 µm. Most therapeutic protein solutions have few particles large enough to cause aperture blockage, while the 2-µm lower limit measurement provides useful information about the subvisible particles in the solution, including the ≥ 10 and ≥ 25 µm particles as required by the compendial criteria. Aperture tubes with nominal diameters ranging from 20 to 2000 µm are available, enabling the measurement of subvisible particles with a potential overall sizing range from 0.4 µm (the lower size limit of the 20-µm aperture) to more than 1000 µm (the upper size limit of the 2000-µm aperture) if required for a specific application.

Calibration. Once the electrolyte and aperture for a given application have been chosen, the instrument should be calibrated, a process to determine the proportionality (i.e., calibration constant) between the equivalent spherical diameter of a particle and the height of the voltage pulse it would be expected to generate. This is achieved by testing particles of known size and analyzing the resulting pulses. The commonly used calibration procedure is to use monosized PSL particle standards with certified sizes. Typically the size of the PSL particles used should be about 10% of the aperture diameter. For instance, 10-µm PSL standard particles can be used for the calibration of a 100-µm aperture. Either a single point or a multipoint calibration procedure can be used.

The calibration constant is system dependent and should be remeasured when changes to the system, such as using a different aperture, are made. In general, even if no change has been made to the system, the simple calibration verification procedure should be run routinely to verify that the instrument and system are performing as expected, as a significant variation or a slow but monotonic drift of the calibration constant could be an indication of problematic instrument performance.

Testing Procedure. A test can be performed in three modes: time, count, and volume. In each mode, the test is complete when the parameter chosen, either run time, total number of particles counted, or volume of sample analyzed, has reached a preset value such as 90 s, 30,000 particles, or 1 mL, respectively. The data are stored and can be analyzed and reported in format appropriate to the mode used, such as particle concentration as a function of particle size, and information such as concentration of the ≥ 10 µm particles can be obtained.

Strengths and Weaknesses

Strengths. Modern ESZ instruments are robust and easy to operate. A sample test can be completed in a matter of a couple of minutes or less. Particle size is measured directly based on its volume, and this measurement result is not sensitive to factors such as particle shape, orientation as it traverses through the aperture, protein concentration, and refractive index; these factors often affect the results obtained from techniques using the interaction of light and the particle such as light obscuration. The size resolution is very high, with up to 400 size channels available for the selected size range. It offers a wide overall sizing range, from 0.4 to about 1000 µm. ESZ systems with enhanced pulse-analyzing and pulse-processing capabilities provide features such as automatic coincidence correction, and possibilities such as differentiating particles of the same volume but different shape.

Weaknesses. One essential requirement of the ESZ technology is that particles have to be stably suspended in a fluid with suitable conductivity. For some products, this can be easily achieved, while for others, it can be very challenging. For some products, it might not be possible to find a solvent that can be used for measurements that does not affect the product stability. Although the technology can offer an overall sizing range from submicrometer to millimeter, each test run with a particular aperture has a limited dynamic size range of ~30×: for example, the 100- μm aperture can be used to measure particles from 2 to 60 μm. To obtain results in a different size range, a different aperture must be used and this could require a different electrolyte solution. Analysis of ≤2 μm particles would require switching to a smaller aperture, and since smaller apertures generally require higher conductivity, a different electrolyte might be needed and the instrument would have to be reoptimized and calibrated. Therefore, multiple measurements obtained under different conditions are necessary to obtain data across a wide size range. The ESZ technique with the currently available instrumentation is also limited in that all operations are manual and require undivided attention of the analyst. Thus, in its current format, this is not a high throughput technique.

How Best to Apply to Protein Pharmaceuticals   One of the biggest challenges in applying the ESZ technology to quantify particles in protein pharmaceuticals is finding the appropriate electrolyte. If PBS is deemed suitable, that is, the product itself and its particles are known to be stable on mixing and/or diluting with PBS, then PBS can be used as the electrolyte at least during the initial studies. A common practice is to take about 200 μL of the product, mix it into 20 mL of filtered PBS, and test the resulting solution. Depending on the sample and the purpose of the study, an aperture can be chosen to provide particle size, concentration, and distribution information in the size range of choice. A common choice is the 100-μm aperture, since its 2–60 μm dynamic sizing range covers most of the traditional subvisible particle size range, including the ≥10 and ≥25 μm as required by the compendia.

Most protein pharmaceuticals, however, are formulated in buffers that are quite different from PBS, with much lower ionic strength (on the order of 10 mM salt), resulting in significantly lower conductivity. These formulations also include tonifying/stabilizing agents other than saline and may be at pH values far away from neutral pH. Changing buffer composition and, in particular, ionic strength could also result in both decrease and increase in the amount of particles measured versus those present under the original conditions. Ideally, formulation buffers rather than PBS should be used as the electrolyte so that the products can be tested as formulated. However, because of their low conductivity, using such formulation buffers as electrolytes often results in increased voltage baseline noise. Therefore, method and technology development efforts are needed to enable the use of formulation buffers as electrolytes. Approaches such as adjusting the electrical current applied or the signal gain setting, reducing the lower dynamic sizing range (e.g., moving the lower sizing threshold from 2 to 3 μm for the 100-μm aperture since small particles generate low voltages and, thus, result in a poor signal-to-noise ratio), or even using a larger diameter aperture (e.g., 200 μm instead of 100 μm) can all be used to improve the data quality. One can also use a "formulation-like" buffer with the same excipients and pH conditions, but with higher ion concentration for increased conductivity. With a combination of such approaches, it is possible to develop a method to measure protein therapeutic products directly in a formulation, or formulation-like environment, and obtain meaningful results for subvisible particles in the micrometer size range.

Apertures with smaller diameters (e.g., 20 µm) are available with the potential to quantify particles as small as 0.4 µm. As discussed in the Section 5.1, this is a size range that has been mentioned to be of increasing interest for protein pharmaceuticals [10]. However, with the currently available ESZ instrumentation, it may be very difficult, if not impossible, to apply these small apertures to directly test protein therapeutic products using their formulation buffers as electrolytes. A smaller aperture requires the electrolyte to be even more conductive, while the conductivity of typical protein formulation buffers is often very low. In addition, because of the polydisperse nature of the protein particles (e.g., particle concentration vs size, as shown in Fig. 5.4), frequent blockage may occur if the aperture diameter is too small.

Another challenge is the sample volume required for routine measurement: even with the smaller version of the sample container, a minimum of about 15 mL of sample solution is needed to ensure that the electrodes and aperture are completely immersed in the liquid sample during the measurement. Using such large volumes of protein solution for a single test is often not feasible, particularly for programs in the early development phase. Therefore, dilution is often used to generate the needed volume for the ESZ measurements. However, if any of the subvisible particles are reversible, and in some rare cases, dilution actually results in the generation of particles, diluting the product could affect the amount of particles present and produce false results.

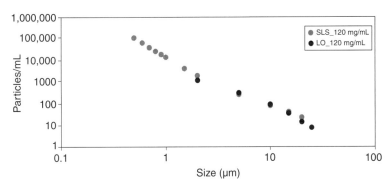

FIGURE 5.4   Particle concentration as a function of size in a protein product, as determined by a static light scattering (SLS) method that covers the size range of ≥ 0.5–20 µm and the modified light-obscuration method with the size range of ≥ 2–25 µm. While the absolute particle concentration values as determined by different techniques in the overlapping size range may (as shown in this case) or may not agree (data not shown), the overall distribution profile and pattern—higher concentrations at smaller sizes—are consistent from different techniques. (*See insert for color representation of the figure.*)

Despite its simplistic nature, it is not always straightforward to apply the ESZ technology to protein pharmaceuticals, particularly if one wishes to make direct measurements of the submicrometer particles in the product as formulated. However, if sufficient and appropriate improvements are made in areas such as the ability to use low conductivity electrolyte solutions, reduced sample volume, and an expanded aperture dynamic size range, it is possible that the ESZ technique can be made into a viable and robust tool for therapeutic protein product subvisible particle characterization.

5.3.2 Flow-Imaging Techniques

The flow-imaging techniques, as described in detail in Chapter 7, achieve particle sizing and counting by recording and analyzing digital images of particles flowing through a confined geometry such as a flow cell. The most important feature of these imaging techniques is that they provide a new dimension to subvisible particle characterization, namely, particle shape and morphology, that is lacking in the other techniques [15], as described in this chapter. Images with high quality can be used as important clues to distinguish particle types and sources, trying to differentiate between amorphous or crystal-like protein particles, air bubbles, silicone oil droplets, and extraneous contaminants. Such information is very useful, sometimes critical, to product development, for root cause determinations, and can also be used to help make product release decisions. This extra dimension of providing particle shape and morphology information in addition to quantitation makes the flow-imaging techniques a very valuable, and in some cases indispensable, technique that is complementary to the compendial methods.

The ability to accurately measure shape and morphology depends on the quality of the images obtained. Higher image quality can be achieved by using better optics with higher magnification, but this often comes at the price of reduced sampling efficiency or throughput. Depending on the purpose of the measurement, it is often necessary to choose the right compromise between image quality and sampling efficiency. Both the instrument manufacturers and end users are actively involved in technology development efforts to improve image quality while maintaining sufficient sampling efficiency, as assessed by the proportion of sample actually measured in relation to the total amount needed to perform the test (e.g., 50% or higher).

5.3.3 Light Scattering Techniques

Light scattering techniques, including both static and dynamic light scattering (SLS and DLS, respectively) and, by extension, laser diffraction, have been used in many ways to characterize particles and protein aggregates, as described in detail in Chapter 3. Here, a brief discussion is provided on using SLS to size and count particles in the submicrometer and micrometer range and to contrast it with the other techniques described thus far.

The operation of this stand-alone SLS system is analogous to that of the light obscuration described previously: liquid sample is introduced to the SLS flow cell by a syringe sampler. A test consists of multiple consecutive runs of a liquid sample with finite volume (such as four consecutive runs of 1 mL for each run). Typically, the first run results are discarded, and the rest is averaged and reported. During the measurement, scattered light produced by particles traveling through the flow cell is collected by a set of parabolic mirrors, focused by lenses onto a photosensitive detector and converted into electrical signals or pulses. For pulses above the baseline noise level, each pulse correlates to a particle and the size of the pulse is proportional to the size of the particle. A calibration curve can be established by running a series of particle calibration standards, usually PSL spheres with narrow size distribution and known sizes, and plotting the resulting pulse sizes versus particle diameters. Particle counting and sizing for a sample of interest can then be achieved by counting the number of the measured pulses and converting the sizes of these pulses into the sizes of the particles via the calibration curve.

One unique feature of this technology is its size range—theoretically from 0.2 to about 20 μm. It can be challenging to make measurements down to the lower size range limit of 0.2 μm for therapeutic protein samples, largely due to the requirement of ultraclean testing environment and the need to highly dilute (e.g., 100×) the test sample to avoid coincident effect and detector saturation. In spite of this, with the right measurement conditions, data of good quality can be routinely obtained for particle size distribution analysis for subvisible particles from 0.5 to 20 μm (Fig. 5.4) using this SLS system, making it one of the very few techniques capable of quantifying particles in the submicrometer size range. One caveat of this measurement is that due to the fact that particle concentration increases with decreased size, dilution (e.g., 1–10 in formation buffer) is often necessary to avoid exceeding the coincidence limit (about 10,000 particles/mL).

A fringe benefit of this dilution requirement is that a relatively small amount (e.g., ≤0.5 mL) of sample is needed for a single test, possibly making this an attractive tool for early development where sample availability is often the factor determining what technique can be employed.

Some of the drawbacks of this technique are that it does not take into consideration factors that could affect SLS such as particle shape and refractive index. Therefore, the sizing and counting results should be regarded as "relative." And since dilution is usually necessary, reliable results can be obtained only from samples that are stable on dilution.

5.4 POTENTIAL USES OF THESE METHODS

In this chapter, the USP methods, light obscuration and microscopy, were first described. Additional techniques to measure subvisible particles, such as the ESZ, flow-imaging, and light scattering techniques, were briefly described to facilitate comparison. The choice of technique to use is dependent on the problem being addressed and where the product is in the development lifecycle. For formulation development and investigational work, typically multiple techniques are used to characterize the particles and determine the underlying root cause of their presence.

Particles in protein pharmaceuticals represent a very heterogeneous population, with a wide size distribution, different shapes and morphologies, different origins and compositions, and existing in different amounts. Current technologies characterize particles based on specific properties such as blocking light or impeding electricity. The results obtained with each technology are dependent on the particular physical principle employed and are limited by the capabilities of measurements using that physical principle. Therefore, each technology and its associated method(s) have their own advantages and limitations, and which technology is the most appropriate for use in a given situation is dictated by the issues being addressed. It is often advantageous to use complementary techniques to verify and augment the results obtained with the individual techniques. A more detailed discussion on the limitations of these particle methods, how to best apply them, and the gaps in the present state of protein therapeutic product subvisible particle characterization is given below.

5.4.1   Comparison of Methods

Of the technologies discussed, light obscuration is probably used most often, in no small part due to its long history of being a compendial method for parenteral subvisible particle testing. The reasons for light obscuration being the workhorse for subvisible particle measurement are manifold. The equipment is relatively inexpensive, there are defined compendial guidelines and acceptance criteria around this measurement, and the measurement process itself is relatively fast. Thus, this measurement is well suited for product development studies such as time point analysis for formulation development, and it is an established lot release method in quality organizations. Collecting data in the small micrometer ranges (e.g., < 10 μm) is being encouraged by the FDA, and this should be considered during development work. One of the biggest limitations of this technology is that the information it provides is limited only to size and amount: it does not provide any information on what the particles may look like or what type of particles they may be. This may be satisfactory for small-molecule parenterals where subvisible particles are often extraneous contaminants, but many of the particles in protein pharmaceuticals are self-associated species of the drug itself, in addition to extraneous material, silicone oil droplets, and microbubbles. Modifications such as expanding the sizing range down to 2 μm and reducing sampling volume are also often necessary to make the method more suitable for protein applications.

The flow-imaging techniques offer results that are rich in information, including shape and morphology, in addition to size and amount. One of the biggest limitations of the flow-imaging techniques is the quality of the particle images obtained, particularly for small particles such as 5 μm or smaller; reliable and robust particle classification based on shape and morphology will be challenging unless the image quality improves.

In addition to its superior sizing resolution, the ESZ technology brings a unique feature in that its results are not affected by the optical properties of the particles and solutions, such as refractive index and particle orientation. The biggest challenge in applying the ESZ technology for protein pharmaceuticals is in finding the appropriate electrolyte solution to enable measurements of the small micrometer or even submicrometer particles without affecting the particle distribution.

The SLS technology as discussed earlier offers the possibility of analyzing particles in the submicrometer particle size range, provided the particle profile of a sample remains constant following dilution with a suitable buffer, such as its formulation buffer.

While each technology has its own strengths and weaknesses, they do share some common features. When appropriately applied, all these techniques count and size subvisible particles and provide similar concentration versus size distribution profiles, such as the plots of light-obscuration and light scattering results shown in Fig. 5.4. This commonality allows the techniques to be used in a complementary manner.

Another common feature is the use of PSL particles by these techniques. For light-obscuration and light scattering techniques, sizing results are reported in the format of equivalent circular (cross section) diameter by assuming that the particles are all spherical and block or scatter light same as their PSL equivalents; the ESZ uses the PSL particles to obtain its calibration constant and reports particle size in the format of equivalent spherical (volume) diameter with no assumption of particle shape. For the flow-imaging-based techniques, even though calibration is not necessary, PSL particles are often used to adjust the system's optics, and the accuracy of the size reported depends on image quality and how well the boundary of the particles can be defined. While results obtained measuring the PSL particles are often comparable across techniques, when the actual protein particles are measured the sizing and concentration results from different techniques follow the same relative trends, but the absolute values can differ by orders of magnitude. This could partially be due to the fact that while the PSL particles are truly spherical and uniform, protein particles are typically of irregular shape with different and varying optical properties such as translucency, refractive index, etc., and protein solutions have optical properties that are dependent on formulation and protein concentration. It should be recognized that this difference does not necessarily represent an error. Rather, it directly relates to the shape and optical properties of the particles and solution and the physical principles used. One potential approach to understand and reduce this difference is to use protein particle standards with known and controlled amount, size, shape, morphology, and optical properties to calibrate across techniques. Currently, such protein particle standards are not available commercially.

Most of the techniques and methods, with perhaps the exception of the SLS system, require a sample volume of about 1 mL or more. This milliliter per test sample volume requirement often makes it prohibitive to do particle testing early on during protein product development, a stage where understanding the propensity of a product candidate to form particles could have maximum impact. Significantly reducing this volume requirement (e.g., to the order of 100 µL/test) is not very feasible due to the hardware configurations (flow cells, etc.) of the current subvisible particle instruments and the necessity of analyzing sufficient sample volume to generate statistically robust results. Since particles in the submicrometer size range exist in much higher concentrations, as shown in Fig. 5.4, it is possible for a (new) technology to use only a fraction of 1 mL sample, a volume much more manageable for early development projects, to generate statistically meaningful results by monitoring the submicrometer particles, an area also of increasing interest due to lack of analytical capacity and potential immunogenicity concerns for these particles.

Another common limitation of these techniques and their associated methods is that the experimental procedures are manual and, therefore, low throughput and labor intensive. Undivided attention and manual execution from the analyst is required for the duration of the testing, from sample preparation to measurement to data analysis and interpretation. Automation for part or whole of the procedure is highly desirable for particle testing to meet the demand of ever quickening pace and increasing complexity of protein therapeutic product development.

One truly crucial aspect of particle characterization that is currently lacking for most of these technologies is to provide chemical identity or classification of the particles. Being able to determine if the particles are proteinaceous (and structure modifications if proteinaceous), silicone oil droplets, or excipients precipitants, is important for root-cause analysis and for process and formulation development. None of the current techniques provides direct information, and to achieve this, new technologies based on principles that can provide particle chemical structure or composition (e.g., Fourier transform infrared spectroscopy (FTIR) spectroscopy) are needed.

5.4.2   Use of These Methods in Protein Pharmaceuticals

For protein products, subvisible particle testing is done primarily to provide guidance on product development and product release. Which techniques and methods to use depends on the purpose of the testing; the methods used need to provide relevant and meaningful information based on which appropriate decisions can be made.

> *Development Testing.*   During product development, the goal of particle testing is often to compare and differentiate between molecules or processes. This includes ranking multiple molecular candidates based on their particulation properties and propensity, assessing the effect of a new process on the particle profile of a product to ensure comparability, or determining the stability of the formulated product. The critical performance parameters of a potential method to be used for this purpose are sensitivity and precision. For example, as demonstrated in Table 5.2, to study the effectiveness of the filtration step in the development process, the compendial light-obscuration method that quantifies the ≥10 and ≥25 µm particles only is not suitable

as it does not show any quantifiable difference between the before and after filtration samples. The concentrations of these subvisible particles in this case are too low to be precisely quantified. The modified method with its expanded size range clearly shows the effectiveness of the filtration steps at removing the particles. While these two methods use the same principle and hardware, the modified (small volume) light-obscuration method takes advantage of the higher particle concentrations at smaller sizes (e.g., 2 μm), which allow the particle amounts to be more precisely quantified. The accuracy, or absolute "correctness," of these results are not important, as long as the measurements are precise, since quantitating the relative difference and comparability is the goal here. Therefore, for product development, any method/technique can be used as long as its been shown to be robust, viable, sensitive, and precise enough to provide the needed information. Since the results are relative, or not "absolute," it is crucial to be consistent and use the same approach and methods as much as possible throughout the product's lifecycle so that results at different development phases can be compared.

In addition to a primary method, it is also a good practice to have at least one secondary method, preferably based on a different principle, to compliment the primary method to either confirm or provide additional information of the particles such as shape or chemical composition. One aspect to consider during development work would be the size of the samples. To gain greater confidence in the measurement, it may be necessary to measure more than one vial for a given lot and/or measure particle profiles across multiple lots to show consistency in the manufacturing process.

Release and Stability Testing. For product release and stability, the purpose of subvisible particle testing is twofold: to determine whether a product conforms with the preset acceptance criteria and is, therefore, suitable to be released and used as protein pharmaceutical, and to determine the stability of the product throughout its shelf life. One aspect of the stability is to detect and determine change at different time points (e.g., every six months), and as discussed earlier, any method/technique with sufficient sensitivity and precision can be used, since the goal is essentially to compare and assess relative difference.

For determining conformity with acceptance criteria, however, since subvisible particle testing results are technique dependent, results by different techniques on the same product may be different; the technique used for conformance testing and for setting acceptance criteria must be the same. Currently, the subvisible particle acceptance criteria used for protein pharmaceuticals are as set by USP <788>, EP 2.9.19, and JP for small-volume parenterals: no more than 6000 and 600 per container for ≥ 10 and ≥ 25 μm particles, respectively, as determined by light-obscuration technique. Therefore, at least for the time being, only light-obscuration-based methods can be used for release testing.

While it is challenging to apply the compendial light-obscuration test (25 mL per test, report ≥ 10 and ≥ 25 µm particles) to protein pharmaceuticals as a release and stability test, it is not feasible to use the compendial method as a development tool. It has been demonstrated that with certain modifications such as improved sample handling, reduced sample volume, and expanded sizing range, a light-obscuration-based method can be used satisfactorily as a release and stability test as well as be applied during development [11].

The compendial subvisible particle limits are set based on historical data and experience with small-molecule parenterals, mainly as a means to control the amount of extraneous contaminants, with capillary occlusion as one of the chief patient safety concerns. With protein pharmaceuticals, the amount of small subvisible particles (e.g., < 10 µm or even submicrometer) and their immunogenic potential (which could be product particle specific) have been recently highlighted as major concerns [10]. To better address these concerns, it may be necessary to set product specific acceptance limits based on development history and clinical experience, rather than the current limits that are uniform and arbitrary for all products. Any of the above-mentioned methods, as long as they are based on sound scientific principles and applications and have been demonstrated to be suitable for the purpose, can be used for development use, for acceptance criteria setting, and after sufficient sample data have been collected, for release and stability testing.

5.5 CASE STUDIES

Key stresses, such as surface interface interactions, thawing a frozen drug substance, or transportation to the clinical site, may induce particle formation, and therefore, understanding a product's particle profile following these stresses is important. In the following section, two case studies are outlined that demonstrate how protein pharmaceuticals (monoclonal antibodies in these cases) responded to these stresses. The first case study describes the role of the formulation in modulating particle formation during freeze/thaw and transportation, while the second study illustrates the importance of particle characterization during process development, in this case a filling step.

5.5.1 Case Study 1: Utility of Light-Obscuration Measurements in Polysorbate Selection during Formulation Development

Formulation development is an important endeavor during product development in the biotechnology industry. The overall goal is to select a formulation that would keep the molecule under consideration stable to various types of stresses that would be encountered during manufacturing, storage, and delivery to the patient. This includes developing a formulation that minimizes protein self-association and the formation of subvisible and visible particles. In this case study, two stresses will be examined, namely, the effects of freeze/thaw and transportation. In each instance, the effect of polysorbate as a stabilizing excipient, for liquid product in vials, will be shown. Polysorbate is an excipient of choice when it comes to shielding proteins from aggregation induced by air–water and ice–water interfaces. Several mechanisms have been postulated to explain the protective action of detergents such as polysorbate [16–19]. Experiments with human growth hormone suggested that polysorbate may bind to hydrophobic regions of the protein molecule during agitation stress, thus minimizing aggregation [18]. Nonionic surfactants can also have the ability to bind to partially unfolded states and reduce interactions that lead to non-native aggregation, a mechanism that probably dominates during freeze/thaw-related protection [19]. Finally, polysorbate can also compete for protein binding to surfaces, thus minimizing surface unfolding and ensuing aggregation [17]. The transportation stress test purposely introduces additional air–water interfaces to examine the stability of the protein under this condition, while the freeze/thaw test introduces ice–water interfaces that could potentially denature the protein.

Figure 5.5 shows the effect of polysorbate on a monoclonal antibody undergoing multiple freeze/thaws. This antibody was placed in a 250-mL carboy, and a profile that mimicked the thawing rate in a 20-L carboy was applied. Freeze/thaw studies were performed by cycling the carboy from a $-30°C$ freezer to room temperature ($15-25°C$) and back. After each cycle, a 5-mL aliquot was taken and particle counts were examined using the light-obscuration method, in formulations in the absence or presence of polysorbate. In both the formulations, particle counts

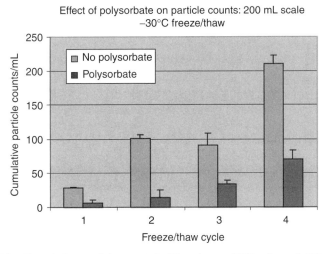

FIGURE 5.5   Cumulative particle counts ($\geq 10\ \mu m$) per milliliter for an IgG2 monoclonal antibody after 1, 2, 3, and 4 rounds of freeze/thaw. Two formulations were tested, one with polysorbate and the other without. It was seen that polysorbate 20 significantly reduced the increase in subvisible ($\geq 10\ \mu m$) particle counts due to freeze/thaw stress.

did increase with each cycle of freeze/thaw, as assessed by monitoring particle counts ≥ 10 μm from the light-obscuration measurements shown in Fig. 5.5. However, the presence of polysorbate significantly suppressed the level of particles, both initially and following each freeze/thaw cycle.

The same antibody filled as a liquid in glass vials was also assessed for its stability toward simulated transportation stress (Fig. 5.6). This antibody was placed in four formulations (marked F1, F2, F3, and F4). In each formulation, polysorbate 20 was tested at four different levels, namely, 0 (no polysorbate), 0.004, 0.008, and 0.012%. The antibody in these formulations was placed on a vibration table that simulated ground and air transportation. Following the simulated transportation stress, these formulations were examined for their particle counts using a modified version of the compendial light-obscuration method. Figure 5.6a shows the amount of particles present that are ≥ 10 μm for these formulations.

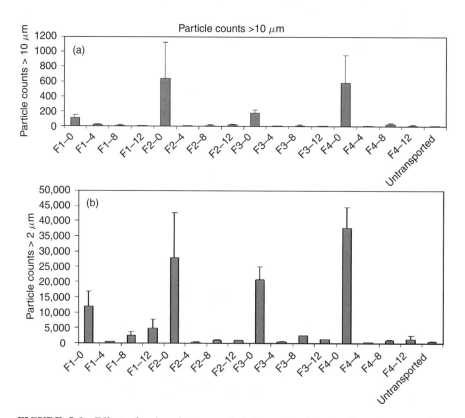

FIGURE 5.6 Effect of polysorbate on subvisible particulate levels on transportation. (a) Light-obscuration counts for ≥ 10 μm particles and (b) Light-obscuration counts for ≥ 2 μm particles for four different base formulations (F1, F2, F3, and F4). Each base formulation contained 0, 0.004, 0.008, or 0.012% polysorbate 20 (denoted by F1-0, F1-4, F1-8, and F1-12, respectively, for the base formulation F1 and so on for F2–F4). The untransported control is also shown.

As seen in this figure, for each formulation, the subvisible particle counts at 10 μm or greater were always higher for the polysorbate-free formulations. This was consistent with the greater level of aggregation that would be expected for proteins that were subjected to air–water interfaces during the transportation stress, without the protection afforded by polysorbate. The errors showed are from averaging two vials tested per formulation. This brings up an interesting point, especially for formulations F2 and F4, where there was seen to be significant variability. Just examining one vial from each formulation might have led the observer to make the interpretation that somehow formulations F1 and F3 were more stable than F2 and F4. However, the large standard deviation in the measurements indicates that this may not necessarily be the case. The source of the variability is not clear and part of it may come from the assay itself. However, in addition, it is possible that the stress experienced by one of the vials may be different from the other vial examined for the same formulation, depending on the location on the vibration table, etc. This could mimic actual product handling conditions, where individual vials in the same lot may be subjected to slightly different amounts of stress.

The effect of transportation stress on ≥ 2 μm particle counts was also examined for the antibody (Fig. 5.6b). Collecting information on these smaller subvisible particles and how they are affected by stress could aid in the development of a stable formulation, while at the same time increase our understanding of both the characteristics of the assay for these smaller subvisible particles as well as the effect of stress on the generation of these subvisible particles. The trend for the 2-μm subvisible particles was similar to that of the 10-μm particles in that all the polysorbate-free formulations showed higher counts than those containing polysorbate 20. In addition, it appeared that F1 was slightly better than F2, F3, or F4, especially in the amounts of subvisible particles in the 0% polysorbate formulations (F1-0 vs F2-0, F3-0, or F4-0). The 2-μm counts did provide an additional piece of information: it appeared that the highest polysorbate 20 level (0.012%) had increased ≥ 2 μm counts compared to that of 0.004% polysorbate 20, especially for F1 (i.e., F1-12 vs F1-4). This was also seen in F3 and F4 to some measure. Thus, monitoring the amounts of the subvisible particles across this size range allowed for a ranking of the formulations, with a 0.004% polysorbate 20 level being preferred for protection against transportation stress. It is unclear at this point why the 0.012% polysorbate 20 had slightly higher counts than that 0.004%. Given that the critical micelle concentration (CMC) of polysorbate 20 in water is 0.0072%, it is possible that the presence of micelles was a contributing factor, but this would need to be explored in greater detail in separate studies.

These types of differences would need to be probed further and resolved during formulation development. However, overall the study clearly revealed that the presence of polysorbate was a stabilizing element in suppressing subvisible particle formation. In this case, it did not appear to matter what the level of polysorbate was, within the ranges tested (0.004–0.012%), as well as the nature of the other formulations for this particular stress.

5.5.2   Case Study 2: Utility of Coulter Counter in Filling Pump-Induced Particulation

This case study concerns the investigation and characterization of particles that were observed in a clinical manufacturing facility while performing a filling operation for an IgG monoclonal antibody [6]. This problem was traced to the use of a positive displacement pump (National Instrument Filmatic pump) that was used in the filling operation. Importantly, this problem occurred right after the filling step, in spite of a filtration step just before entering the filling apparatus, thus implicating the filling operation. The questions raised in this study included the mechanism underlying particle formation and characterization of the size distribution and structural features of the observed particles.

The authors assessed particle size using two instruments, a Beckman Z1 Coulter counter and a Beckman LS230 particle sizer. For model particle testing and heterogeneous nucleation experiments, nanoparticles were obtained from Argonide Corporation, with an average particle size of 100 nm. In the case of the Beckman Z1 counter, a majority of particles in the product samples were found to be present in the lower size range of the instrument, namely 1.5–3 μm, and there were relatively few particles beyond 10 μm. The Beckman LS 230, which has a lower limit of 0.04 μm, showed that 99% of the total number of particles were in the 0.25–0.95 μm range. Thus, these protein particles were found to be very small in size compared to foreign particles that are typically expected to be in the ≥10 and ≥25 μm ranges.

On the basis of the observation that every vial that underwent the filling operation contained a few visible particles, the authors hypothesized that nano- and microparticles shed from the contact surfaces of the filling pump were responsible for nucleating the association of protein molecules to form a particle large enough to be detectable. FTIR data from isolated particles indicated the presence of protein, although the structure of the antibody was slightly perturbed from the native state. The second evidence that indicated a direct participation of protein molecules was the ∼20-fold lower level of particles observed in placebo samples. In separate experiments, the authors showed using elemental analysis that this low, basal level of particles was probably due to stainless steel shedding from the pump. To then directly test for the ability of stainless steel particles to nucleate protein particulation, the authors mixed a protein solution that did not contain particles with a solution containing stainless steel particles sized at 0.1 μm. A large increase in particles in the 1.5–3 μm range was observed in a matter of hours, as determined by the Coulter counter, while a ∼4% drop in the level of soluble IgG in solution was indicated by SEC. Intriguingly, the number of particles found in this larger range (1.5–3 μm, compared to the 0.1 μm size of the stainless steel bead) was similar in number (30,000) to the starting level of stainless steel beads, suggesting that the growth in particle size was due to several layers of IgG adsorbing on to these particles. These observations suggested a shedding of stainless steel material from the displacement pump, which served as a nucleus to drive protein association to form particles in the 1–10 μm range. Presumably, these particles coalesced together to appear visually detectable while dissociating during the quantitative measurement. Possibly, light scattering effects may also have rendered them barely visible. In summary, this case study illustrated how the manufacturing process can play a role in generating protein particles, and how particle-sizing measurements, coupled with other characterization techniques such as chemical identification, can be used to arrive at the root cause underlying the problem. At this point, it is unclear what effect the dilution required to analyze the results with the Coulter counter might have had on the final size of the heteronucleated particles.

5.6 SUMMARY AND FUTURE DIRECTIONS

5.6.1 Summary

In this chapter, we have discussed the techniques available for subvisible particle quantification and characterization, with particular emphasis on the compendial light-obscuration method. All these techniques are based on different fundamental measurements, have different strengths and weaknesses and can therefore be used as complementary methods. For all these methods, sample handling is the key to their successful use for protein pharmaceuticals, and care must be taken to remove microbubbles and to avoid generating or dissociating particles during the experimental manipulations.

The light-obscuration methods can be used on the formulated drug product without any manipulations, have a range of $\sim 2-150$ µm, and can determine only the concentration and size distribution. In addition, the method was originally written for small-molecule therapeutics and requires some modification in terms of volumes used and sample handling before it can be successfully applied to protein pharmaceuticals during development in addition to stability and lot release. This method does not provide any information on the nature of the particles being counted. In addition, dilution with buffer may be required for high protein concentration formulations. The ESZ technique measures the volume of the particle directly, rather than calculating it based on interactions with light, and can potentially analyze particles as small as 0.4 µm. However, the analysis may require dilution of the sample into a buffer that can carry a defined charge, and this can affect the particle distribution profile. Static light scattering, though more commonly used to characterize submicrometer particles, can be used to quantify subvisible particles from about 0.5 to 20 µm. It reports concentration and size distribution and very often requires dilution with formulation buffer. The flow-imaging methods, in contrast to all the other techniques available, provide information on the morphology and size of the subvisible particles based on the analysis of captured images. The quality of the analysis depends in part on the quality of the optics and the amount of the sample analyzed. The analysis can often occur on the drug product without dilution unless the protein concentration is very high.

During process and formulation development, material is limited and the ability to get precise and consistent results using very little material is the key. Determining the size distribution profile as well as obtaining some information that can be used to guide further development is the focus. This information can be invaluable for choosing the product candidate and also to help guide decisions around process steps and formulation composition. For lot release and stability, the amount of material is no longer as limiting, and the focus shifts to the robustness of the method and the ability to obtain comparable results in different laboratories and on different lots. The light-obscuration method remains, at present, the technique most amenable for use for routine lot release and stability testing to demonstrate conformance with the current compendial requirements. However, for this method to be applied to protein pharmaceuticals throughout the product lifecycle, some modifications are required.

5.6.2   Future Directions

The development and improvement of the techniques described here, as well as other novel approaches, is continuing. The ultimate goal would be an automated high throughput method using very little material that allows direct analysis of the protein solution with no dilution. This technique, or combination of techniques, should provide not only a robust, repeatable concentration and size distribution analysis but also information on the morphology and optical properties of the particles and their identity.

The current compendial limits on the subvisible particles ≥ 10 and ≥ 25 μm were set based on historically safe levels in small-molecule parenterals, and the application to protein pharmaceuticals delivered by other routes is slightly arbitrary. Accumulating sufficient data to understand the lot-to-lot and sample-to-sample variability in subvisible particles, the effect of delivery device and route of administration, and the historical patient exposure to particles in the clinic should allow for the setting of specifications that are meaningful for protein pharmaceuticals. If specifications are ever to be set, they would have to be specific to the drug under consideration and the method being employed, as opposed to being universal.

An important gap in our current knowledge is the potential role that protein particles might play in the safety and efficacy of products, including possible immunogenicity. Studies are underway to probe this relationship, made possible in part by the development of the techniques described above. Understanding the underlying mechanism of particulation should allow the development of more robust protein pharmaceuticals that have decreased the tendency to aggregate.

REFERENCES

1. Chi EY, Krishnan S, Kendrick BS, Chang BS, Carpenter JF, Randolph TW. Roles of conformational stability and colloidal stability in the aggregation of recombinant human granulocyte colony-stimulating factor. Protein Sci 2003;12:903–913.

2. Murphy R, Amos T, editors. Misbehaving proteins: protein (mis) folding, aggregation, and stability. Springer-Verlag New York, Inc; 2006.

3. Mahler H-C, Friese W, Grauschopf U, Kriese S. Protein aggregation: pathways, induction factors and analysis. J Pharm Sci 2009;98:2909–2934.

4. Weiss WF, Young TM, Roberts CJ. Principles, approaches, and challenges for predicting protein aggregation rates and shelf life. J Pharm Sci 2009;98:1246–1277.

5. Dobson CM. Principles of protein folding, misfolding and aggregation. Semin Cell Dev Biol 2004;15:3–16.

6. Tyagi AK, Randolph TW, Dong A, Maloney KM, Hitscherich C, Carpenter JF. IgG particle formation during filling pump operation: a case study of heterogeneous nucleation on stainless steel nanoparticles. J Pharm Sci 2009;98:94–104.

7. Narhi LO, Cao S, Jiang Y, Benedek K, Shnek D. A critical review of analytical methods for subvisible and visible particles. Curr Pharm Biotechnol 2009;10:373–381.

8. Knapp JZ. Overview of the forthcoming PDA task force report on the inspection for visible particles in parenteral products: practical answers for present problems. PDA J Pharm Sci Technol 2003;54:218–232.

9. USP General Chapters: <788>. Particulate matter in injections. Pharmacopeial Forum 2009;28:1930, USP32–NF27.

10. Carpenter JF, Randolph TW, Jiskoot W, Crommelin DJA, Middaugh CR, Winter G, Fan Y-X, Kirshner S, Verthelyi D, Kozklowski S, Crouse KA, Swann PG, Rosenberg A, Cherney B. Overlooking subvisible particles in therapeutic protein products: gaps that may compromise product quality. J Pharm Sci 2009;98:1201–1205.

11. Cao S, Jiang Y, Narhi L. A light-obscuration method specific for quantifying subvisible particles in protein therapeutics. USP Pharmacopeial Forum 2010;36(3):824–834.

12. Coulter, WH. US patent 2,656,508. 1953.

13. Grover NB, Naaman J, Ben-Sasson S, Doljansk F. Electrical sizing of particles in suspensions. I. Theory. Biophys J 1969;9:1398–1413.

14. Harfield JG, Knight P. Experimental evidence of the linear response of the Coulter counter. In: Stanley-Wood NG, Allen T, editors. Particle size analysis 1981. Chichester: Wiley Heyden; 1982. pp. 199–208.

15. Sharma D, King D, Moore P, Oma P, Thomas D. Flow microscopy for particulate analysis in parenteral and pharmaceutical fluids. Eur J Parenter Pharm Sci 2007;12:97–101.

16. Chou DK, Krishnamurthy R, Randolph TW, Carpenter JF, Manning MC. Effects of Tween 20 and Tween 80 on the stability of Albutropin during agitation. J Pharm Sci 2005;94:1368–1381.

17. Randolph TW, Jones LS. Surfactant-protein interactions. Rational design of stable protein formulations. In: Carpenter JF, Manning MC, editors. Volume 13, Pharmaceutical biotechnology New York: Kluwer Academic/Plenum Publishers, New York; 2002. pp. 159–175.

18. Bam NB, Cleland JL, Yang J, Manning MC, Carpenter JF, Kelley RF, Randolph TW. Tween protects recombinant human growth hormone against agitation-induced damage via hydrophobic interactions. J Pharm Sci 1998;87:1554–1559.

19. Kreilgaard L, Jones LS, Randolph TW, Frokjaer S, Flink JM, Manning MC, Carpenter JF. Effect of Tween 20 on freeze-thawing- and agitation induced aggregation of recombinant human factor XIII. J Pharm Sci 1998;87:1597–1603.

6 Detection of Visible Particles in Parenteral Products

RONALD SMULDERS

Analytical Method and Validation, Merck Manufacturing Division, Oss, The Netherlands

HANS VOS

Biological and Sterile Product Development, Schering Plough Research Institute, Oss, The Netherlands

HANNS-CHRISTIAN MAHLER

Pharmaceutical and Device Development, Pharma Technical Development Biologics Europe, F. Hoffmann-La Roche Ltd., Basel, Switzerland

6.1 INTRODUCTION

Protein pharmaceuticals have become an important part of modern therapeutics. Of the top 50 pharmaceutical companies, 30 are currently involved in biologics, and 27% of the US Food and Drug Administrations new drug approvals in 2009 were for biologic license applications [1]. Owing to their limited stability in the gastrointestinal tract and relatively low absorption upon oral, pulmonary, or nasal administration, most protein pharmaceuticals are "parenteral products," that is, sterile dosage forms administered by injection, infusion, or implantation [2–4]. In most cases, the product is either in liquid or dried (mostly lyophilized) form, in either vials or prefilled syringe. Since terminal sterilization techniques such as autoclaving, γ-irradiation, gas or chemical sterilization are typically not applicable to such sensitive molecules, protein drug products are manufactured using aseptic unit operations and sterile filtration [5]. Aseptic manufacturing follows current good manufacturing practices (cGMP) requirements. The requirement to use products for injection or infusion being "essentially free of visible particles" is both a GMP and pharmacopeial requirement. The presence of visible particulate matter is one of the top 10 reasons for the recall of parenteral products. Therefore,

Analysis of Aggregates and Particles in Protein Pharmaceuticals, First Edition.
Edited by Hanns-Christian Mahler, Wim Jiskoot.
© 2012 John Wiley & Sons, Inc., Published 2012 by John Wiley & Sons, Inc.

during the manufacture of parenteral preparations, great effort and care is taken to monitor, control, and minimize potential sources of particulate contamination to obtain products that are safe for use in patients. Interestingly, protein pharmaceuticals may contain or develop aggregated protein during manufacturing, storage, or use. In some cases, the aggregated protein may even be large enough to be detected visually. Thus, visual control of protein parenterals especially is an area of current discussion. In this chapter, we discuss requirements for visible appearance of protein parenterals, and we give examples of how visual testing is performed and implemented into the manufacturing and analytical process.

6.2 CURRENT REGULATORY REQUIREMENTS AND EXPECTATIONS

Since the 1930s and 1940s, when antibiotic parenteral products were widely used, concerns were raised on the optical quality of those products: at that time, even the optical quality of soft drinks was superior to that of parenteral products. Because of clinical concerns, it was desirable to use parenteral products free of "flecks, haze, or other particulate contaminations." Thus, the U.S. National Formulary (NF) VI contained for the first time the recommendation that these products should be "essentially free of visible particles."

All units intended for parenteral preparation are required to undergo visual inspection for particulates and other foreign matter and should be inspected to the extent possible [6]. Every container that shows evidence of visible particulates should be rejected.

The European Pharmacopeia (EP) and US Pharmacopeia (USP) require parenteral products to be "essentially free" and "practically free" of visible particles, respectively. The term essentially/practically free has led to confusion in the industry on how the term should be interpreted as a real limit. This will be discussed in the following sections.

The EP monograph "monoclonal antibodies for human use" in its current version requires these products to be "without visible particles." The recent monograph update will include the addition "unless otherwise justified and authorized." This statement is interesting, as a parenteral product of a therapeutic protein is generally not different from any other parenteral product, maybe excluding the fact that intrinsic proteinaceous particles may occur. However, the addition reflects the fact that the minimization of particles and defects should be a driver for continuous formulation and process improvement but that "zero defects" are probably not a workable acceptance criterion for visible particles because of current processing capability and packaging components. This is also reflected by the term practically/essentially free in the monograph for parenteral preparations.

Recently, Madsen et al. elaborated on what practically/essentially free may mean and suggested that the term shall reflect that "not more than 1 unit from 60 units inspected shall contain visible particles" [7]. However, this suggestion does not include a definition on the number of particulates per contaminated container. The future will show whether more specific definitions of practically/essentially free are possible.

6.3 SOURCES OF VISIBLE PARTICULATES

Particulate contaminations of injections and infusions were defined by the EP and USP as consisting of "extraneous, mobile undissolved particles, other than gas bubbles, unintentionally present in the solutions" [8,9]. Particulate matter in a sterile product may come from [10]

1. the solution itself and its ingredients, including the active pharmaceutical ingredient;
2. the production process and its variables, such as the environment, equipment, and personnel;
3. the product's packaging; and
4. the preparation of the product before administration (i.e., manipulating the product, the environment in which it is prepared).

The source of particles can be *extrinsic* or *intrinsic* to the process. Material or substance that is inherent to the manufacturing process is defined as *intrinsic*. An extrinsic source is material or substance that is not inherent to the manufacturing process. Particles may be visible or subvisible.

Common sources of particulates found during final visual inspection are [11]

1. lint/fibers
2. glass
3. product-related, for example, particles originating from the formulation or components thereof (e.g., protein precipitation, excipient incompatibilities, or insolubilities)
4. rubber
5. metal and
6. extrinsic protein (e.g., of human source).

The current methods to inspect for visible particulates typically do not readily allow identification of those contaminants. Thus, units that are sorted out during visual inspection typically do not undergo identification. However, in case, the rejection rate is abnormal during visual inspection, identification studies may be a part of the root-cause investigation. Such an investigation (and also subsequent process improvements) can be very challenging, not only because particles may originate from complex interaction effects (Section 6.7.1) but also because particle identification often requires a "forensic" approach. That is, the amount of particles in terms of mass is typically extremely low (picogram to nanogram range) and several hints need to be collected to unravel the real identity. First, microscopy or sole visual description may already help, as, for example, particles may be fiberlike (which may be a cellulose fiber) or amorphous (which may be protein derived). Second, particles would need to be isolated by either filtration or centrifugation. Both preparation methods include the risk of potential contamination of the analyte with extrinsic particulates and/or alteration of the analyte itself. For example, in many cases, particles in a protein formulation may not easily be centrifuged due to formation of gels. Methods such as Fourier-Transform Infrared Spectroscopy (FT IR) or Raman may be used to record structural spectra of the isolated particles, trying to compare these with known spectra (databases), to come up with suggestions of structure and thus identity. Adequate control samples and reference spectra are also of utmost importance. In summary, identification attempts typically have a forensic nature and thus are considered helpful for root-cause analysis, but they are not regularly applied for Quality Control (QC) release analytics.

6.4   CLINICAL CONCERNS WITH VISIBLE PARTICULATES

While there still seems to be a lack of sufficient clinical data to incriminate particles as origin of significant clinical complications on parenteral administration, it is believed that particulate matter may present a clinical hazard and should be absent from injectable solutions [12]. Specifically, clinical concerns with visible particulates—also depending on indication, treatment frequency, and duration—are

- mechanical obstruction with lung as the target and
- injection site reactions, phlebitis, and granuloma.

No controlled studies are known that have analyzed potential adverse reactions as a function of particles of different sizes and nature. Thus, only some anecdotal information obtained from the examination of studies of intravenous (IV) drug abusers indicate potential safety concern. For example, indications for pulmonary foreign body emboli and granulomas were observed in drug abusers [13–17] Furthermore, emboli seemed to have been caused by cotton fibers, talcum, and cellulose in IV drug abusers [18]. Complications in drug abusers related to inflammatory material, for example, IV talc or cotton wool may include interstitial lung granuloma [15] and variable degrees of fibrosis [19].

Infusion of large quantities of particulate matter has been associated with an increased incidence of phlebitis [20]. Reports of infusion phlebitis (injection site reactions) were decreased with the use of filters or filter needles. In a repeated double-blind study of 146 patients, a significant reduction in the incidence of infusion phlebitis was seen when patients were administered IV fluids filtered through an in-line 0.45-μm filter [21]. Other studies have supported this finding [22]. Injection site granulomas potentially related to the presence of particles have been reported in drug abusers [14].

A number of studies have also been performed in animals, for example, using latex and glass particles (100–440 μm), which indicated that IV administered particles are distributed mainly in lungs and to a lesser extent in liver and spleen [23,24]. It has been reported that glass spheres with diameters 20–40 times the average diameter of the lumina of the capillaries (particle size up to 390 μm) can travel to the lungs by means of noncapillary channels [23]. Uptake of particles can also depend on charge, with negatively charged material being taken up by the liver and positively charged material being initially accumulated in the lung and later in the spleen [25].

The risk of thromboembolic events is patient dependent and may increase, for example, with age, cancer, cardiac failure, and infection [26]. The route of parenteral administration is also considered relevant: there are very few reports of adverse reactions from particles given by intramuscular (IM) injection [27]. Potential adverse events from IM administration of a product with particles could include local injection site reactions such as pain, swelling, and inflammation. Potential adverse reactions from IV administration of a product with foreign particles could be more serious including damage to blood vessels or embolic events and anaphylactic, allergic, and immune-mediated reactions. Experience with various sizes of massive particle load for embolization is of limited relevance as parenteral drug would usually not be developed for the arterial route.

Interestingly, review of the medical literature for visible particles does not clearly indicate a clear relationship between particle composition and patient risk. However, biodegradable particles, for example, may be better tolerated as these would be cleared from the body. In addition, if visible particulates would consist of or contain protein, this may lead to increased risk of immunogenicity of the product [28,29].

In summary, visual inspection is a method and process to ensure adequate quality of the injectable. The essential absence of visible particles is an important quality attribute. However, only little if known about adverse effects specifically related to particles and/or certain types or sizes of particles administered parenterally to humans. No direct clinical evidence for adverse reactions of parenterally administered particles exist that direct which types or sizes of particulates are a safety issue. Anecdotal studies and data are available, highlighting potential relevance for mechanical obstruction of vessels and site reactions. Thus, particles currently remain a relevant quality attribute.

6.5   DETECTION OF VISIBLE PARTICLES

Filled containers of parenteral products are inspected individually for contamination or other defects. Visual inspection needs to be done under suitable and controlled conditions of illumination and background. Thus, the EP suggests a black/white panel for visual testing using at least 1000–3750 lux of illumination, the Japanese Pharmacopeia (JP) at least 1000 lux.

Operators doing the inspection need to pass regular eyesight checks and have to be allowed frequent breaks from inspection. The USP <1> describes that the "inspection process shall be designed and qualified to ensure that every lot of parenteral preparations is essentially free from visible particles" and that "qualification of the inspection process shall be performed with reference to particulates in the visible range of a type that might emanate from the manufacturing or filling process." Thus, operators are frequently, for example, every 6 or 12 months, trained with (product-specific or product-unspecific) training sets, typically containing 200–1000 units.

The detection of visible particles is based on (statistical) probability. The probability of detection increases with increasing particle size. Analysis of inspection results pooled from several studies involving different groups of inspectors (under lighting and background conditions accepted to EP 2.9.20) shows that the probability of detection for a single 50-μm particle in clear solution in a 10-mL vial with diffuse illumination between 2000 and 3000 lux was slightly >0% (Fig. 6.1). This probability increased to approximately 40% for a 100-μm particle and became >95% for particles that were 200 μm and larger [13].

Visibility may depend on [30]

- operator's eyesight and eye fatigue
- type of particle (transparency, size, density, and shape)
- illumination intensity and light conditions
- magnification
- observation time
- type of background inspected against
- distance from samples
- type (manual and automated) and speed of rotation
- fill volume and primary packaging material used
- location of particulate (e.g., floating in solution or stuck to wall).

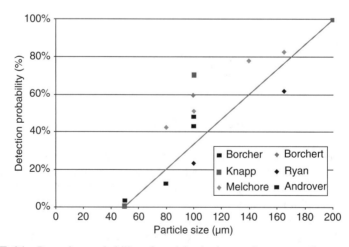

FIGURE 6.1   Detection probability of particles by human inspectors. *Source:* Modified from Shabushnig [31]. *(See insert for color representation of the figure.)*

Thus, the sensitivity of different visual inspection methods may differ. Additionally, inspection by different operators (using a single method) shows variation [31] and equipment conditions can be a source of variation (e.g., light intensity typically diminishes over use time). Finally, it is noteworthy that the visual inspection conditions/procedures may induce instabilities, especially in protein products. It is known that both light and mechanical stress may lead to protein precipitation and aggregation [30]. Thus, it may be wise to test the impact of the visual inspection conditions on the product, especially when considering to use brighter light conditions, longer inspection times, and when applying container spinning. In other words, visual inspection methods may actually require some development and validation and should not a priori be seen as generic procedures.

6.5.1   Visual Inspection Using the Black/White Box

The inspection method described in the EP includes a vertical matt black panel and a vertical nonglare white panel next to it (Fig. 6.2). An adjustable lamp holder is included, with shaded, white light source and a diffuser (two 13-W fluorescent tubes, each 525 mm in length are suitable). Illumination at the viewing point is between 2000 and 3750 lux for clear glass material. Higher values are preferable for colored glass and plastic containers. No specific pharmacopeial guidelines, methods, or criteria exist for such containers, apart from the statement mentioned above.

For inspection, the individual container is gently swirled or inverted, making sure that no air bubbles are introduced. The solution is then observed in front of the white and black panel for a specified amount of time (e.g., 5 s). In case of the presence of any particles, this needs to be documented and recorded.

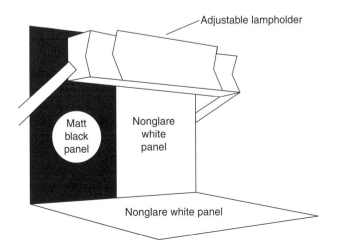

FIGURE 6.2   EP cabinet for visual inspection.

6.5.2   Visual Inspection Using Other Inspection Devices

The visual inspection process may be supported by certain devices or machines for economic (efficiency) or ergonomic (convenience for the operators) reasons. Just to name a few, visual inspection devices may be

- cold-light lamps (e.g., Schott)
- video-camera-enabled systems (e.g., APK Keyence)
- manual, semiautomatic, or automatic inspection devices with automated container spin (e.g., Seidenader)
- polarized light inspection devices (e.g., Optima).

When using, for example, a manual table-top Seidenader inspection machine, the units to be inspected are manually placed on the machine (rolling tubes). The containers are rotated by the machine. Using a concentrated light beam and optionally also magnification lenses, any particles potentially present in the container solution are rotated and can be detected in the light beam by a trained operator.

For the reasons mentioned earlier (Section 6.5), the inspection procedure itself or the use of certain equipment or inspection devices may have a pronounced impact on rejection rates (Section 6.7.2). For this reason, it is recommended to evaluate performance of visual inspection methods and establish acceptance criteria for visual inspection in an early development stage. Furthermore, developers should be keen on the various inspection methods used throughout process upscaling (e.g., from clinical to commercial scale) and (site-to-site) transfers. Especially for (protein) products that are prone to form intrinsic particles over time or products that contain nonstandardized particles (e.g., flaky particles that easily scatter light), visual inspection procedures need to be established carefully to prevent major problems at the time of product release and/or long-term storage.

6.5.3   Automatic Inspection Devices

Automatic inspection systems provide a high detection rate of inspection with usually good reliability. For vials and ampoules (≤ 10 mL), the automatic inspection rate is 12,000–24,000 units/h, whereas the rate of a manual process (single operator) is only 500–1,000 units/h. The principle of automatic inspection devices is based on either light blockage or image analysis. As to the latter, which is a more advanced technique, cameras take multiple images of a container via an oscillating mirror. Images are then analyzed and moving particles are recognized. Next to that, the images also allow screening on glass cracks, cosmetic defects, and misalignment or lack of stoppers.

Although the use of an automatic inspection device may sound attractive from an efficiency and consistency perspective, it should be realized that for each individual product an automatic inspection process needs to be developed and validated against human operators. Development strategies for automatic inspection processes typically comprise definition of a product-specific test set. That is, extensive manual inspection is applied to a regular product batch to identify units with a high rejection probability (e.g., more than 70%). Subsequently, the settings of the automatic inspection device are chosen in such a way that units with a high manual rejection probability are also rejected during an automatic process. After the development and validation of an automatic inspection process, the human factor is still not excluded. Following 100% automatic inspection of a routine product batch, a manual (operator-based) AQL (acceptable quality-level) test is performed on a subset of the batch to verify the accuracy of the automatic inspection process.

In summary, automatic visual inspection is perfectly suitable as a high throughput technique. However, development and validation needs to be done in a product-specific way and does require substantial time and effort. For this reason, especially high volume products may benefit from an automatic inspection process.

6.6   PROCESS OF VISIBLE PARTICLE INSPECTION

Visible particle inspection occurs during manufacturing and also potentially during release and stability of a parenteral drug product. Figure 6.3 shows a potential process flow with highlighted visual inspection of a liquid drug product.

It needs to be mentioned that "visual inspection" is not solely focusing on "particulates" in the product. Actually, the inspection takes place to ensure that a number of critical, major, or minor/cosmetic defects are not included in the "good part" of the batch, which will be released for human use. Typical defects sorted out during inspection include cracks in the vial (critical, because potential impact on maintaining sterility of the product), issues with caps, etc.

Following 100% inspection, an AQL inspection may be performed. The purpose of AQL testing is to confirm that the process under scrutiny produces product that is "essentially free of visible particles" after 100% visual inspection according to well-established probabilistic decision criteria. AQL is used to decide if a lot may be acceptable. The sample size to be tested during AQL (the number of primary packaging containers such as vials to be reinspected visually) depends on the batch size and can be based on statistical evaluations, for example, according to DIN ISO 2859. AQL limits in the range of 0.1–0.6% are typically used for "particulate" defects, which may be classified as "major defect."

The release of batch does not solely depend on AQL testing. Even if the visual inspection method can discriminate the "good part" of the batch unequivocally, a high number of rejects is not acceptable from a quality perspective. In modern sterile facilities, the rejection rate is usually below 1–2%, depending on the product and process and batch history. Acceptable rejection rates and, thus, required yield may be included in the manufacturing batch records. Incidentally, the rejection rate may be (much) higher than the acceptance criterion (e.g., between 5% and 10% instead of <1%) and then a root-cause investigation is

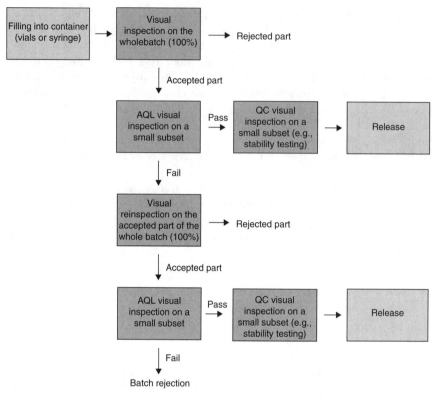

FIGURE 6.3   Process flow with focus on visual inspection of a liquid drug product.

required. High rejection rates may result in batch rejection, but sometimes, it may be decided to do a reinspection (e.g., in case neither the batch records nor the particle identification studies point toward irregularities).

The GMP drug product release specifications in many cases contain "visible particles" or "appearance." Either an additional inspection on a small subset of the batch is performed during QC testing or the specifications refer to the 100% inspection and/or AQL. As visible particles may also form during subsequent storage, for example, because of induction of visible protein precipitate, visual inspection does also make sense during stability testing. However, it should be realized that visual inspection on a small subset of the batch (e.g., 10–50 units) can detect "significant" particle contaminations (e.g., caused by protein precipitation over time) but not the presence of particles with a low detection probability.

In addition, more complex sterile products such as lyophilizates and suspensions are subjected to "100% inspection," and in principle, the same methods and inspection devices can be used. Containers with large particulates (e.g., fiber structures) or other critical/major defects will be rejected and not included in the "good part" of the batch. In the case of lyophilizates, inspection for visible particles after reconstitution is obviously more challenging. This is because (i) the lyophilization process step is an additional unit operation potentially adding to particulate contaminations; (ii) to detect visible particles, reconstitution of the lyophilizate is required, again potentially contaminating the samples; and (iii) visual inspection of reconstituted lyophilizates can only be performed on a small subset of the batch and statistical power is lacking to detect particles with a low detection probability. Visual inspection of reconstituted lyophilizates is normally done during QC testing. The reconstitution procedure for lyophilizates should be carefully designed, closely reflecting the actual clinical practice and avoiding potential environmental contaminations and needs to be laid down in a standard operating procedure.

Visual inspection cannot be replaced by testing for "subvisible particles." This is because in "visual inspection" also other endpoints than solely particles are tested. Furthermore, there are a number of examples where product showed "visible particles" but did not show significant increase in subvisible particles (Section 6.7.3). This is easily imaginable as a single large cellulose fiber, for example, may easily be seen during visual inspection but not by a light-obscuration measurement (subvisible particles).

"Visual inspection" for protein particles also cannot be replaced by analysis of soluble aggregates, for example, using Size-exclusion HPLC (SE-HPLC). Typically, insoluble precipitation that may be observed in "visual inspection" cannot be seen in SE-HPLC as this material is not even able to enter the column. The analysis of the "total area under curve%" (AUC) has thus been recommended by some authors to serve as an indirect measure of insoluble aggregates. However, there are a number of examples from the authors where "visible protein precipitation" has occurred without a major change in AUC of SE-HPLC.

6.7 CASE STUDIES

6.7.1 Case 1: Effect of Product Solution on Detection of Extrinsic Particles

Production and treatment of primary packaging materials as well as the manufacture of the final product contribute to the presence of extrinsic particles. Detection of these particles obviously depends on the size and number of the particles, but there may also be interaction effects that significantly impact the visibility of these particles. Namely, depending on container materials and the formulation matrix, extrinsic particles may have the tendency to remain on container surfaces, and as a result, they may cause variable rejection rates during routine visual inspection. This is illustrated by the following case in which adsorption of extrinsic particles to stopper materials was studied in the presence of two different vehicles, that is, water for injection (WFI) and product solution. Batches were prepared in a GMP facility, and visual inspection was performed by qualified operators. As listed in Tables 6.1 and 6.2, the vehicle had a pronounced effect on the detection of particles, which were identified as cellulose fibers and protein particles (not product related). The conclusion of this head-to-head experiment was that the

TABLE 6.1   Table Repeated Visual Inspections of a WFI Batch

Contact Between Stopper and Solution during Autoclaving	Rejection Rate after Different Holding Times (%)		
	Day 4	Day 6	Day 8
No	1.0	0.4	0.0
Yes	1.8	0.4	0.0

TABLE 6.2   Repeated Visual Inspections of a Product Batch

Contact Between Stopper and Solution during Autoclaving	Rejection Rate after Different Holding Times (%)		
	Day 3	Day 5	Day 7
No	1.4	0.2	0.0
Yes	8.1	17.4	18.9

TABLE 6.3   Number of Particles Extracted from Stoppers

Size and Number of Stoppers per Test (Equals 300 cm^2)	Extraction Fluid	Number of Particles >25 μm
22 Stoppers 13 mm	Water	13
	Polysorbate solution	49
	Product solution	29
10 Stoppers 20 mm	Water	11
	Polysorbate solution	44
	Product solution	44

product matrix actually induces extraction of extrinsic particles from the stopper surface into the solution during the autoclaving process.

This result was confirmed by a controlled laboratory experiment (performed by technicians specialized in particle studies), in which ready-to-sterilize stoppers (packed in bags) were incubated with WFI, polysorbate solution (detergent, 0.3 mg/mL), and product matrix. Subsequently, the "extraction fluids" were filtered, and the number of particles on the filters was determined by microscopic counting. Table 6.3 shows that ready-to-sterilize stoppers for GMP manufacture indeed contain particles and that there is a clear effect of the "extraction fluid" on the extraction of these particles.

6.7.2   Case 2: Effect of Visual Inspection Method on Detection Probability

Companies sometimes use manual methods for "100% visual inspection" that differ from the method as described in the EP. Decisions to use alternative methods may be driven by ergonomics (more convenience), efficiency (higher throughput), and/or higher sensitivity. Typically alternative methods are then cross validated

TABLE 6.4   Visual Inspection of Product with In-House and EP Methods

VI Method	Sample	Accepted (%)	Rejected (%)
In-house	Total batch	60	40
Ph. Eur.	"Good part" of the batch[a]	95	5
	"Bad part" of the batch[a]	96	4

[a] As established with the in-house visual inspection method.

against the compendial method using commercial test sets comprising defined spherical particles (ranging from 50 to 400 μm) made of glass, stainless steel, or polystyrene. Although good results may be obtained with these test sets, it should be recognized that particles in real products may have different shapes and properties (e.g., flaky instead of spherical) and this may strongly influence light scattering during the visual inspection process. In other words, especially if nonstandardized particles are present, the inspection procedure (e.g., observation time, swirling method, etc.) and illumination conditions may have a profound impact on the rejection rate. This is illustrated in the following case in which a liquid protein product was initially inspected with an in-house method. The in-house cabinet had two light sources and samples were illuminated both from above and below. In contrast, the EP cabinet has only one light source that illuminates the product from above. On "100%" visual inspection of a large GMP batch (nearly 20,000 units), a rejection rate of 40% was observed with the in-house method due to particle contamination. Surprisingly, in-depth particle identification studies did not reveal any indication that the batch had an atypical particle load (i.e., both accepted and rejected vials only contained very low amounts of typical particles such as cellulose fibers). Subsequently, it was decided to perform a reinspection on the "good" and "bad" part of the batch using the EP method. As listed in Table 6.4, the EP method did not confirm the "good" and "bad" parts and the absolute rejection rate was much lower (near 5%). One may explain these results by a time effect (i.e., particles may appear or disappear over time), but in this case, it was very obvious (based on additional studies) that the in-house method was much more sensitive with regard to particle detection than the EP method.

6.7.3   Case 3: Poor Relationship between Visual Inspection Data and Laser Obscuration Data

Especially, for protein products that are prone to form intrinsic particles, one may hypothesize that large visible particles are formed on agglomeration of small subvisible particles. In other words, it would not be fully irrational to assume that the results of subvisible particle analysis are somehow indicative for the outcome of visual inspection. However, in practice, it is very difficult to establish a clear relationship between subvisible and visual data. This is illustrated by the following case in which a protein product was subjected to manual visual inspection. The confirmed rejected and accepted vials of this protein product were

TABLE 6.5   Subvisible Particle Analysis on Rejected and Accepted Vials

Particles Size(μm)	Average Number of Subvisible Particles per Unit		
	Rejected Vials[a]	Accepted Vials[a]	Compendial Criterion
≥2	3692	5611	n/a
≥5	756	758	n/a
≥10	193	140	<6000 per container
≥15	41	55	n/a
≥20	17	33	n/a
≥25	8	25	<600 per container
≥50	0	7	n/a
≥100	0	1	n/a

[a]As established by manual visual inspection.

then subjected to laser obscuration analysis. As listed in Table 6.5, the average (subvisible) particle load of rejected vials was certainly not higher than that of the accepted vials.

6.8   SUMMARY

Protein products are used parenterally and thus need to be inspected for visible particles. Visible particulates may be intrinsic or extrinsic to the product and can be regarded as a quality and cleanliness parameter of parenteral manufacturing. However, protein pharmaceuticals may also undergo aggregation that can lead to protein precipitates. These precipitates may be detected at very low levels during visual inspection.

Different methods for visual inspection exist and are applied during manufacturing of parenteral products to inspect 100% of filled containers and to reject the ones containing particulates or other defects, as required by cGMP and the pharmacopeias. The detection of particulates, however, is a probabilistic event, which is impacted by a number of operator and equipment parameters.

Although the experimental part of visual inspection is very basic, the complexity of data interpretation should not be underestimated. Unfortunately, there are currently no alternatives for visual inspection that fully exclude the human factor. For this reason, we recommend to address the performance of visual inspection methods thoroughly during product development and transfers, using adequate statistical control (e.g., AQL testing) whenever possible to warrant consistency and reliability of the inspection process.

REFERENCES

1. Bain B, Shortmoor J. Pharma market trends. Pharm Technol 2010;34:38–45.
2. Antosova Z, Mackova M, Kral V, Macek T. Therapeutic application of peptides and proteins: parenteral forever?. Trends Biotechnol 2009;27:628–635.

3. Andrade F, Videira M, Ferreira D, Sarmento B. Nanocarriers for pulmonary administration of peptides and therapeutic proteins. Nanomedicine 2011;6:123–141.

4. Park K, Chan Kwon I, Park K. Oral protein delivery: current status and future prospect. React Funct Polym 2011;71:280–287.

5. Restetzki L, Mahler H-C. Drug product manufacturing of therapeutic proteins In: Mahler H-C, Luessen H, Borchard G, editors. Protein pharmaceuticals-formulation, analytics & delivery (APV PharmaReflexions). Editio Cantor Verlag (ECV); 2009. ISBN 3-87193-382-1.

6. USP. USP/NF general chapter <1> Injections. 2008.

7. Madsen RE, Visual Inspection of Parenterals Advisory Panel Meeting. 2010.

8. European Pharmacopoeia. 2.9.20. Particulate contamination: visible particles. 2008.

9. USP. USP/NF general chapter <788> Particulate Matter in Injections. 2008.

10. Turco S. *Sterile Dosage Forms*. 4th ed. Philadelphia: Lea & Febiger; 1994.

11. Shabushnig JG. Hot Topics in the visual inspection of injectable products. 2009.

12. Akers MJ, Larrimore DS, Guazzo DM. Parenteral quality control: sterility, pyrogen, particulate and package integrity testing. New York: Marcel Dekker; 2003.

13. Madsen RE, Cherris R, Shabushnig JG, Hunt DG. Visible particulates in injections—a history and a proposal to revise USP general chapter Injections (1). Pharmacopeial Forum 2009;35:1383–1387.

14. Burton JF, Zawadzki S, Wetherell HR, Moy TW. Mainliners and blue velvet. J Forensic Sci 1965;10:466–472.

15. Douglas FG, Kafilmout KJ, Patt NL. Foreign particle embolism in drug addicts: respiratory pathophysiology. Ann Intern Med 1971;75:865.

16. Richman S, Harris RD. Acute pulmonary edema associated with Librium abuse. Radiology 1972;103:57–58.

17. EFPIA 2009. Proposed acceptance criteria for visible particles in parenteral solutions for submission to EDQM. Draft EFPIA proposal for comments.

18. Jorens PG, Van Marck E, Snoeckx A, Parizel PM. Nonthrombotic pulmonary embolism. Eur Respir J 2009;34:452–474.

19. Rubin R, Strayer DS. Rubin's pathology. Philadelphia: Lippincott Company. 5th ed; 2007.

20. Avis KE, Lachman L, Lieberman HA. Parenteral drug administration: routes, precautions, problems, complications, and drug delivery systems. In: Pharmaceutical dosage forms: parenteral medications. New York: Marcel Dekker; 1992.

21. DeLuca PP, Rapp RP, Bivins B, McKean HE, Griffin WO. Filtration and infusion phlebitis: a double-blind prospective clinical study. Am J Hosp Pharm 1975;32:1001–1007.

22. Turco SJ. Infusion phlebitis: a review of the literature. Parenterals 1987;5:1–8.

23. Prinzmetal M, Ornitz EM, Simkin B, Bergman HC. Arteriovenous anastomoses in liver, spleen and lungs. Am J Physiol 1948;152:48–52.

24. Illum L, Davis SS, Wilson CG. Blood clearance and organ deposition of intravenously administered colloidal particles. The effects of particle size, nature and shape. Int J Pharm 1982;12:135–146.

25. Wilkins DJ, Myers PA. Studies on the relationship between the electrophoretic properties of colloids and their blood clearance and organ distribution in the rat. Br J Exp Pathol 1966;47:568–576.

26. Nutescu EA. Assessing, preventing and treating venous thromboembolism: evidence-based approaches. Am J Health Syst Pharm 2007;64:S5–S13.

27. Shabushnig JG. Visual inspection of injectable products: more than sorting good from bad. 2005.

28. Rosenberg AS. Effects of protein aggregates: an immunologic perspective. AAPS J 2006;8:E501–E507.

29. Carpenter JF, Randolph TW, Jiskoot W, Crommelin DJA. Overlooking subvisible particles in therapeutic protein products: gaps that may compromise product quality. J Pharm Sci 2009;98:1201–1205.

30. Mahler HC, Friess W, Grauschopf U, Kiese S. Protein aggregation: pathways, induction factors and analysis. J Pharm Sci 2009;98:2909–2934.

31. Shabushnig JG. PDA Annual Meeting. 1995.

7 Characterization of Aggregates and Particles Using Emerging Techniques

HUI ZHAO, MANUEL DIEZ, ATANAS KOULOV, MARIOLA BOZOVA, MARKUS BLUEMEL, and KURT FORRER

Analytical Research and Development of the Process Science and Production Department, Novartis Pharma AG, Basel, Switzerland

7.1 INTRODUCTION

In the last 30 years, protein pharmaceuticals have become a major focus in the pharmaceutical industry. Significant therapeutic targets have been met, and biotechnology has become the fastest growing pharmaceutical sector. However, together with their unique advantages, protein pharmaceuticals present their own challenges. For example, one of the major factors determining the stability and quality of protein-based drugs is their propensity to aggregate during manufacturing processes including cell culture, purification, formulation, filling, during storage, or under physical stress (elevated or reduced temperatures, shaking, pH, etc.) [1–3]. Protein aggregates can differ in structure, size, solubility, and reversibility and can occur covalently or noncovalently [4]. As protein aggregates may have potential in affecting efficacy, immunogenicity, pharmacokinetics, pharmacodynamics, and quality profiles of a drug product, protein aggregation needs to be assessed and closely monitored [5–9] (Chapter 1).

Protein aggregation poses significant analytical challenges. Aggregates are usually not well defined, that is, they span a continuous and large range of sizes—from several nanometers to hundreds of micrometers. Since this size range is impossible to cover using a single analytical technique, complementary methods are needed for the measurement and/or quantification of aggregates. A brief overview of some of these techniques is presented in Fig. 7.1. Size-exclusion chromatography (SEC) is the most commonly used analytical method for quantification of relative small soluble aggregates in a limited size range. It is easy to

Analysis of Aggregates and Particles in Protein Pharmaceuticals, First Edition.
Edited by Hanns-Christian Mahler, Wim Jiskoot.
© 2012 John Wiley & Sons, Inc., Published 2012 by John Wiley & Sons, Inc.

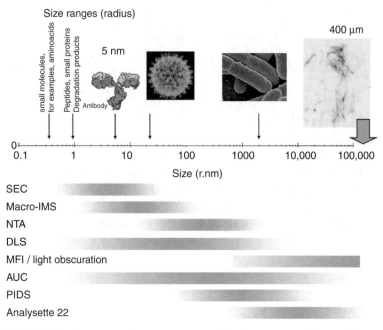

FIGURE 7.1   Aggregate size ranges covered by the corresponding techniques.

use and has abilities to measure proteins and protein aggregates with high sample throughput. In most cases, SEC provides information on soluble aggregates with high precision. However, the accuracy of SEC results may be influenced by nonspecific interaction of proteins and protein aggregates to chromatographic materials such as columns, column frits, and tubings in the high performance liquid chromatography (HPLC) [10–12]. As discussed in Chapter 2, it is necessary to confirm the accuracy of the SEC results using other analytical orthogonal techniques, such as analytical ultracentrifugation (AUC), a useful tool for the characterization of proteins and protein aggregates [13–15], which has been used to support results obtained by SEC [16,17]. In this chapter, macroion mobility spectrometry (macro-IMS) is introduced as an alternative tool for confirming the SEC results.

Dynamic light scattering (DLS) and static light scattering (SLS) are used to measure the hydrodynamic diameter and the average molecular weight, respectively, of protein aggregates/particles (Chapter 3). Both DLS and SLS, however, have limitations in quantification of protein aggregates/particles. Light obscuration (LO), on the other hand, is capable of quantitatively measuring particles in the subvisible range, but cannot differentiate protein aggregates/particles from foreign particles, as explained in Chapter 5. Thus, there is an increasing need for additional analytical techniques to complement the conventional analytical techniques such as SEC, AUC, DLS, and LO and to measure a broader size range of protein aggregates and subvisible/visible protein particles.

In recent years, a number of emerging techniques have become available for the measurement of aggregates or subvisible particles in the size ranges that are not or poorly covered by the conventional analytical techniques such as SEC, AUC, DLS/SLS, and LO (Fig. 7.1). In this chapter, examples of using three emerging techniques (macro-IMS for the size range of 3–65 nm, flow imaging (e.g., microflow imaging (MFI)) for the size range of 1–100 µm, and nanoparticle tracking analysis (NTA) technology for the range of 10 nm–1 µm) are illustrated for the characterization and quantification of protein aggregates and/or subvisible/visible protein particles in the size ranges bridging the conventional analytical techniques (Fig. 7.1). Theories and general applications of other potential emerging techniques based on laser light scattering (e.g., polarization intensity differential scattering (PIDS) for the size range of 40 nm–2000 µm [18] (Beckman Coulter Inc.,: AN-12622A), Analysette 22 NanoTec for the size range of 300 nm–300 µm [19] (Fritsch GmbH)) for the analysis of particles are also briefly discussed (Fig. 7.1).

7.2 MACRO-IMS FOR CHARACTERIZATION OF PROTEINS AND PROTEIN AGGREGATES

7.2.1 Introduction to Macro-IMS

Macro-IMS is a new tool that was first introduced by Kaufman and coworkers in analyzing macromolecules such as large proteins and aggregates in the mass range of 8 kDa–80 MDa (diameters of ~3–65 nm) [20]. Since macro-IMS can measure the sizes of proteins and protein aggregates within the measurement range of SEC, it has potential to be used as a method for confirming results of the SEC method.

Macro-IMS is a successor of gas-phase electrophoretic mobility molecular analysis (GEMMA), which has already been used in many research areas such as analyzing structure and stoichiometry of noncovalent biocomplexes, whole viruses, and binding of antibodies to viruses [21–29]. Macro-IMS is inexpensive, easy to operate at near atmospheric pressure, and the analysis can be done within very short time. It is also capable of measuring proteins and protein aggregates with sizes that are too large for SEC and mass spectrometry analysis (e.g., a protein complex with a mass higher than 200 kDa), while providing better resolution than that by light scattering techniques.

7.2.2 Principle of Macro-IMS

A typical macro-IMS setup consists of a charge-reduced electrospray ionization (ESI) source, an ion mobility drift cell, and a macroion/nanoparticle detector (Fig. 7.2). Analytes in liquid phase are converted into gas-phase ions by nano-ESI. The resulting multiply charged ions are charge reduced by bipolar air molecules generated by an α-beam (e.g., emitted from a Polonium-210 source) primarily to neutral and singly charged macroions, which are separated

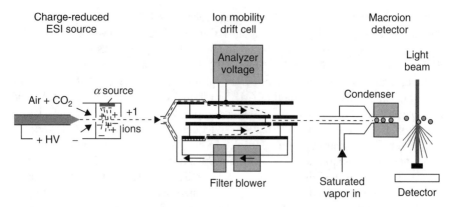

FIGURE 7.2   Schematic representation of macro-IMS. *Source:* © Copyright TSI Incorporated, Shoreview, MN, USA.

by size according to their electrical mobility in the drift cell [30]. The macroion detector is an ultrafine condensation particle counter (UCPC), which condenses and counts macroions by light scattering using a laser-diode light source and a diode photodetector.

The electrical mobility of a particle is defined by its ability to move under the influence of an electric field. In an electric field, a particle experiences two forces: an electric and a drag force. When both forces are equal, the electrical mobility, Z_p, of the particle can be calculated using Equation 7.1

$$Z_p = \frac{n \cdot e \cdot C}{3 \cdot \pi \cdot \mu \cdot D_p} \tag{7.1}$$

where n is the number of elementary charges on the particle, e the elementary charge (1.6×10^{-19} C), C, the Cunningham slip correction, $C = 1 + Kn \cdot [1.142 + 0.558 \cdot e^{\frac{-0.999}{Kn}}]$, $Kn =$ Knudsen Number $= \frac{2\lambda}{D_p}$, λ the gas mean free path, μ the gas viscosity (dyne·s/cm^2) poise, and D_p the particle diameter (cm);

$$\Delta Z_p = \frac{q_a}{q_{sh}} \cdot \Delta Z_p^* \tag{7.2}$$

The mobility bandwidth, ΔZ_p, that is, the small range of particles that are extracted at a certain voltage from the drift cell, depends on the aerosol flow rate through the classifier, q_a, the sheath air flow rate, q_{sh}, and the set mobility ΔZ_p^* (Eq. 7.2). Using Equations 7.1 and 7.2, the electrical mobility of particles can be converted into particle diameters and masses (see Macro-IMS User's Manual, TSI Inc., Shoreview, MN).

7.2.3   Case studies of Macro-IMS

7.2.3.1   Sample Preparation for Macro-IMS Analysis of Monoclonal Antibodies   Different monoclonal antibody (mAb) drug product or drug substance solutions (Novartis Pharma AG) with different concentrations were used. They were diluted with 20 mM ammonium acetate, pH 9.0 (except where stated otherwise), to a concentration range of 7.5–15 µg/mL (50–100 nmol/L). The samples were measured directly after dilution.

7.2.3.2   Sample Preparation for Macro-IMS Analysis of Large Protein Aggregates   Different batches of protein X (Novartis Pharma AG) were used for analysis. The protein lyophilisates were reconstituted in water (Riedel-de Haën) (2 mg/mL), dialyzed against 20 mM ammonium acetate buffer, pH 9.0, for 4 h at room temperature. After dialysis, the samples were filtered through a 5.0-µm pore membrane and measured undiluted.

7.2.3.3   Sample Preparation for Macro-IMS Analysis of Viruslike Particles
Different batches of viruslike particles (VLPs) (Novartis Pharma AG) were used for analysis. All sample solutions were diluted with 20 mM ammonium acetate buffer, pH 6.8, to a concentration of 0.1 mg/mL (30 nmol/L) and dialyzed against 20 mM ammonium acetate, pH 6.8, for 4 h at room temperature. The samples were measured directly after dialysis.

7.2.3.4   General Instrumental Setting for Macro-IMS Analysis   For all analyses, a TSI macro-IMS system, consisting of a charge-reduced nanoelectrospray unit (model 3480C), a nano-differential mobility analyzer (DMA) (model 3085C), a control platform (model 3080C), a nanoparticle detector (model 3776C), and a manager software (version 390063C), was used. The instrument was calibrated using a mixture of five proteins with known molecular masses (High Molecular Weight Calibration Kit, GE Healthcare). The effective density and the transport time from the DMA to the detector were adjusted until all measured masses were within ±10% of the theoretical masses of the five proteins at both high and low flows. Fused silica capillary tubes (24 cm long, 25 µm ID, and 150 µm OD) with cone-shaped tips were used for the analysis of mAbs and protein aggregates. Fused silica capillary tubes (24 cm long, 30 µm ID, and 150 µm OD) with a larger inner diameter (30 µm ID) were used for the analysis of VLPs. The capillaries were equilibrated with the sample solutions for 5–15 min before measurements. The capillary tubes can be cleaned by 2% acetic acid and 50% Acetonitrile in H_2O and reused for the next measurement.

7.2.3.5   Specific Instrumental Setting and Data Handling for Macro-IMS Analysis of Monoclonal Antibodies   The ESI source was operated in the stable "cone jet" mode at a voltage of 1.75–1.90 kV until stable sprays were reached. The samples were introduced into the electrospray chamber by a gauge pressure of 0.4 psi, resulting in a flow rate of 7.1 nL/min. Immediately after highly charged primary droplets were formed at the tip of a capillary, they were transported by a sheath flow of clean air (1.5 L/min) and CO_2 (0.1 L/min) to the ionization chamber and subsequently to the DMA. A coaxial flow of filtered air (20 L/min) was used to transport the ions within the DMA. The voltage in the DMA was varied from 48 to 1039 V, which allowed separation of ions with molecular weights from 10 to 1000 kDa. The spray and separation occurred at room temperature and atmospheric pressure. An inlet flow of 1.5 L/min was used to pull the ions from the DMA into the detector for the measurements. For each measurement of mAbs, six scans were recorded and summed up to one macro-IMS spectrum in the selected mass range.

For data analysis, mass spectra plotted using raw counts (y_i) versus mass intervals (x_i), average masses, and peak heights of each individual peak are available for data evaluation using the software from the manufacturer (TSI Inc.). The software, however, cannot be used for the calculation of peak areas. For the determination of impurities (e.g., for mAbs), it is necessary to know peak areas of the impurity peaks and main peaks. Mass intervals (x_i) and raw counts (y_i) obtained from the macro-IMS measurements were, therefore, exported to Microsoft Excel and plotted as XY-scatter plots. The peak area of each individual peak was calculated by summing up areas of all channels (A_i). The peak area of each channel was determined using Equation 7.3. The channel (i) stands for the range of molecular masses collected in each time interval at defined voltages.

$$A_i = y_i \cdot (x_{i+1} - x_i) + 0.5 \cdot (y_{i+1} - y_i) \cdot (x_{i+1} - x_i) \qquad (7.3)$$

where A_i is the area of channel i ($i = 1, 2, \ldots, n$), x_i the mass assigned to channel i, and y_i the raw counts in channel i.

7.2.3.6 Specific Instrumental Setting for Macro-IMS Analysis of Large Aggregates

The ESI source was operated in the stable "cone jet" mode at voltages between 2.3 and 2.6 kV until stable sprays were reached. The samples were introduced into the electrospray chamber by a gauge pressure of 3.7 psi, resulting in a flow rate of 66 nL/min. Similar as the analysis for the mAbs, a sheath flow of clean air (1.5 L/min) and CO_2 (0.1 L/min) was used to transport macroions to the ionization chamber (DMA). Since large aggregates with high molecular masses were expected, the coaxial flow of filtered air in the DMA was reduced to 6 L/min to allow larger macroions migrating at low velocities to reach the exit gap. The voltage in the DMA was varied from 10 to 9985 V, which allowed separation of ions with molecular weights from 5.4 kDa to 220 MDa. An inlet flow of 0.3 L/min was used to pull the ions from the DMA into the detector for the measurements. For each measurement, five scans with a duration of 1 min were recorded and summed up to one macro-IMS spectrum in the selected mass range.

7.2.3.7 Specific Instrumental Setting for Macro-IMS Analysis of Viruslike

Particles   The ESI source was operated in the stable "cone jet" mode at voltages between 2.3 and 2.6 kV until stable sprays were reached. The samples were introduced into the electrospray chamber by a lower gauge pressure of 1.2 psi as a wider capillary diameter was used. A sheath flow of clean air (1.0 L/min) and CO_2 (0.4 L/min) was used to transport macroions to the DMA. A coaxial flow of 20 L/min of filtered air was used to transport the ions within the DMA. The voltage was varied from 10 to 9880 V, which allows separation of ions with molecular weights from 0.86 kDa to 30 MDa. An inlet flow of 1.5 L/min was used to pull the ions from the DMA into the detector for the measurements. For each measurement, five scans with a duration of 1 min were recorded and summed up to one macro-IMS spectrum in the selected mass range.

7.2.3.8 Size-Exclusion Chromatography Analysis of Monoclonal Antibodies

SEC was performed on mAbs using a 4.6×300 mm^2 TSK gel super SG3000SW size-exclusion column (Tosoh Bioscience) with a flow rate of 0.2 mL/min. A 150 mM sodium phosphate buffer, pH 6.5, was used as mobile phase. The mAbs were diluted to 5 mg/mL using 15 mM sodium phosphate buffer before the analysis.

7.2.3.9 Dynamic Light Scattering Analysis of Monoclonal Antibodies   A

Zetasizer nano-ZS light scattering system (Malvern Instruments) was used for DLS measurement. The samples were diluted with placebo solutions to a concentration of 6.0 mg/mL before the analysis. The sample solutions were irradiated by a 4 mW He–Ne laser, and the scattered light was detected by an avalanche photodetector. Five measurements of each sample were recorded. Malvern Dispersion Technology Software was used for data acquisition and data evaluation.

7.2.3.10 Analytical Ultracentrifugation Analysis of Monoclonal Antibodies

The mAb samples were diluted to 0.5 mg/mL using 150 mM sodium phosphate buffer, pH 6.5, and loaded into cells with two c-channel charcoal–epon center-pieces with 12-mm optical path length. The dilution buffer was loaded into the reference channel of each cell. The loaded cells were placed into an AN-60Ti ana-lytical rotor, loaded into Beckman–Coulter analytical ultracentrifuge. The rotor was first brought to 3000 rpm and then to 40,000 rpm, the final speed. Scans were recorded at 40,000 rpm every 4 min for 5.7 h. The data were evaluated using the SEDFIT software [31].

7.2.3.11 Results and Discussion of Macro-IMS

Method Development for Macro-IMS Analysis of Monoclonal Antibodies. Volatile buffers such as ammonium formate and ammonium acetate at different pH values were evaluated for macro-IMS measurements of mAbs. Such volatile buffers are needed for ESI of the analytes. All buffers, except for ammonium formate, pH 2.0, had a conductivity of approximately 2 mS/cm, which is expected to generate stable sprays. In the initial study, the antibody samples were diluted to 50 nmol/L (7.5 µg/mL) using ammonium formate or ammonium acetate buffers at pH 2.0, 4.0, 6.0, 8.0, and 9.0 and analyzed at a mass range from 10 to 2000 kDa. It took ~20, 45, >60, 30, and 5 min for the detector to detect mAbs in buffers at pH 2.0, 4.0, 6.0, 8.0, and 9.0, respectively. At pH values below or near the pI values (~8.0) of the antibodies, the mAbs were slightly positively charged or neutrally charged, whereas the silanol groups on the inner surface of the capillary were negatively charged, and the mAbs had to first be adsorbed to the capillary walls before moving up to the tip of the capillaries, reaching stable sprays and further being detected by the detector. At pH 9.0, however, both the antibodies and inner surface of the capillary were negatively charged, and nearly no adsorption of antibodies to the capillary walls took place. Therefore, it did not take long (about 5 min) for the mAbs to migrate to the tip of the capillary and to have detectable signals. Similar degradation profiles were shown for the same sample freshly prepared using different ammonium acetate buffers at different pHs, indicating that no artificial degradation products were induced by the buffers during sample preparation. A PVA-coated capillary was also tested during the method development. As expected, it took only a few minutes for the mAbs to be detected as mAbs had no interactions with the inner surfaces of the PVA-coated capillary. Surprisingly, the PVA-coated capillaries induced the formation of artificial aggregates (data now shown). In addition, the PVA-coated capillaries with cone-shaped tips are not yet commercially available and need to be prepared individually, which poses a potential risk of poor reproducibility of the method. Fused silica capillaries and 20 mM ammonium acetate buffer at pH 9.0 were, therefore, used for macro-IMS analysis of mAbs.

During the development of the method, the impact of the gauge pressure on the formation of artificial aggregates was also explored. The gauge pressure is needed for the introduction of samples into the electrospray chamber. On the basis of literature, a decrease in the gauge pressure across the capillary results in a reduction of the sample flow and proportionally a smaller droplet size [28,29]. Therefore, if the aggregates are real, changes of the gauge pressure should not result in any changes in the amount of aggregates. However, if the aggregates are artificial, a twofold decrease in the gauge pressure would result in an approximately twofold increase in the amount of aggregates. We started with a gauge pressure of 3.7 psi, which was suggested by the equipment vendor, for the analysis. As shown in Fig. 7.3, gradual reduction of the gauge pressure from 3.7 to 0.4 psi led to a decrease in the amount of aggregates for the same sample. Similar results were obtained for several different mAbs, suggesting that the gauge pressures did, in fact, induce the formation of the aggregates (e.g., dimers). To avoid the formation of such artificial aggregates, a gauge pressure of 0.4 psi, the lowest limit for the macro-IMS instrument, was used for all macro-IMS analyses of mAbs.

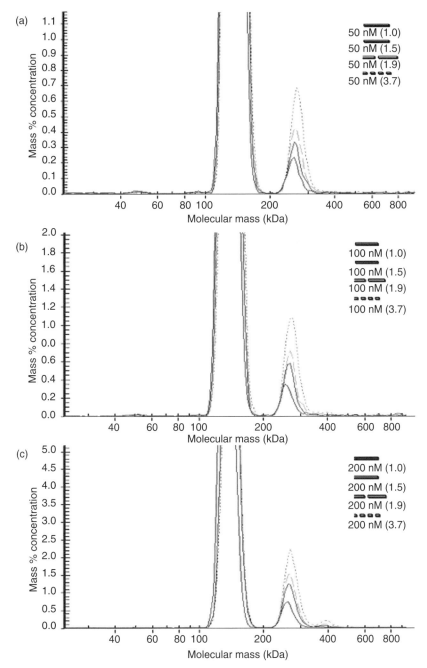

FIGURE 7.3   Macro-IMS spectra of a mAb (IgG1) at (a) 50 nmol/L, (b) 100 nmol/L, and (c) 200 nmol/L using gauge pressures of 1.0, 1.5, 1.9, and 3.7 psi. (*See insert for color representation of the figure.*)

Linearity of Macro-IMS Analysis for Monoclonal Antibodies.   Linearity of the method was tested using antibodies with a concentration of 1.5–150 µg/mL (10–1000 nmol/L). Peak areas were calculated using an average of three replicate scans of 1 min in a range of 10–1000 kDa. At a concentration of 1.5 µg/mL (10 nmol/L), only the monomer peak was detected (roughly 99% of the total protein). The amounts of product-related impurities (around 1% of the total protein) were undetectable as they were below the limit of quantification (LOQ) of the instrument. The linear range for the macro-IMS analysis of mAbs was from 1.5 to 150 µg/mL (25–300 nmol/L), where the peak areas increased proportionally to the concentrations (Fig. 7.4).

At higher concentrations, the dimeric peak increased overproportionally with the concentration. Multimer peaks (trimers, tetramers, etc.) started to appear, which was consistent with what has been previously observed for other proteins [27,29]. With increases in protein concentrations, two antibody monomers have

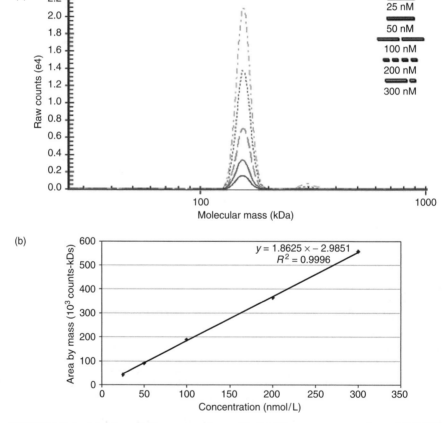

FIGURE 7.4   (a) MacroIMS spectra of a mAb (IgG1) at a concentration of 25–300 nmol/L. (b) Linearity for the main monomeric peak of the antibody at a concentration of 25–300 nmol/L. (*See insert for color representation of part (a).*)

high possibilities to be captured in one droplet and mistakenly counted as a dimer, which leads to an overestimation of dimers and so as well for the larger aggregates. Additionally, at higher concentrations, especially when the number of particles oversaturated the detector (limit: 3×10^5/ mL gas), the detector can no longer count accurately, which may result in false estimation of the amounts of both monomers and lager aggregates. To consider all factors and data, we have generated using different mAbs, 15 µg/mL (100 nmol/L) was chosen for further macro-IMS analysis of mAbs.

Repeatability of Macro-IMS Analysis for Monoclonal Antibodies.   The repeatability of the method was assessed by calculating the relative standard deviation of 18 separate runs, an average of five scans of 1 min over the range from 10 to 2000 kDa, performed by three different operators on three different days (Fig. 7.5). The relative standard deviations of the mass percentages of the monomer and dimer peaks were 0.13% and 7.6%, respectively.

Macro-IMS versus SEC and AUC Analysis of Monoclonal Antibody mAb1 (IgG1).   Macro-IMS was used to analyze a mAb (mAb1) lyophilisate after storage at 5 and 25°C for 36 months. Three measurements were recorded for each sample, and a mean value was calculated and used for data evaluation. The macro-IMS data were compared to the data from SEC and AUC analyses (Table 7.1).

Two fragments with masses of 54 kDa (Fc) and 108 kDa ((Fab')$_2$) and one aggregation product with a mass of 292 kDa (dimer) were detected by macro-IMS analysis (Fig. 7.6a) [32]. Fragmentation in the hinge region (e.g., the formation of Fc and (Fab')$_2$ fragments) and aggregation (e.g., the formation of dimer) are commonly seen degradation pathways for antibodies, thus often closely monitored. The profiles of the degradation products observed in the macro-IMS spectra of these tested samples were consistent with the data from SEC and AUC analyses (Fig. 7.6b,c) [32]. The (Fab')$_2$ fragment peak was well resolved from the intact mAb peak using macro-IMS, while it was not detectable at low levels by SEC since it was not well resolved from the main antibody peak. Therefore, macro-IMS has better accuracy in the estimation of the (Fab')$_2$ fragment, especially at low levels, compared to that of the SEC method. The accuracy of such a measurement is not concentration dependent as higher concentration could only potentially induce the formation of artificial aggregates, but not fragments.

All three methods (macro-IMS, SEC, and AUC) showed similar trends for the estimation of the aggregates, primarily dimers (Table 7.1). No significant differences in the amounts of fragments (i.e., Fc and (Fab')$_2$) were detected. These data indicate that the macro-IMS method could be used as a potential alternative method to confirm the SEC results. However, it is noticeable that the amounts of dimer detected in the control sample using macro-IMS were consistently and reproducibly higher than those from SEC. One possible explanation for this discrepancy is that the amounts of aggregates may have been underestimated by SEC due to interaction of the aggregate to the column or the column frits, as

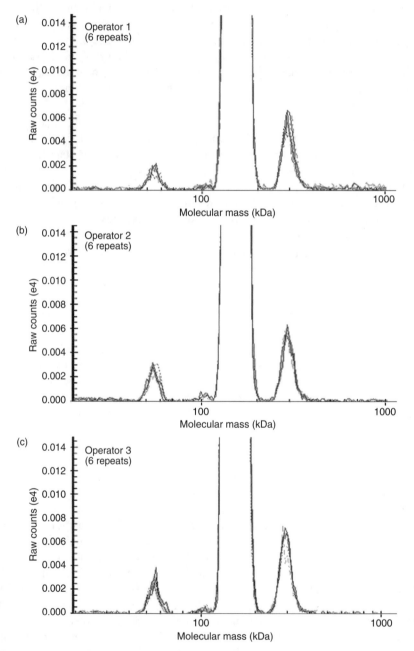

FIGURE 7.5 (a–c) Overlays of six macro-IMS spectra from three operators run on three separate days. (*See insert for color representation of the figure.*)

TABLE 7.1   Percentages of Dimers in mAb1 (IgG1) after Storage at 5 and 25°C for 36 Months Estimated by Macro-IMS in Comparison to SEC and AUC Analysis

	Macro-IMS	SEC	AUC
Control	2.0 ± 0.06%	0.8	0.5
5°C, 36 M	2.2 ± 0.16%	0.9	1.1
25°C, 36 M	4.0 ± 0.17%	4.1	4.3

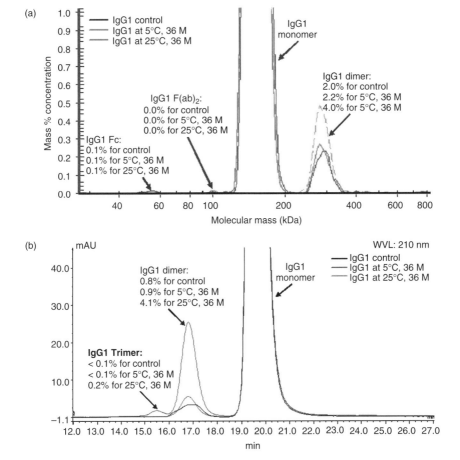

FIGURE 7.6   (a) Macro-IMS analysis of an antibody (IgG1) lyophilisate in vial after storage at 5 and 25°C for 36 months. (b) SEC analysis of an antibody (IgG1) lyophilisate in vial after storage at 5 and 25°C for 36 months. (c) AUC analysis of an antibody (IgG1) lyophilisate in vial after storage at 5 and 25°C for 36 months. (*See insert for color representation of parts (a) and (b)*.)

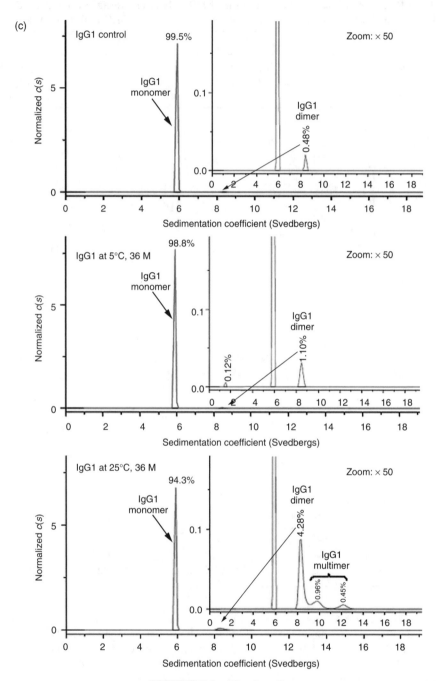

FIGURE 7.6 (*Continued*)

has been observed for other proteins [33]. Another possible explanation is that the amounts of dimers in the samples may have been slightly overestimated by the macro-IMS analysis, as two antibody monomers may have been captured in one electrospray droplet and counted mistakenly as a dimer. As indicated earlier, the gauge pressure also induces the formation of low amounts of artificial aggregates, even though it was adjusted to the lowest possible level for the instrument (Fig. 7.3).

To check the feasibility of using macro-IMS in detecting antibody aggregates with larger sizes, mAb1 was stressed under an acidic condition (pH 3.3) at 50°C for 2 h. The amounts of aggregates in the control and stressed sample were analyzed by both SEC and macro-IMS. As shown in Fig. 7.7a, the total amounts of aggregates increased significantly from 0.67% (control) to 72.1% in

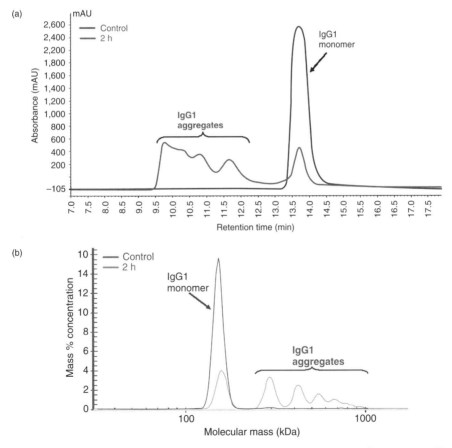

FIGURE 7.7 (a) SEC analysis of an antibody (IgG1) drug substance after stress at pH 3.3 at 50°C for 2 h compared to a control sample. (b) Macro-IMS analysis of an antibody (IgG1) drug substance after stress at pH 3.3 at 50°C for 2 h compared to a control sample.

the stressed samples by SEC, but aggregates larger than dimers were not well resolved. Macro-IMS, however, showed well-separated dimer, trimer, tetramer, etc. in the spectrum of the stressed sample (Fig. 7.7b). The total amounts of aggregates increased significantly from 1.7% (control) to 67.4%, and the percentages of each individual aggregate species could be quantified separately. These data indicate that macro-IMS is not only useful for the confirmation of the SEC results but also shows its own advantage of resolving antibody oligomers (trimers, tetramers, etc.).

Macro-IMS versus DLS Analysis of Monoclonal Antibody mAb2 (IgG1).   An IgG1 mAb (mAb2) in a liquid formulation was tested by macro-IMS and DLS after storage at 40°C for six months. The macro-IMS spectra and the size distribution profiles from the DLS analysis for the stressed sample and reference are shown in Fig. 7.8a,b, respectively.

According to macro-IMS analysis (Fig. 7.8a), the intensities of the fragment peaks (Fc and F(ab′)$_2$), as well as the number and the intensities of the aggregate peaks (dimer, trimer, tetramer, etc.), increased significantly in the stressed sample compared to the reference. All peaks resulting from degradation (fragments and aggregates) of the antibody were very well separated from the main monomeric peak. By the DLS analysis, a broadened main peak at 5.0 nm (radius) and a less intense peak at 30 nm (radius) were observed for the stressed sample compared to the reference (Fig. 7.8b). Broadening of the main peak indicates the presence of oligomeric mAb species (e.g., dimers, trimers, etc.) besides the monomer. DLS was certainly not able to resolve and quantify the aggregates. In contrast, these oligomeric species were well resolved from the mAb monomer by macro-IMS.

Macro-IMS Analysis of Large Soluble Protein Aggregates.   Macro-IMS can also be used to measure the size of large soluble protein aggregates. One example of using macro-IMS for the analysis of large protein aggregates is illustrated in Fig. 7.9. The protein X was used for the analysis. The monomeric protein X has a molecular weight of 27 kDa and has a high tendency to form both covalently and noncovalently linked large aggregates. Difficulties in reproducibility were encountered during the development of an SEC method for the protein under native conditions. Macro-IMS was, therefore, used to measure the size distribution of the protein X aggregates during formulation development and assess batch-to-batch consistency and comparability of the protein X during production.

As shown in an example of macro-IMS analysis of protein X (Fig. 7.9), the size distribution of two representative batches of protein X manufactured at site A in 2000–2003 and four representative batches manufactured at site B in 2005–2007 were compared. The protein batches manufactured at site A showed one major population of aggregates with molecular masses of about 5 MDa, whereas batches produced at site B contained two populations of aggregates with molecular masses of ~270 kDa and 20 MDa. The aggregates in the later batches produced at site B apparently had much larger masses than those produced earlier at site A. The macro-IMS data were very reproducible (when analyzed

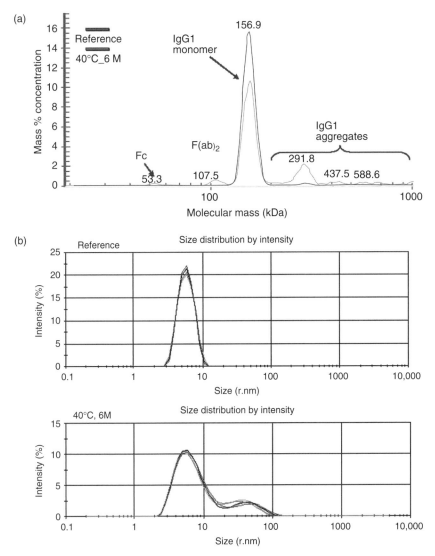

FIGURE 7.8 (a) Macro-IMS and (b) DLS analysis of an antibody (IgG1) liquid in syringe after storage at $40°C$ for six months.

by three different analysts) and consistent with the data from other analyses such as nonreducing sodium dodecyl sulfate–polyacrylamide gel electrophoresis (SDS-PAGE) and native peptide mapping, which also showed a higher number of larger aggregates and more diversity in disulfide bond linkages in the later batches (data not shown). Therefore, macro-IMS is also suitable for the analysis of large aggregates with more complexities.

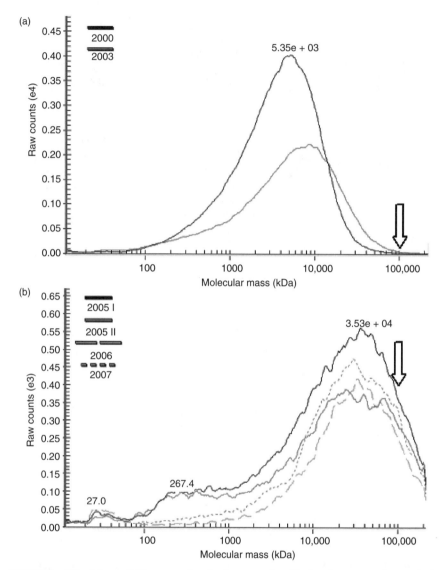

FIGURE 7.9 Macro-IMS spectra of the protein X batches manufactured in 2000–2003 (a) and in 2000–2007 (b).

Macro-IMS Analysis of Viruslike Particles.   Macro-IMS was also used for the determination of sizes of intact VLPs. To avoid clotting of capillaries, capillaries with a larger ID (30 μm) were used. As shown in Fig. 7.10, all seven different batches of VLPs showed the same molecular mass of 3.3 MDa, which was consistent with the VLP's theoretical molecular mass of 3.4 MDa. A dimer peak with a molecular weight of 7.00 MDa was also found for all batches. The

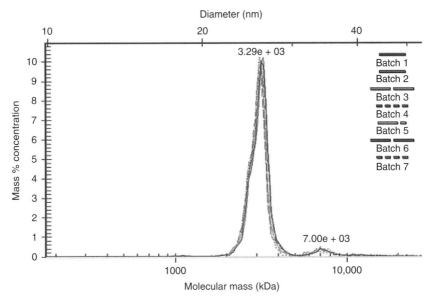

FIGURE 7.10 Macro-IMS spectra of different batches of VLPs.

intensities of the dimer peaks were also similar for all batches. The macro-IMS method is, therefore, a fast and excellent tool for measuring the size of VLPs.

7.2.4   Summary of Macro-IMS

Macro-IMS was shown to be an excellent tool for monitoring degradation products (e.g., fragments and aggregates) of mAbs, large protein aggregates, and VLPs. Macro-IMS analyses revealed similar levels of degradation products, including aggregates, as SEC, indicating that macro-IMS could be used as a method for confirming SEC results. Macro-IMS also demonstrated a better resolving power in separating small soluble aggregates (e.g., dimers, trimers, and tetramers) from the main monomeric peak of antibodies than SEC and DLS. Additionally, compared to SEC, macro-IMS does not expose proteins to large solid–liquid interfaces, thereby avoiding potential in underestimation of aggregate levels.

The major drawback of the macro-IMS technique is that the samples must be significantly diluted (e.g., to 15 μg/mL (100 nmol/L) for the analysis of mAbs) to have the number of particles not exceeding the upper detection limit of the instrument. Using such diluted samples has potentials in leading to dissociation of noncovalently linked protein aggregates and, thus, underestimation of the amounts of aggregates. Another drawback is the need of volatile buffers. Buffer exchange poses another potential risk of changing aggregation profiles. In addition, macro-IMS has potentials in generating artificial aggregates especially at higher protein concentrations, although such artifacts were minimized to the lowest possible level during the method development.

In the development of protein pharmaceuticals, it is, however, very important to use more than one technique to assess the biophysical characteristics of a molecule. In this respect, macro-IMS clearly showed its potential of being a complementary technique to other currently available analytical techniques such as SEC, AUC, and DLS in the analysis of mAbs, large aggregates, and VLPs.

7.3   FLOW MICROSCOPY FOR CHARACTERIZATION OF PROTEIN AGGREGATES AND PARTICLES

7.3.1   Introduction to Flow Microscopy

Until recently, only a small number of analytical techniques were available to measure protein particles with sizes in the micrometer range (Fig. 7.1). In the past, the Coulter counter and LO were practically the only technologies, which provided quantitative information on these particles in terms of number and size distribution. Since LO provides only the number and size of particles but no information regarding their natures, this technique is unable to discriminate air bubbles (e.g., in high viscosity mAb formulations) and silicon oil droplets (e.g., in prefilled syringes) from proteinaceous aggregates. Flow microscopy is one of the recently emerged techniques for measurements of subvisible particulates ranging from one to several hundreds of micrometers (Fig. 7.1). This includes subvisible particles of both proteinaceous and nonproteinaceous nature. The technology represents a significant advance in the field of subvisible particle measurements as it offers increased sensitivity and the digital images collected during flow microscopy measurements not only allow detailed analysis of the size and number of particles but also provide quantitative information about their shape and relative transparency. Thus, flow microscopy offers a possibility to better discriminate protein particles and particles from other sources (e.g., silicon oil) from the production and packaging process. In addition, flow microscopy allows better and more detailed characterization of proteinaceous particulates.

Currently, two flow microscopy instruments are commercially available—MFI (Brightwell Technologies Inc., Ottawa, Ontario, Canada) (Fig. 7.11) and flow particle image analysis (FPIA) (Malvern Instruments Limited, Malvern, UK). Theoretically, the two instruments should provide similar information on subvisible particles. In the following sections, characterization of aggregates and particles using MFI is addressed. All data were collected using an MFI system, but the general considerations should be valid for both instruments.

7.3.2   Principle of Microflow Imaging

In flow microscopy, bright-field images are captured in successive frames as a continuous sample stream passes through a flow cell positioned in the field of view of a microscopic system (Fig. 7.11). Each image is analyzed in real time by the system software. MFI images are analyzed by creating a database consisting of particle count, size, transparency, intensity, and shape. This database

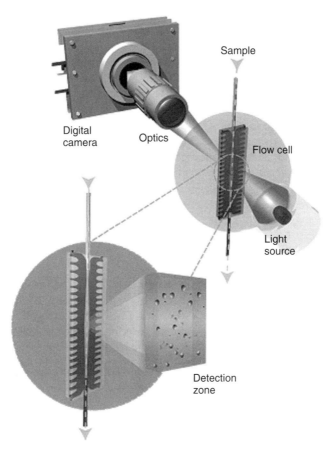

FIGURE 7.11 Schematic representation of the MFI instrument configuration. *Source:* © Copyright Brightwell Technology Incorporated, Ottawa, Ontario, Canada.

can be digitally interrogated by the application software to produce parameter distributions, scatter plots, and isolate particle subpopulations of interest (e.g., spherical particles being probably silicone oil droplets in a prefilled syringe). Particle images are then available for verification and further analysis.

Instrument operation of MFI is straightforward, and no calibration is necessary. A standard bench top configuration uses a simple fluidics system, by which each sample is drawn gently directly from a pipette tip or larger container through the flow cell by a peristaltic pump. Measurements of concentration and size are absolute and can be verified using particle standards with known sizes and concentrations. Sample volumes range from about 0.25 mL to tens of milliliters, depending on the needs. Images displayed during operation provide immediate visual feedback on the nature of a given particle population. MFI measurements are accurate, repeatable, and considered sensitive to near-transparent particles (see below).

7.3.3   Materials and Methods of MFI Analysis

All tested protein sample solutions were subjected to high temperature (55°C) and shaking stress (14,000 rpm) for 10 min using a thermoshaker (Eppendorf AG, Germany). The samples (1000 µL each) were degassed before each analysis by exposing them to vacuum (20 mbar) for 30 min. All samples were measured undiluted. LO measurements were carried out on a PAMAS SBSS C low-volume LO analyzer (PAMAS GmbH, Germany).

MFI measurements were carried out on a DP4100 system (Brightwell Technologies) using a low magnification flow chamber (Model BP-4100-FC-UN) and 0.2 mL/min sample flow. Image optimization routine was performed for each sample using an aliquot filtered via a 0.22-µm syringe filter. The performance of the instrument was verified using NIST Traceable Particle Concentration Standards, for example, 3000/mL, sizes 2, 5, 10, and 25 µm (Duke Scientific Corporation catCC25-PK).

7.3.4   Results and Discussion of MFI

One of the main features of flow microscopy is its capability of distinguishing particles with different characteristics by aided microscopic control. For example, by using MFI, the digital images of particles collected during the course of an experiment can be visualized on a computer screen, and consequently, the presence of particular particles (e.g., fibers or oil droplets) with distinct characteristics (e.g., shapes and sizes) can be identified (Fig. 7.12). Thus, MFI provides additional layers of information and features, which allow better characterization of samples. In addition to the manual mode by looking at the images of particles on the computer screen, MFI provides sophisticated image analysis, which allows quantitative analysis of characteristics (e.g., shape, size, and transparency) of particles found in a given sample. For example, the distribution of spherical (bubbles and droplets) or fibrillar particles with different sizes can be evaluated by plotting the aspect ratio and/or circularity versus the size of the particles. Creating such scatter plots with information on characteristics (transparency, equivalent circular diameter, perimeter, circularity, aspect ratio, and maximum Feret diameter) of all particles is fairly easy and straightforward. The data processing is automated and provides in-depth analysis of particles.

After the advent of flow microscopy techniques, questions regarding the accuracy of LO were raised. For example, MFI measurements often show higher numbers of particles for the same sample compared to that of LO (Fig. 7.13). The amounts of particles in the larger size range in this particular sample agreed well using both techniques, while differences were observed for the particles with smaller sizes (below 5 µm). This discrepancy was found consistently using different proteins and conditions, that is, MFI always gave a higher readout in numbers of particles in the sub-5-µm size bins than that by LO. The extent of these discrepancies seems to vary depending on the individual proteins and protein formulations (Fig. 7.14). As the accuracy of sizing of MFI and LO was nearly identical using latex beads with certified size and concentration (data not

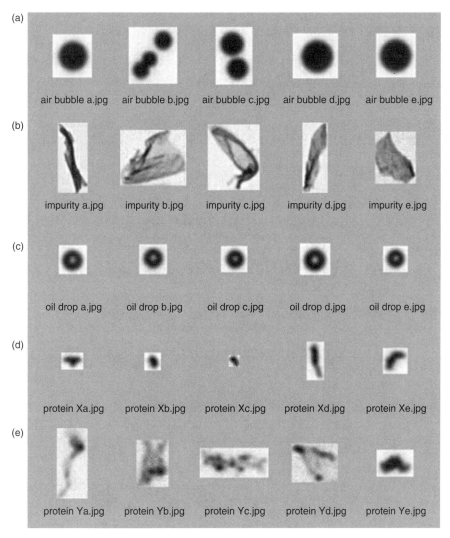

FIGURE 7.12 Examples of different particles found in solutions of protein pharmaceuticals: (a) air bubbles, (b) glass shards, (c) silicon oil droplets, and (d and e) protein aggregates.

shown), it became important to identify the factors that could potentially cause such discrepancies. It has been previously reported that transparency of the particles, that is, the difference in refractive indices between these particles and the solvent (placebo) may be one of the potential causes [34].

After extensive testing, we noted that the relative transparency of the particles was indeed the cause for the disagreement between these two techniques in the smaller size range. As shown in Fig. 7.15, there is a strong correlation between

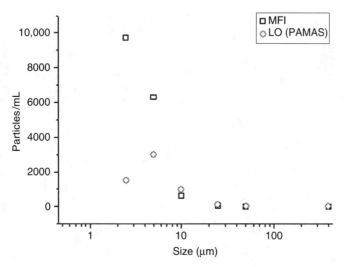

FIGURE 7.13   Size distribution of particles in solution of protein 1 on severe shaking stress measured by LO and MFI.

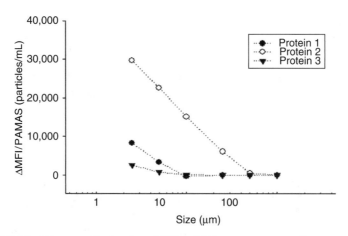

FIGURE 7.14   Discrepancies between MFI and LO measurements. Shown are the particle concentrations (by size) in solutions of three different proteins subjected to severe shaking stress.

the transparency of particles and the difference of particles counted by MFI or LO in three representative stressed protein products (averaged by size bins 2.0–2.5, 2.5–5.0, 5.0–10, 10–25, 25–100, and 100–400 μm). The more transparent the particles were, the larger was the difference between the counts of MFI and LO. The data set presented here also shows that the two techniques were well aligned for measurements of particles with a transparency of up to about 700 (the Brightwell MFI term is "object intensity") on a scale of 1–1023. However,

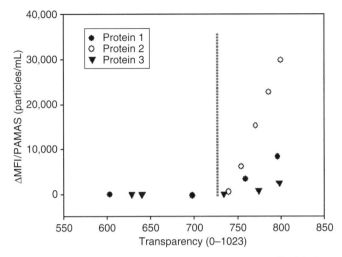

FIGURE 7.15 Differences in particle concentrations correlate well with the transparency of particles. Three different proteins were subjected to shaking stress (Fig. 7.13).

for particles with transparency higher than 700, the number of particles counted diverged. In all cases, MFI showed higher numbers than that by LO. The strong dependence on the type of proteins used may have been originated from differences in the morphological characteristics of the particles formed by the different proteins. While some proteins have highly elongated fibrillar structures, others form much more circular particles. The fibrillar particles are often more transparent than the circular ones. This observation can be explained with different mechanisms that presumably underpin the aggregation processes, which highly depend on factors such as protein sequence, structure, buffer, stress conditions, etc.

7.3.5 Summary of MFI

Flow microscopy is a novel method for quantification of subvisible particles, which offers new and exciting technical capabilities. For example, the digital images collected by MFI can be useful in identifying the presence of different types of particles (protein aggregates, rubber, glass shards, silicon oil droplets, etc.). The sophisticated software offered by MFI provides an opportunity for analyzing images automatically and assessing particle characteristics such as aspect ratio and transparency in a quantitative manner. In addition to its novel capabilities, MFI also offers unprecedented sensitivity in measurement of particles in the low micrometer size range. This technique is particularly sensitive to detecting highly transparent proteinaceous particles of sub-5 μm size. Such sensitivity may give a significant advantage to MFI over the classical LO technology in monitoring quality of protein pharmaceuticals. Owing to increasing requests by health authorities on monitoring/quantifying subvisible particles in therapeutic protein products [9,35], we anticipate that emerging techniques such as flow microscopy techniques will become increasingly important for the evaluation of particles throughout the pharmaceutical biotech industry.

7.4 NANOPARTICLE TRACKING ANALYSIS FOR CHARACTERIZATION OF PROTEIN AGGREGATES AND PARTICLES

7.4.1   Introduction to NTA

NTA is a novel technology for direct visualization of the movement of individual particles in the size range 10–1000 nm. It tracks the movements of the particles on a particle-by-particle basis. Although the NTA technology is still very new and has not yet been widely used, there have been already some applications in different areas. For example, NTA has been used for the visualization and characterization of VLPs [36], pigments, carbon nanotubes [37], nanocolloids and particles [38] in material sciences, drug delivery [39,40], and other fields. NTA also shows potential in detecting large aggregates/particles in protein solutions as discussed later.

7.4.2   Principle of NTA

The NTA system (LM10) consists of a laser, a sample chamber, an objective (×20, 0.25 NA), and a CCD camera (Marlin F033B) (Fig. 7.16). The currently available system has an objective (×20 magnification) with a field of view of ~100 × 80 μm and can detect protein aggregates/particles with sizes larger than 10 nm. The particles with sizes smaller than the laser wavelength (635 nm) appear as point scatterers as they cannot be optically resolved by the microscope. The intensity of light scattered by a particle is highly dependent on many factors such as illumination, polarization, sizes and shapes of particles, and refractive index difference between that of the particles and the dispersion medium.

Particles that diffuse into the laser light beam by Brownian motion are visualized by a CCD camera in real time (30 pics/s). The camera is mounted on an optical microscope, which is aligned orthogonally to the laser beam. The movement of each individual particle is traced through a series of pictures, which results in particle trajectories that can be further analyzed by the particle-tracking software. For each trajectory, the diffusion coefficient is determined from the mean square displacement using Equation 7.4. The diffusion coefficient is then used to calculate the sphere-equivalent hydrodynamic radius (r_h) (Eq. 7.5).

$$\overline{(x, y)^2} = 4D_t \tag{7.4}$$

where $\overline{(x, y)^2}$ is the mean square displacement and D_t the diffusion coefficient;

$$D_t = \frac{k_b \cdot T}{6\pi \eta \cdot r_h} \tag{7.5}$$

where k_b is the Boltzmann constant, T the temperature, and η the viscosity.

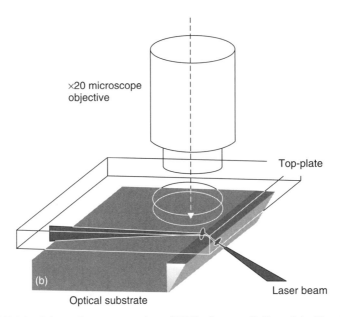

FIGURE 7.16   Schematic representation of NTA. *Source:* © Copyright NanoSight Ltd, UK.

Size distribution of particles can be obtained by NTA for even very heterogeneous samples. A total of 300–3000 pictures (10–100 s) are often needed for the calculation of the size distributions of such heterogeneous samples. Individual trajectories can be recorded with a time resolution of 33 ms. The number of particles in the field of view should not exceed 100 (about 2×10^9 particles/mL), so that trajectories of different particles would not overlap. Acquisition of a trajectory of each individual particle stops when the particle diffuses out of the field of view or when it is too close to an adjacent particle (Fig. 7.17). NTA visualizes the Brownian motion of particles as a two-dimensional projection, whereas the particles themselves move randomly in three dimensions. Equation 7.6 is, therefore, used to calculate the mean square displacement by reducing one dimension from Equation 7.7, which would be used for a freely moving spherical particle. If the particle is not spherical, a correction is also needed for the determination of the hydrodynamic radius.

$$\overline{(x, y)^2} = \frac{2k_b \cdot T \cdot t}{3\pi\eta \cdot r} \tag{7.6}$$

$$\overline{(x, y, z)^2} = \frac{k_b \cdot T \cdot t}{\pi\eta \cdot r} \tag{7.7}$$

7.4.3   Materials and Methods of NTA

Theoretically, for NTA analysis, protein solutions in any buffer can be used directly. To avoid potential risks of external contamination, preparation of

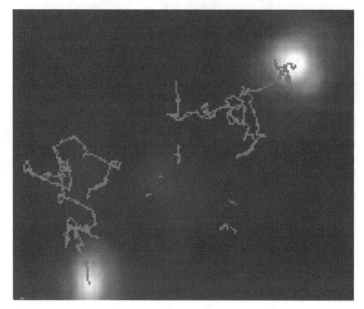

FIGURE 7.17   Signals and trajectories of two particles by NTA. *Source:* © Copyright NanoSight Ltd, UK.

samples using a laminar flow hood for sample handling is recommended. Dilution of samples (e.g., IgM and IgG) is necessary only if the number of particles in the field of view exceeds ~100 (corresponding to about 2×10^9 particles/mL). Antibodies (IgG and IgM) (150 mg/mL) in 20 mM histidine, pH 6.0, were measured by both NTA and DLS. NTA images were recorded for 10–20 s with a time resolution of 33 ms. A microscope objective with a × 20 magnification and a CCD camera (Marlin F033B) were used for all NTA measurements. The trajectories were extracted from the recorded images and the size distributions of aggregates and particles were calculated using the NanoSight software (NTA 2.0). DLS data were recorded by a Zetasizer Nano (Malvern) and the NNLS (Non-Negative Least Squares) fit was used for the determination of the distribution of particles (see chapter on dynamic light scattering (plus chapter reference)).

7.4.4   Results and Discussion of NTA

7.4.4.1   Accuracy of NTA Analysis   The accuracy of the NTA technique depends on the number and size of particles and the time used for the measurement. The supplier's recommended range for a NTA measurement is $10^7 – 10^9$ particles/mL. For a homogeneous sample, the NTA measurement is very reproducible. For example, the standard deviation of three individual measurements of polystyrene beads (e.g., particle size of 97 nm) was around 0.6%. A solution containing 10^9 particles/mL and a time of 10 s were used for the measurement. When the measurement time is too short or the concentration of the particles is too high, the individual track lengths become shorter and, consequently, size determination of particles less accurate. For a very heterogeneous sample, the size distribution histogram derived from trajectories of a smaller population of particles is statistically less robust (or reproducible) because the number of particles (thousands) used per NTA analysis is orders of magnitude lower than that with other analytical methods such as DLS.

7.4.4.2 NTA Analysis of Protein Aggregates   An IgG1 antibody that tends to form large aggregates was used for the NTA analysis. Large aggregates or particles with different sizes in the range of 30 and 300 nm were detected in the IgG1 antibody solution. The size distribution histogram accumulated from individual particle trajectories of the IgG1 aggregates is shown in Fig. 7.18a. For comparison, the size distribution of the same sample was also analyzed by DLS (Fig. 7.18b). Similar to the NTA results, peaks containing large aggregates were also found by the DLS analysis. These data indicate that, in principle, both the DLS and NTA techniques can be used to detect such populations of large aggregates ranging up to several hundred nanometers.

Both NTA and DLS were also used to measure size distribution of aggregates in an IgM antibody sample (Fig. 7.19a,b). Again, large aggregates with different sizes (up to several hundred nanometers) were detected in the tested sample by the NTA measurement (Fig. 7.19a). For the DLS measurement, besides the main monomer peak ($\sim$13 nm), an aggregate peak (around 100 nm) with a relatively high intensity was also detected. Even though there was only a small percentage of aggregates present in the solution, the intensities of light scattered by these aggregates were high due to its correlation to the particle radius (intensity $\sim r^6$).

Although the size range measured by NTA and DLS are overlapping and they both measure the intensity of light scattered by molecules in solution, information obtained from the two techniques is quite different. For DLS, information regarding the diffusion of particles is derived from an autocorrelation of the recorded light scattering intensity–time trace of a large number of particles, and the hydrodynamic radius is calculated from the autocorrelation by an exponential curve fitting (Chapter 3). For samples containing protein mixtures or different population of aggregates, a multiexponential curve fitting (e.g., CONTIN or NNLS algorithm) is needed for data analysis. In contrast, the NTA approach does not give an average on particle sizes, but it tracks the Brownian motion of individual particles in a liquid suspension. The histogram regarding size distribution of particles is accumulated particle by particle. No sophisticated fitting algorithms are needed for data analysis. One major advantage of NTA over DLS is its capability of resolving very heterogeneous samples. Particles with all sizes (small or large) can be measured by NTA simultaneously. Information regarding size of each individual particle is given by the intensity and step length within the trajectory (Figs. 7.18a and 7.19a). Particles with similar radii (e.g., a mixture of 100- and 200-nm beads) can also be resolved by NTA (data not shown). DLS, on the other hand, is biased in measuring heterogeneous samples, and small particles, even at high abundance, may not be detectable in the presence of large particles by DLS

(a)

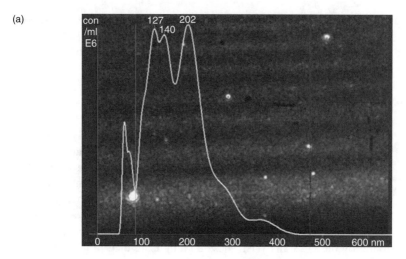

(b)

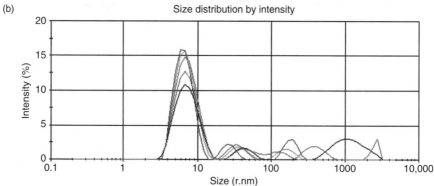

FIGURE 7.18   (a) A representative NTA image and corresponding size distribution of IgG aggregates and (b) size distribution of IgG aggregates by DLS. (*See insert for color representation of part (a)*.)

(Figs. 7.18b and 7.19b). Another advantage of NTA over DLS is its ability of quantifying particles with given sizes. Individual particles (e.g., oil droplets or air bubbles) that are not sample related can be manually excluded for data analysis.

NTA also has some disadvantages compared to DLS. For example, molecules with sizes smaller or equal to IgG1 antibody monomer are not detectable by NTA. NTA can only measure a sample with a concentration of $10^7 - 10^9$ particles/mL, while DLS can measure samples at a much broader concentration range.

7.4.5   Summary of NTA

The NTA technology is an additional valuable tool for characterization of large aggregates/particles in the size range of 10–1000 nm. NTA tracks the Brownian motion of particles in a liquid suspension on a particle-by-particle basis. Its main

(a)

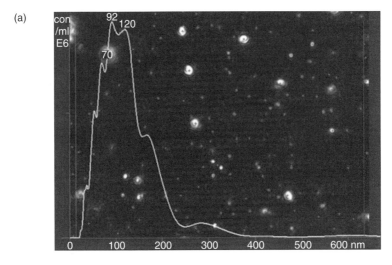

(b)

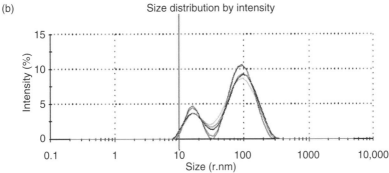

FIGURE 7.19   (a) A representative NTA image and corresponding size distribution of IgM aggregates and (b) size distribution of IgM aggregates by DLS. (*See insert for color representation of part (a).*)

advantage over DLS is that it is suitable to measure heterogeneous samples. NTA may, thus, develop to become a complementary technique to the currently available analytical techniques for analyzing/quantifying large aggregates and submicron particles.

7.5   OTHER EMERGING TECHNIQUES

Emerging light scattering techniques such as PIDS (Beckman Coulter Inc., AN-12622A) and Analysette 22 (Fritsch GmbH) have also become available for detecting aggregates and particles in the recent years. PIDS is an LO technique that can measure particles in the size range of 40 nm–2000 µm (Beckman Coulter Inc., AN-12622A) [18]. A sample solution is sequentially illuminated with vertically and horizontally polarized light at several wavelengths (e.g., 450, 600, and 900 nm). When the light beam is polarized either in vertical or in horizontal direction, the light polarized vertically shows a scattering pattern different from that of the light polarized horizontally. A more distinguished fine structure can be revealed by the difference, which makes it possible for the PIDS technique to measure particles with small sizes. Since the PIDS signal is dependent on particle size relative to the wavelength of light, a particle size distribution can be obtained by the measurement of the PIDS signals at several wavelengths. Overall, PIDS is capable of quantifying particles with sizes smaller than 1 μm. However, up to date (January 2010), no application of this technique on proteins has been published, and a relative large sample volume is needed for the analysis.

Analysette 22 is a laser light scattering technique for the measurement of particles in the size range of 300 nm–300 μm [19] (Fritsch GmbH). This is achieved through the use of a second laser beam that is directed at the sample from behind, allowing for the detection of the back-scattering light. An addition of the second laser light is necessary for measurements of particles in a broader range. Analysette 22 is capable of measuring not only the size distribution but also the shape of particles simultaneously. However, a relatively large sample volume is usually needed for measurements using Analysette 22. Until date, there is not yet any publication on the analysis of proteins using the instrument (January 2010).

7.6 SUMMARY

In the past few years, macro-IMS, flow microscopy, NTA, and other techniques have emerged to complement the conventional analytical techniques such as SEC, AUC, LO, and DLS/SLS for the analysis of aggregates/particles and to cover a broader size range for measurement (Fig. 7.1). Examples of using macro-IMS, MFI, and NTA in analyzing aggregates and particles were illustrated and discussed.

Macro-IMS is a fast, inexpensive, and reliable technique, which showed better resolution in separating fragments and small aggregates of mAbs, compared to SEC and DLS. Macro-IMS has also demonstrated its capabilities of analyzing large protein aggregates and VLPs. The analysis is very gentle and, therefore, allows the measurement of intact aggregates even for noncovalently linked aggregates. The macro-IMS technique, however, requires buffer exchange and extensive sample dilution, which could potentially lead to changes of aggregation profiles and underestimation of the amounts of aggregates. In addition, macro-IMS has potential to generate artificial aggregates, although this can be minimized to the lowest possible level during method development.

Flow microscopy offers new and exciting technical capabilities in distinguishing different types of aggregates/particles and assessing particles with different characteristics quantitatively. MFI is highly sensitive in detecting particles (sub-5 μm in size) and measuring particles in the low micrometer size range. Such sensitivity and especially the fact that it visualizes particles may give an advantage to MFI over the classical LO technology. Cautions have to be taken during sample preparation of MFI. Potential contamination of foreign particles needs to be avoided. NTA is a novel technology for direct visualization of the movement of individual particles in a range of approximately 10–1000 nm in solution. It tracks the movements of the particles on a particle-by-particle basis. It has an advantage over DLS in its capability of measuring heterogeneous samples both qualitatively and quantitatively. More importantly, NTA can be used to distinguish particles with similar sizes, but having different refractive indices (data not shown). One drawback of NTA is that it cannot detect molecules with sizes smaller or equal to IgG1 antibody monomer. In addition, it has a relatively small dynamic range of $10^7–10^9$ particles/mL.

Overall, these emerging techniques are promising in analyzing and monitoring aggregates and particles in the size range that poses great challenges to the pharmaceutical biotech industry.

Acknowledgments

This work was supported by Margit Jeschke, the head of the analytical research and development of the process science and production. We thank Markus Smolny for performing Macro-IMS analysis for a study using different gauge pressures and Sadrine Hammer for the SEC analysis of mAb1. We also thank Vinita Marathe and Rene Strehl who did the DLS and MFI analysis, as well as John Philo who performed the AUC analyses. We also thank Axel Zerrath from TSI Inc. and Robert Carr from NanoSight Inc. for their technical support.

REFERENCES

1. Manning MC, Patel K, Borchardt RT. Stability of protein pharmaceuticals. Pharm Res 1989;6:903–917.

2. Chi EY, Krishnan S, Randolph TW, Carpenter JF. Physical stability of proteins in aqueous solution: mechanism and driving forces in non-native protein aggregation. Pharm Res 2003;20:1325–1336.

3. Cromwell ME, Hilario E, Jacobson F. Protein aggregation and bioprocessing. AAPS J 2006;8(3):E527–E579.

4. Andya JD, Hsu CC, Shire SJ. Mechanisms of aggregate formation and carbohydrate excipient stabilization of lyophilized humanized monoclonal antibody formulations. AAPS Pharm Sci 2003;5(2):E10.

5. Schellekens H. Factors influencing the immunogenicity of therapeutic proteins. Nephrology. Dial Transplant 2005;20 Suppl 6:vi3–vi9.

6. Hermeling S, Crommelin DJ, Schellekens H, Jiskoot W. Structure-immunogenicity relationships of therapeutic proteins. Pharm Res 2004;21:897–903.

7. Robbins DC, Hirshman M, Wardzala LJ, Horton ES. High-molecular-weight aggregates of therapeutic insulin: in vitro measurements of receptor binding and bioactivity. Diabetes 1988;37:56–59.

8. Maislos M, Bialer M, Mead PM, Robbins DC. Pharmacokinetic model of circulating covalent aggregates of insulin. Diabetes 1988;37:1059–1063.

9. Carpenter JF, Randolph TW, Jiskoot W, Crommelin DJA, Middaugh CR, Winter G, Fan YX, Kirshner S, Verthelyi D, Kozlowski S, Clouse KA, Swann PG, Rosenberg A, Cherney B. Overlooking subvisible particles in therapeutic protein products: gaps that may compromise product quality. J Pharm Sci 2009;98:1201–1205.

10. Kamberi M, Chung P, DeVas R. Analysis of non-covalent aggregation of synthetic hPTH (1-34) by size-exclusion chromatography and the importance of suppression of non-specific interactions for precise quantitation. J Chromatogr B: Analyt Technol Biomed Life Sci 2004;810:151–155.

11. Link GW, Keller PL, Stout RW, Banesm AJ. Effect of solution used for storage of size-exclusion columns on the subsequent chromatography of peptides and proteins. J Chromatogr 1985;331:253–264.

12. Chirino AJ, Mire-Sluis A. Characterizing biological products and assessing comparability following manufacturing changes. Nat Biotechnol 2004;22:1383–1391.

13. Laue T. Analytical ultracentrifugation: a powerful 'new' technology in drug discovery. Drug Discov Today: Technol 2004;1:309–315.

14. Philo, JS Analytical ultracentrifugation. In: Jiskoot W, Crommelin D, editors. Methods for structural analysis of protein pharmaceuticals. Arlington (VA): AAPS Press; 2005. pp. 379–412.

15. Berkowitz SA. Role of analytical ultracentrifugation in assessing the aggregation of protein biopharmaceuticals. AAPS J 2006;8(3):E590–E605.

16. Laue T. Biophysical studies by ultracentrifugation. Curr Opin Struct Biol 2001; 11:579–583.

17. Lebowitz J, Lewis MS, Schuck P. Modern analytical ultracentrifugation in protein science: a tutorial review. Protein Sci 2002;11:2067–2079.

18. Keck CM, Müller RH. Size analysis of submicron particles by laser diffractometry-90% of the published measurement are false. Int J Pharm 2008;355:150–163.

19. Sforzini A, Bersani G, Stancari A, Grossi G, Bonoli A, Ceschel GC. Analysis of all-in-one parenteral nutrition admixtures by liquid chromatography and laser diffraction: study of stability. J Pharm Biomed Anal 2001;24:1099–1109.

20. Kaufman SL, Skogen JW, Dorman FD, Zarrin F, Lewis LC. Macromolecule analysis based on electrophoretic mobility in air: globular proteins. Anal Chem 1996;68:1895–1904.

21. Moore JM, Patapoff TW, Cromwell ME. Kinetics and thermodynamics of dimer formation and dissociation for a recombinant humanized monoclonal antibody to vascular endothelial growth factor. Biochemistry 1999;38:13960–13967.

22. Loo JA, Berhane B, Kaddis CS, Wooding KM, Xie Y. Electrospray ionization mass spectrometry and ion mobility analysis of the 20S proteasome complex. J Am Soc Mass Spectrom 2005;16:998–1008.

23. Rofougaran R, Vodnala M, Hofer M. Enzymatically active mammalian ribonucleotide reductase exists primarily as an $\alpha6\beta2$ octamer. J Biol Chem 2006;281:27705–27711.

24. Kaddis CS, Lomeli SH, Yin S, Berhane B, Apostol MI, Kickhoefer VA, Rome LH, Loo JA. Sizing large proteins and protein complexes by electrospray ionization mass spectrometry and ion mobility. J Am Soc Mass Spectrom 2007;18(7):1206–1216.

25. Seefeldt MB, Ouyang J, Froland WA, Carpenter JF, Randolph TW. High pressure refolding of bikunin: efficacy and thermodynamics. Protein Sci 2004;13:2639–2650.

26. Hogan CJ, Kettleson EM, Ramaswami B, Chen DR, Biswas P. Charge-reduced electrospray size spectrometry of mega- and gigadalton complexes: whole viruses and virus fragments. Anal Chem 2006;78:844–852.

27. Laschober C, Wruss J, Blaas D, Szymanski W, Allmaier G. Gas phase electrophoretic molecular mobility analysis of size and stoichiometry of complexes of a common cold virus with antibodies. Anal Chem 2008;80:2261–2264.

28. Tan P, Kennedy S, Zerrath A. Mass analysis from kilodaltons to megadaltons using macroion mobility spectrometry. Curr Trends Mass Spectrom 2007;26–29.

29. Basa LJ, Lancaster K, Shyong BJ, Tan P, Katta V. Stoichiometry of antibody aggregates and complexes measured by macroion mobility spectrometry. ASMS Poster 2007.

30. Bacher G, Szymanski W, Kaufman S, Zollner P, Blass D, Allmaier G. Charge-reduced nanoelectrospray ionization combined with differential mobility analysis of peptides, proteins, glycoproteins, noncovalent protein complexes and viruses. J Mass Spectrom 2001;36:1038–1052.

31. Schuck P. Size-distribution analysis of macromolecules by sedimentation velocity ultracentrifugation and Lamm equation modeling. Biophys J 2000;78:1606–1619.

32. Zhao H, Bozova M, Smolny M, Tour K, Diez M, Lam HT, Bluemel M, Forrer K. MacroIMS as an emerging technique for characterization of protein aggregates. 2010. Forthcoming.

33. Gabrielson JP, Brader ML, Pekar AH, Mathis KB, Winter G, Carpenter JF, Randolph TW. Quantitation of aggregate levels in a recombinant humanized monoclonal antibody formulation by size-exclusion chromatography, asymmetrical flow field flow fractionation, and sedimentation velocity. J Pharm Sci 2006;96:268–279.

34. Huang CT, Sharma D, Oma P, Krishnamurthy R. Quantitation of protein particles in parenteral solutions using micro-flow imaging. J Pharm Sci 2009;98:3058–3071.

35. European Medicines Agency, Committee for Medicinal Products for Human Use. Guideline on development, production, characterization and specifications for monoclonal antibodies and related products. London; 2008.

36. Moser M. Emerging analytical techniques to characterize vaccines. Proceeding of international conference on Vaccines Europe; Brussels; 2008 Dec.

37. Trushkevych O, Collings N, Hasan T, Scardaci V, Ferrari AC, Wilkinson TD, Crossland WA, Milne WI, Geng J, Johnson BFG, Macaulay S. Characterization of carbon nanotube–thermotropic nematic liquid crystal composites. J Phys D: Appl Phys 2008;41:125106–125117.

38. Barcikowski S, Manjon AM, Chichkov B, Brikas M, Raciukaitis G. Generation of nanoparticle colloids by picosecond and femtosecond laser ablations in liquid flow. Appl Phys Lett 2007;91(8):083113. Nanoscale Science and Design.

39. Ghonaim HM, Li S, Blagbrough1 IS. Very long chain N4, N9—diacyl spermines: non-viral lipopolyamine vectors for efficient plasmid DNA and siRNA delivery. Pharm Res 2009;26:19–31.

40. Nassar T, Rom A, Nyska A, Benita S. Novel double coated nanocapsules for intestinal delivery and enhanced oral bioavailability of tacrolimus, a P–gp substrate drug. J Control Release 2009;133:77–84.

SECTION II
Methods Used to Characterize Protein Aggregates and Particles

8 Ultraviolet Absorption Spectroscopy

REZA ESFANDIARY and CHARLES RUSSELL MIDDAUGH

Department of Pharmaceutical Chemistry, University of Kansas, Lawrence, Kansas, USA

8.1 INTRODUCTION

Owing to recent advances (e.g., the invention of diode-array detectors and improved spectral analysis), interest has been renewed in the utility of ultraviolet (UV)-absorption spectroscopy to study protein conformational alterations and aggregation. As described in this chapter, UV-absorption spectroscopy is a rapid, nondestructive, high resolution, and inexpensive alternative to other commonly used spectroscopic techniques for protein studies. Herein, a brief discussion of the light absorption phenomenon, instrumentation, protein chromophores (intrinsic and extrinsic), and different modes of data analysis (zero-order and derivative analysis) is provided. The major focus of this chapter is, however, on the utility of UV-absorption spectroscopy for the analysis of protein aggregates both indirectly (i.e., by the identification of major and subtle protein conformational alterations as well as dynamic fluctuations) and directly (i.e., turbidity measurements in both thermodynamic and kinetic modes). Absorption spectroscopy is shown to have much to offer for structural analysis of proteins and other macromolecules in the context of their aggregation behavior.

8.2 THEORETICAL BACKGROUND

Light is a mixture of oscillating magnetic and electric fields and is described quantum mechanically as photons of energy (E) according to

$$E = h\nu = hc/\lambda \tag{8.1}$$

Analysis of Aggregates and Particles in Protein Pharmaceuticals, First Edition.
Edited by Hanns-Christian Mahler, Wim Jiskoot.
© 2012 John Wiley & Sons, Inc., Published 2012 by John Wiley & Sons, Inc.

where h is Planck's constant and λ, ν, and c are the wavelength, frequency, and speed of light, respectively. Light of certain defined frequencies absorbed by a chromophore can promote an electron from its ground electronic state to an excited state. The promotion occurs only if the energy of the incident light is equivalent to the energy gap between the chromophore's two electronic states. An absorption spectrum is obtained by continuously changing the wavelength of the incident light and monitoring the changes in the amount of light absorbed. A typical absorption plot is described by the degree of absorption (arbitrary unit) on the y-axis versus wavelength (nanometer) on the x-axis. Following absorption, the excited electrons return to the ground state through either a radiative (i.e., fluorescence or phosphorescence) or a nonradiative (i.e., primarily heat generating in the case for UV-absorption spectroscopy) process.

8.2.1   The Beer–Lambert Law

The relationship between the absorption of light and the amount of absorbing chromophore present follows two basic rules that when combined are known as the *Beer–Lambert law*. Lambert's law states that the fraction of light absorbed is independent of the incident light intensity and that each successive layer of the medium absorbs an equal fraction of the light passing through it. Mathematically, this is expressed according to

$$A = \mathrm{Log}_{10}(I_0/I) = kl \tag{8.2}$$

where A is the measured absorbance signal, l is the length of the light pass, k is a constant described by Beer's law (see below), and I_0 and I are the intensity of the incident and transmitted light, respectively. Beer's law states that the amount of light absorbed is proportional to the number of chromophore molecules through which the light passes. The constant k is, therefore, proportional to the chromophore's concentration (c) and is described as $k = \varepsilon c$, where ε is the absorption of a one molar (M) solution of chromophore over a 1-cm pathlength ($\mathrm{M}^{-1}/$ cm) and is often referred to as the *molar extinction coefficient*. Therefore, Equation (8.2) can be rearranged as

$$A = \mathrm{Log}_{10}(I_0/I) = \varepsilon c l \tag{8.3}$$

which is known as the *Beer–Lambert law*. Thus, according to Equation (8.3), absorption of a chromophore is linearly proportional to its concentration. Deviations from the Beer–Lambert law, however, frequently occur and can introduce significant artifacts in absorption measurements, which are discussed in detail later in this chapter (Section 8.10). Also note that scattered light, which can be incorrectly interpreted as absorption, does not obey this linear response.

8.2.2 Instrumentation

Most spectrophotometers contain four basic components: a light source, sample holder (which can be temperature controlled), light dispersion device, and detector. An effective light source should be able to produce and maintain stable light intensity of low noise for extended periods of time over the desired wavelengths of interest. A commonly used source is a combination of deuterium and tungsten–halogen lamps. Either a combination of the two lamps into a single source or the ability to automatically switch between the two during spectral collection is used for coverage of the full UV/Vis range (typically 190–600/800 nm). The cell holder that can contain one or more (typically 1–8) quartz or glass cuvettes is often positioned in a temperature-controlled block (either Peltier based or water jacketed). Dual-beam designs in which the reference and sample cells are measured simultaneously to minimize the time-dependent fluctuations of incident light intensity are also available. The high quality and reproducibility of data of modern commercially available single-beam spectrophotometers, however, has at least partially eliminated the need for multibeam-based instruments.

An important factor governing acceptable spectral resolution is the design of the light dispersion/detector systems, optimization of which is crucial for high resolution derivative absorbance spectroscopy (see below). In the more common system, light is passed through an entrance slit and focused on a dispersion device (today usually a diffraction grating and in the past a prism) from which a narrow fraction is passed through an exit slit to the sample and then to the detector, commonly a photomultiplier tube (PMT). In the early 1990s, the availability of diode-array instruments enhanced the effective spectral resolution significantly. A diode-array detector consists of an array of photodiodes set at fixed intervals (usually 0.5–2.0 nm) that can simultaneously detect the full-light spectrum. In such a device, the entire spectrum of light is transmitted through the sample and passed into an entrance slit of a polychromator to the dispersion device and eventually to the multidiode detector. Although the natural resolution of such a system is not high, the collected spectrum can be further enhanced mathematically through interpolation algorithms (Section 8.7.6) to produce very high resolution results.

High throughput microplate-reader-based spectrophotometers are also available and are widely used in protein pharmaceutical preformulation studies. Modern day systems are often monochromator based and have the ability to measure absorbance, fluorescence, and luminescence. The plate-reader-based systems, however, are often less sensitive compared to the cuvette-based instruments and provide less flexibility in temperature control. Absorption spectroscopy can be used to obtain a wide variety of information related to the aggregation behavior of proteins and is the subject of the remainder of this chapter.

8.3   INTRINSIC CHROMOPHORES

8.3.1   Aromatic Side Chains

Proteins display a broad peak in the 250- to 300-nm region of their UV spectrum. This is composed of multiple overlapping bands arising primarily from the aromatic residues phenylalanine, tyrosine, and tryptophan. These signals are in large part due to $\pi \rightarrow \pi^*$ transitions involving the electrons of their aromatic rings [1]. The indole side chain of tryptophan absorbs strongly ($\varepsilon_{280 \text{ nm}} = 5540$) with a maximum peak at $\sim$280 nm and a less intense transition, usually observed as a shoulder in proteins at $\sim$292 nm (both corresponding to $\pi \rightarrow \pi^*$ transitions). Alterations of the tryptophan absorption spectrum can occur due to oxidation of the indole moiety [2,3]. For example, oxidation of tryptophan to kynurenine is distinguished by the appearance of a strong absorbance band at longer wavelengths near 365 nm in a region over which tryptophan itself shows no absorption [4]. Modification of tryptophan (e.g., oxidation induced by N-bromosuccinimide) has been used to measure the solvent accessibility of these residues [5].

The absorption of tyrosine is less intense ($\varepsilon_{280 \text{ nm}} = 1480$) with maximum absorbance seen at $\sim$276 nm ($\pi \rightarrow \pi^*$) with two small shoulders at $\sim$267 and 280 nm. Tyrosine is even more susceptible to structural modifications than tryptophan with the phenolic side chain susceptible to ionization [6], iodination [7], chlorination [8], and oxidation [3]. The ionization of the phenol side chain of tyrosine results in a large redshift of the absorption maxima from 222 and 275 to 242 and 295 nm, respectively. A considerable hyperchromic effect also occurs on ionization [6]. In addition, phenolic compounds undergo large redshifts and intensification of their absorbance bands on iodination [7]. Finally, cross linking of tyrosine residues can occur to form di-tyrosine-linked dimers [9–11]. This often results in alteration of the tyrosine absorption spectrum as indicated by the appearance of a new peak near $\sim$320 nm [12].

The benzene side chain of phenylalanine exhibits the weakest transition ($\varepsilon_{258nm} = 197$) and is present in the 250- to 270-nm region ($\pi \rightarrow \pi^*$), usually appearing as multiple subtle inflection points (due to vibrational fine structure) in the near-UV region of proteins, with a peak centered near 260 nm. When analyzing zero-order spectra, the weak absorbance of phenylalanine is often at least partially obscured by the presence of tyrosine and tryptophan residues requiring derivative analysis for resolution of its contribution. As discussed below, the sensitivity of the absorption bands of the three aromatic side chains to their local protein environment make them especially useful in the study of conformational changes.

8.3.2   The Peptide Group

The most frequent chromophore present in any protein is the amide group of the peptide backbone. It contains two major transitions with the first strongly absorbing at 195 nm ($\pi \rightarrow \pi^*$) and a second weaker transition occurring at $\sim$220 nm ($n \rightarrow \pi^*$). With α-helix, β-sheet, and random coil secondary structure

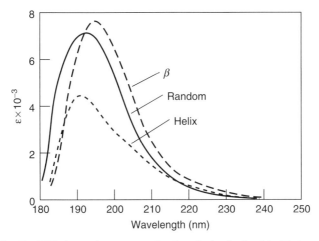

FIGURE 8.1   Far-UV-absorption spectra of poly-L-lysine hydrochloride in aqueous solution: random coil; pH 6.0, 25°C; α-helix, pH 10.8, 25°C; and β-sheet, pH 10.8, 52°C. *Source:* Adapted from Rosenheck and Doty [13].

each exhibiting distinct absorbance characteristics in the far-UV region, in the past, the spectral characteristics of peptide group was used to study protein secondary structure [13] (Fig. 8.1). Interpretation of such data is, however, difficult due to extensive spectral overlap and interference by inorganic ions and dissolved oxygen below 200 nm [5]. The latter requires purging of the spectrophotometer with nitrogen, a capability not usually available in commercial instrumentation. The availability of other sensitive and higher resolution techniques (e.g., circular dichroism and FTIR spectroscopy) for use in protein secondary structural analysis has essentially eliminated the use of UV-absorption spectroscopy for this application.

8.3.3   Disulfide Bonds and Other Chromophores

A nonaromatic amino acid contributing appreciably in the 250- to 300-nm region of the protein absorption spectrum is the disulfide-bridge form of cysteine (i.e., cystine) [14]. Other residues such as methionine and histidine absorb weakly in the lower wavelength regions, but their contributions are usually obscured by the much stronger absorption bands of the peptide backbone and the aromatic side chains [5].

8.4   EXTRINSIC CHROMOPHORES

In addition to a variety of intrinsic chromophores that contribute to the absorption spectrum of proteins, a number of different extrinsic chromophores absorb in the near-UV region, often with absorption characteristics sensitive to the polarity of their surrounding environment. Therefore, comparison of their absorption spectra in the free and protein-bound states has been employed as a tool to study protein conformation, the nature of binding sites, binding stochiometry, and kinetics.

8.4.1 Divalent Metal Cations

The most prevalent class of extrinsic chromophores in proteins is the divalent metal cations (e.g., iron, copper, cobalt, cadmium, and terbium). These often possess spectra that are sensitive to their local protein environment and their own oxidation states [15]. Investigation of alterations in their absorption spectra in protein-bound states has frequently been used to study protein ion-binding capacities [16] as well as coordination geometries [17].

8.4.2 Dyes and Coenzymes

A number of dyes show strong absorption bands in the near-UV and visible regions and have been used in studies of proteins. Concentration-dependent binding studies of Congo red (CR) to the amyloid fibrils seen in Alzheimer's disease have been used as a tool for the detection of amyloidogenesis [18,19]. Large redshifts of the major absorption band of Thioflavin T (ThT) on binding to amyloid fibrils have also been employed to detect fibril formation [20]. Their use has now been extended to studies of a many proteins as a general probe of intermolecular β-sheet formation. Coenzymes comprise another class of useful extrinsic chromophores. For example, the reduction of nicotinamide adenine dinucleotide (NAD) to NADH results in the formation of a strong absorbance band at $\sim$340 nm, which is used to study the kinetics of a wide variety of enzymatic reactions [21,22].

8.5 DATA ANALYSIS

8.5.1 Zero-Order Spectra

The application of UV-absorption spectroscopy to proteins was initiated more than half a century ago by analysis of "zero-order spectra" at relatively low resolution [1]. Zero-order spectra represent the raw data of absorption versus wavelength collected by the spectrophotometer. In the case of proteins, the zero-order spectrum typically consists of a strong absorbance below 210 nm from the amide group of the peptide backbone followed by a weaker transition in the 250- to 300-nm region, composed of multiple overlapping bands from the aromatic residues phenylalanine, tyrosine, and tryptophan [23]. As discussed earlier, the utility of the amide backbone peak has been of limited use due to interferences from inorganic ions and dissolved oxygen. It is well recognized, however, that peak shifts in the spectra of the aromatic residues can reflect even quite subtle protein structural perturbations due to their sensitivity to the polarity of the surrounding environment. Until the last few decades, however, the utility of the spectrum of the aromatic residues was fairly limited due to the extensive overlap of their absorption peaks and, subsequently, only major structural changes such as protein-unfolding events were extensively studied. This has changed significantly with the development of high resolution derivative spectroscopy.

8.5.2 High Resolution Derivative Spectroscopy

Derivatization of zero-order data in the 250- to 300-nm region of the UV spectrum of proteins resolves the overlapping peaks of phenylalanine, tyrosine, and tryptophan to allow both quantitative and qualitative analysis of the contribution of each class of residues to the overall protein spectrum. Limitations in early spectrophotometers permitted detection of only 0.5- to 1-nm shifts of the absorbance derivative peaks [24]. Following advances in instrumentation, especially the availability of diode-array detectors and supplementation of the derivative analysis with interpolation algorithms [25,26], the resolution of the absorption bands of each of the three aromatic residues has been greatly enhanced. In some cases, resolution as high as 0.01 nm can be obtained from second-derivative spectra generated by fitting the data to a cubic function using a multiple (typically nine) data point filter and a fifth-degree Savitzky–Golay polynomial supplemented with 99 interpolated points between each raw data point. This provides a powerful tool for probing protein conformational alterations by monitoring derivative peak position shifts of the aromatic residues as a function of a number of environmental conditions. The intensity of such derivative peaks and their ratios has also been used as a quantitative probe of the number of phenylalanine and tryptophan residues in a protein [27]. These signals can also be employed to measure Tyr/Trp ratios and as a qualitative measure of solvent polarity surrounding aromatic side chains [28]. Because derivative analysis is not sensitive to broad spectral components, artifacts such as light scattering effects do not significantly perturb the determination of derivative peak positions [25].

Figure 8.2 illustrates the high resolving power of derivative analysis (a) in which the broad, low resolution zero-order absorption peaks of the three aromatic residues (b) have been deconvoluted to their component peaks exhibited as minima in second-derivative plots.

8.6 DIFFERENCE SPECTRA

8.6.1 Difference Spectroscopy

Before the advent of high resolution derivative analysis, difference spectroscopy was the method of choice to study protein conformational alterations at higher resolution and with less experimental noise than zero-order analysis. Its applications included analysis of protein thermal unfolding [29,30], formation of enzyme–substrate complexes [31], binding of small molecules [32], determination of chromophore environment [33], protein–protein association and dissociation [33], and enzyme action [34]. A difference spectrum is generated by the

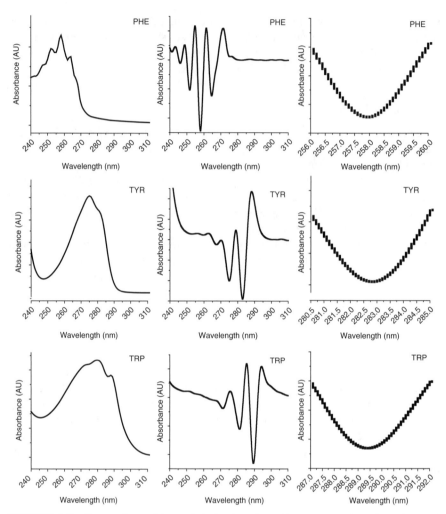

FIGURE 8.2 Zero-order and second-derivative absorption spectra of N-acetyl-X-ethyl ester derivatives of phenylalanine (PHE), tyrosine (TYR), and tryptophan (TRP). The column on the far right is a zoom-in plot of the most intense derivative peak for each residue, illustrating the resolving power of second-derivative analysis when used in conjunction with diode-array data acquisition and curve-fitting algorithms. The ordinate axis is presented in arbitrary units.

subtraction of a reference spectrum from a sample spectrum in which both contain a protein of identical concentration but under different solution conditions [33]. Alterations are detected on perturbation of the sample using, for example, a chaotropic agent or extremes of pH, temperature, ionic strength, or other environmental alterations. Despite the wide spread use of this technique in the past in both zero-order [35] and derivative formats [36], data interpretation can be very complex since changes in the shape, position, and intensity of the sample and reference peaks all contribute to the difference spectrum. A general guideline, however, suggests that negative values in the difference spectra are indicative of peak shifts to lower wavelengths or increases in the polarity of the chromophore microenvironment. Positive values are usually thought to reflect shifts to longer wavelengths (i.e., redshifts).

8.6.2 Solvent Perturbation Spectroscopy

Solvent perturbation spectroscopy, an early application of difference spectroscopy, has been used to study alterations in a protein's UV spectra as a result of changes in the surrounding solvent, in the absence of protein conformational alterations [37]. Employing this technique, only surface-exposed chromophores in direct contact with the surrounding solvent molecules contribute to the difference spectrum, essentially providing a comparative average measure of a given chromophore's exposure level to solvent. Low to moderate concentrations of non-structural altering perturbants (e.g., 20% ethylene glycol, glycerol, sucrose) induce shifts in chromophore UV spectra. Difference spectra are then generated with reference to the fully unfolded protein induced by chemical unfolding agents such as urea, guanidine hydrochloride, and disulfide reducing agents. When employing this technique, proper selection of perturbant size is crucial since smaller perturbants can penetrate into a protein's matrix more readily and interact with buried chromophores, contributing to the signals observed. Special double sectored cells are available to facilitate solvent perturbation analysis.

8.7 INDIRECT MEASURES OF PROTEIN AGGREGATION

Aggregation of proteins is a phenomenon of biological, biomedical, and pharmaceutical interest. In particular, the nature of any early events leading to the formation of nonnative species that may serve as precursors of aggregation sensitive species is critical to our understanding of protein association events. The older view of protein aggregation often postulated the association of extensively unfolded states [38,39]. More recently, the role of folding/unfolding intermediates has taken precedent [40,41]. Detection of such altered states as precursors of protein aggregation is, therefore, thought to be of paramount importance in the prevention and inhibition of protein aggregation. High resolution second-derivative UV-absorption spectroscopy of aromatic amino acids provides a very sensitive and powerful tool for the detection of subtle as well as more extensive protein conformational alterations for this purpose and is discussed in more detail later.

8.7.1 Studies of Protein Conformational Alterations (Static Properties)

With the availability of diode-array detectors and employing high resolution second-derivative analysis supplemented with interpolation algorithms, the absorption bands of each of the three aromatic residues can often be deconvoluted with a resolution of approximately 0.01 nm. This provides a very sensitive tool with which to probe protein conformational alterations in which the average polarity of the microenvironment surrounding the aromatic side chains and their level of exposure to solvent are detectably altered on protein structural changes. By monitoring the individual shifts of the derivative peak positions of these residues, fairly detailed information can be obtained regarding the conformational alterations of proteins as a function of a variety of solution conditions such as pH, temperature, ionic strength, presence of solutes. In general, peak shifts to lower wavelengths (i.e., blueshifts) are indicative of the increased exposure of aromatic side chains to a more polar solvent environment, whereas shifts to longer wavelengths (i.e., redshifts) imply increased burial and less solvent exposure of these groups. Employing this technique, shifts as small as 0.1 nm or less and as large as 6 nm have routinely been correlated with protein structural alterations [42,43].

An example of the sensitivity of second-derivative analysis and its utility in studies of protein conformational alterations is shown in Fig. 8.3, in which the burial of one or more of the aromatic side chains on induced structural alterations of the FKBP protein due to binding of a ligand, FK520, are manifested as redshifts in the derivative peaks (Fig. 8.3b). Increases in peak intensities in both zero-order and second-derivative spectra on binding of the ligand are also evident.

8.7.2 Empirical Phase Diagrams (EPDs)

Deconvolution of the overlapping peaks of the three aromatic residues by second-derivative analysis results in multiple distinct peaks in the near-UV region. Although potentially up to three peaks for each aromatic residue could be seen, five to seven are usually resolved. Considering the dispersal of the aromatic residues throughout the three-dimensional structure of proteins and the sensitivity of these peaks to protein structural alterations, analysis of such peak shifts as a function of a variety of solution conditions such as pH, temperature, and ionic strength can provide a global picture of a protein's behavior in solution. Some further information is possible since phenylalanine residues are typically buried, tyrosines are located interfacially, and tryptophans are fairly randomly dispersed. The large amount of data generated by such studies, however, can make interpretation slightly difficult. One practical approach to integrating such large sets of data is to construct what is known as an *empirical phase diagram* (*EPD*) in which the individual peak positions of the aromatic residues at each set of coordinates (e.g., at specific temperature and pH combinations) are used to construct an N-dimensional vector (N refers to the number of different pieces of data, in this case wavelength position). Details of the mathematical theory and calculation process can be found elsewhere [44], but in brief, projectors of each individual vector are calculated and summed into an $N \times N$ density matrix containing N sets of eigen values and eigenvectors. The individual vectors at each coordinate are truncated into three-dimensional vectors and reexpanded into a new basis set consisting of the three eigenvectors corresponding to the three largest eigen values. The resultant three-dimensional vectors are then converted into a color plot

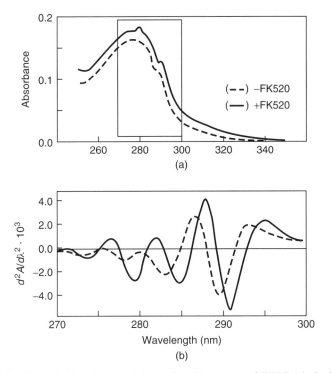

FIGURE 8.3   Normal (a) and second-derivative (b) spectra of FKBP (dashed line) and FKBP-FK520 complex (solid line). Part of the zero-order spectrum (a) used in the second-derivative calculation (b) is enclosed in a box. Increases in peak magnitudes in both zero-order and second-derivative spectra on binding of the ligand are evident. *Source:* Adapted from Mach et al. [25].

with each vector component corresponding to a color using an arbitrary RGB (red, green, and blue) color system. When analyzing EPDs, regions of continuous color define uniform structural physical states within the limit of resolution of the techniques employed. More importantly, abrupt changes in color identify alterations in the physical state of the protein over the conditions examined (Fig. 8.4). It should be emphasized that EPDs are not thermodynamic phase diagrams in which equilibrium exists between different phases and must always be interpreted with this in mind. At least partially irreversible structural alterations and/or aggregation clearly prevent any type of rigorous thermodynamic analyses.

The utility of the EPD approach was originally illustrated in studies of bovine granulocyte colony stimulating factor (bGCSF) conducted over a wide range of pH and temperature [44]. Distinct phases are identified based on the uniformity of the color blocks in the EPD (Fig. 8.4) and by further reference to the raw spectroscopic data (which can include other experimental methods). For example, the red region (pH 4, 10–60°C) contains soluble aggregates, whereas the phase

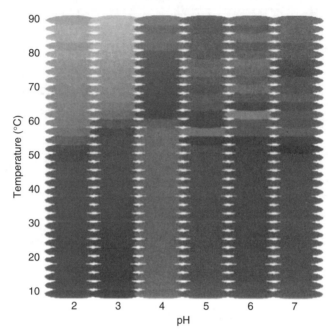

FIGURE 8.4   Temperature–pH phase diagram of bGCSF based on second-derivative absorbance data. Six distinct phases are observed: (1) pH 2–3, T 10–55°C; (2) pH 2–3, T 55–90°C; (3) pH 4, T 10–60°C; (4) pH 4, T 60–90°C; (5) pH 5–7, T 10–50°C; and (6) pH 5–7, T 50–90°C. Blocks of continuous color represent single phases, conditions under which the raw data-derived vectors behave similarly. The colors are arbitrarily chosen. *Source:* Adapted from Kueltzo et al. [44]. (*See insert for color representation of the figure.*)

between pH 5–7 and 50–90°C contains aggregates as well as extensive amount of precipitate.

EPDs can also be generated employing multiple other techniques, each sensitive to certain feature of protein structure. For example, combinations of circular dichroism, intrinsic and extrinsic fluorescence, as well as static and dynamic light scattering generate an EPD sensitive to changes in protein secondary, tertiary, and quaternary structural alteration as well as aggregation tendencies. EPDs are a rapid and efficient approach to display complex data sets and have been effectively employed as a pharmaceutical formulation tool for a wide variety of other macromolecular systems including peptides, proteins, recombinant protein-based vaccines, viruses and viruslike particle (VLP)-based vaccines, DNA and bacterial vaccines, and gene delivery vectors [44–59].

8.7.3   Studies at High Protein Concentration

With an increasing number of protein therapeutics being formulated at high concentrations (e.g., 5–100 mg/mL), challenges arise due to the tendency of proteins to aggregate more extensively. With a few simple modifications, similar high resolution second-derivative analysis can be employed at very high protein concentrations [60,61] (>100 mg/mL). At moderately high concentrations, short pathlength cells in the range of 10–1000 μm are available. To reduce the possibility of excessive scattering at ultrahigh concentrations, short pathlength cuvettes (as small as 1 μm) can be created by simply placing microliter volumes of protein samples on a quartz plate and sliding a second plate across it in a manner that allows the capillary action of the solution to fill the space between the plates. The protein concentration is then calculated from the measured absorbance value employing the Beer–Lambert law (corrected for the pathlength). This approach appreciably reduces the local heterogeneous distribution of the sample, allowing equal amount of light to interact with each chromophore (Section 8.10.2). Such measurements can be combined with techniques such as front surface fluorescence, FTIR spectroscopy, and differential scanning calorimetry to provide comprehensive analyses of highly concentrated protein solutions and suspensions over a very wide range of conditions.

8.7.4 Studies of Protein Dynamic Properties

Proteins are known to undergo a wide variety of internal motions of various magnitudes. Such rapid fluctuations in structure are thought to play a major role in protein stability and aggregation behavior. The complex interrelationship between protein dynamics and stability as well as function has been reviewed [62]. Such studies suggest that the analysis of protein flexibility in conjunction with their static properties provides a particularly valuable description of their properties. Thus, techniques that detect both time-averaged extensive and subtle conformational alterations of proteins, as well as those that detect internal motions, are critical for a comprehensive picture of protein behavior. A variety of methods have been used to measure various aspects of protein structure related to dynamic behavior. These techniques include isotope (H/D) exchange monitored by infrared spectroscopy, mass spectrometry, and nuclear magnetic resonance (NMR) spectroscopy as well as methods such as red edge shift spectroscopy, solute fluorescence quenching, ultrasonic spectroscopy, pressure perturbation scanning calorimetry, and molecular dynamics simulations. Recent investigations have demonstrated that high resolution second-derivative UV-absorption spectroscopy of aromatic amino acids can also be used as a qualitative probe of protein dynamics using the two different approaches described later.

8.7.5 Cation–π Interactions as a Probe of Protein Dynamics

By analogy to solute-based fluorescence quenching of proteins, Lucas et al. developed a UV-spectroscopy dynamic-based analyses by employing the spectral shifts induced by cation (Na^+, Li^+, and Cs^+)–π interactions in proteins as a function of increasing cation size and concentration [23]. Small cations were found to be more effective at inducing spectral shifts due to their ability to diffuse through a protein's matrix and make contact with the aromatic side chains. In some cases, interpretation of such effects can be difficult due to specific interactions between the cations (and perhaps accompanying counteranions) and proteins [23].

8.7.6   Temperature-Dependent Second-Derivative Absorbance Spectroscopy of Aromatic Residues as a Probe of Protein Dynamics

Plots of the temperature-dependent second-derivative peak positions of the aromatic residues have measurable slopes below protein-unfolding temperatures [44]. Experimental and computational studies suggest that such shifts are sensitive to the dielectric properties of the surrounding microenvironment as well as local motions of the aromatic side chains [63]. Considering the contribution of solvent penetration (due to protein dynamic motions) to the high polarizabilities and high dielectric constant values observed in protein interiors [64], a direct correlation between such slopes and hydration of the buried aromatic residues in protein cores appears to exist. Preliminary studies do indeed support this idea and suggest that temperature-dependent second-derivative peak shifts of the aromatic side chains can, in principle, be used as a qualitative probe of protein dynamics [63].

8.8   DIRECT MEASUREMENT OF PROTEIN AGGREGATION

In addition to the ability of UV-absorption spectroscopy to detect alterations in protein conformation and dynamic fluctuations, both of which could lead to protein aggregation, this technique has been widely employed to directly probe protein aggregation as well as analyze aggregation kinetics and identify the presence of intermediates and the underlying mechanisms involved. Such analyses often include time-dependent turbidity measurements to monitor the formation of aggregates or probing time-dependent protein monomer loss. Herein, we use the term *aggregation* to refer to any process including fibrillation, polymerization, gelation, etc. that leads to the formation of multimeric nonnative protein species.

8.8.1   Turbidity Measurements

Turbidity (τ) is defined as

$$\tau = -\ln(I/I_0) \tag{8.4}$$

where I_0 and I are the intensity of the incident and transmitted light, respectively. The measured optical density (OD) signal is related to turbidity according to

$$\tau = 2.303 \, \text{OD} \tag{8.5}$$

Note that $\text{OD} = A + S$, where S is the light extinction due to scattering and any other process that blocks light from being detected. Thus, when $A = 0$, the OD is the loss due to scattering under common circumstances. Furthermore, τ is a coefficient that reflects attenuation of the light passing through the sample. Such attenuation of light is often due to the presence of larger particles (i.e., multimers and aggregates) approaching $1/50–1/20$ or above of the wavelength of incident light in size. To reiterate, in the presence of such scattering contributions, the raw spectrum (Fig. 8.5, solid line) is referred to as *OD spectrum* and contains both absorbance and scattering signals. In the case of Rayleigh scattering ($\lambda <$ $1/20\lambda_i$), the scattered light is approximately proportional to the inverse fourth power of the incident wavelength. Therefore, it exhibits a gradual decrease (i.e., negative slope) in the OD signals (Fig. 8.5, dotted line) as a function of increasing wavelength in the nonabsorbing region of the spectrum (>320 nm). To obtain true absorption signals (Fig. 8.5, dashed line), the effect of light scattering must be subtracted from the total spectrum (Section 8.10).

A parameter commonly used to correct for turbidity (i.e., light scattering) effects is the aggregation index (AI) parameter defined according to the following equation:

$$AI = A_{350}/(A_{280} - A_{350}) \times 100 \tag{8.6}$$

where A_{280} and A_{350} are the measured absorbance at 280 and 350 nm, respectively. The AI parameter is usually more informative than just measuring OD_{350}, since it also corrects for protein content [65]. Most commercially available

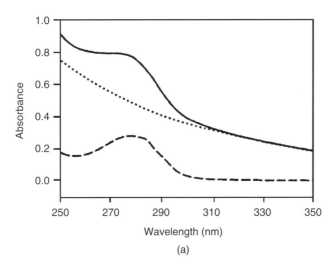

(a)

FIGURE 8.5 Near-UV spectrum of a 0.1 mg/mL solution of conjugates of polyribosyl ribitol phosphate and outer membrane protein complexes from Neisseria meningitidis PRP-OMPC (solid line). The light scattering contribution is removed by the subtraction of the extrapolated data (dotted line) from a linear plot of log OD versus log λ between 320 and 350 nm, and the resultant corrected spectrum is shown as the dashed line. Note the lack of OD in corrected spectrum above 310 nm. *Source:* Adapted from Mach et al. [25].

spectrophotometers are equipped with built-in algorithms that can be programmed to correct for scattering effects.

Although introducing significant difficulties in interpretation of absorbance data, light scattering (i.e., turbidity) has the potential to provide information concerning the association of proteins (i.e., oligomerization and aggregation). Thus, an increase in OD signals in the nonabsorbing region of a protein's UV spectrum (>320 nm) is typically taken as indicative of aggregation (i.e., the appearance of some form of larger species).

A classical example of this phenomenon involves studies of time-dependent deoxyhemoglobin S gelation as determined by monitoring turbidity signals at 700 nm. Figure 8.6 shows the effect of temperature on deoxyhemoglobin S gelation rate in which both the onset and extent of gelation are shown to be temperature dependent. Increasing temperature shortens the characteristic lag phase associated with this nucleation-dependent mechanism (Section 8.8.3). It also increases the extent of gelation as detected by larger OD values as a function of increasing temperature [66].

Another example involves studies of actin filament formation in which actin exhibits distinct filament formation pathways in the presence and absence of calcium or magnesium. In the absence of these divalent cations, actin filament formation proceeds via an exclusive nucleation–elongation event with short lag times and a slow approach to the final equilibrium phase (Fig. 8.7a). In the presence of calcium or magnesium, however, a nucleation–elongation–fragmentation process (in which new filaments are also formed by the addition of the fragmented

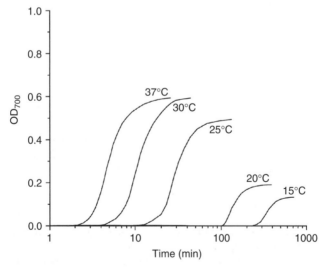

FIGURE 8.6 Effect of temperature on the rate of aggregation of deoxy Hb-S. Hemoglobin (0.09 g/dL) in 1.8 M phosphate buffer, pH 7.34. The protein was heated from $0°C$ to the temperature indicated in the figure. *Source:* Adapted from Adachi et al. [66].

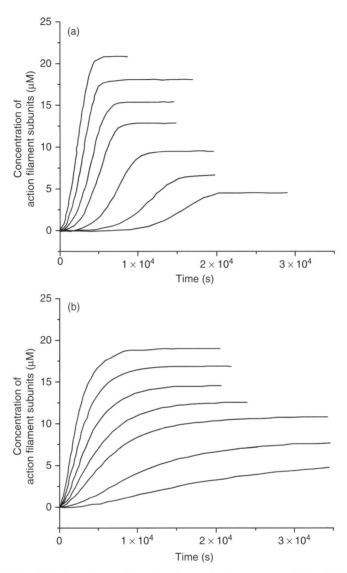

FIGURE 8.7 (a) Polymerization kinetics of actin in the presence of 40 mM KCl. Total actin concentrations 7.4, 9.6, 12.4, 14.2, 16.2, 18.4, and 20.5 μM. (b) Polymerization kinetics of actin in the presence of 0.6 mM MgCl$_2$ and 0.5 mM EGTA. Total actin concentrations 6.7, 8.5, 11.5, 14.9, 17.3, 20.3, and 22.9 μM. *Source:* Adapted from Wegner et al. [67].

filaments) is shown to exist [67] in which long lag phases of polymerization are followed by strongly increasing polymerization rates to reach the final equilibrium stage (Fig. 8.7b).

The aforementioned studies and many others available in literature show that by studying the shape and characteristics of kinetic-based turbidity plots as a function of variety of variables (e.g., protein monomer concentration, temperature, incubation time, pH, ionic strength, presence of additives), information regarding the underlying mechanisms involved in protein aggregation can be obtained. More detailed quantitative analysis of protein aggregation mechanisms is often achieved by associated mathematical treatment and modeling of such data. A description of mathematical models and computational methods used to predict a variety of different protein aggregation pathways is beyond the scope of this chapter and can be found elsewhere [68].

Aggregation kinetics of a wide variety of proteins have been studied employing turbidity measurements. A few examples include studies of the effect of sucrose on the aggregation of recombinant basic fibroblast growth factor [69], the effect of dianions on the aggregation of alcohol dehydrogenase [70], the effect of pH and protein concentration on the aggregation kinetic rates of cryoglobulins [71], the effect of pressure and temperature on amyloid fibril formation [72], the effect of silicone oil on protein aggregation [73], and the effect of low temperatures on the cold-induced precipitation of a variety of monoclonal cryoglobulins [71].

Kinetic-based turbidity measurements can be used in protein pharmaceutical preformulation studies [74–76], in a high throughput mode employing plate-reader-based spectrophotometers to screen a large number of solution conditions and solutes based on their inhibitory effect on protein aggregation. Percent inhibition of aggregation (%IA.) is typically quantitatively estimated according to the following equation:

$$\%\text{IA} = 100 - [\text{OD}_{350(\text{Sample})}/\text{OD}_{350(\text{Ref})}] \times 100 \qquad (8.7)$$

where $\text{OD}_{350(\text{Sample})}$ and $\text{OD}_{350(\text{Ref})}$ are the changes in the OD of the protein at a certain wavelength above 320 nm (350 nm in this case) in the presence and absence of a given solution stress variable over similar incubation times, respectively.

Employing turbidity measurements, protein aggregation can also be monitored as a function of a variety of solution conditions in a nonkinetic manner. The most common such use is to monitor protein thermal unfolding/aggregation from which the onset and/or midpoint of unfolding/aggregation transition temperatures can be estimated.

Figure 8.8 illustrates the pH-dependent aggregation behavior of FGF20 [77] in which shifts of the temperature of aggregation onsets to lower values are observed as a function of decreasing pH. This demonstrates the enhanced aggregation tendencies of FGF20 at more acidic pH values. The following decrease in OD signals at higher temperatures after an initial increase is indicative of protein precipitation out of solution and therefore out of the path of the incident light. Thermal aggregation of a wide variety of proteins has been studied employing this approach [61,74,77,78]. Such studies are also employed in protein pharmaceutical preformulation studies in which the stabilizing effect of a certain solution variable or solute on the onset and extent of thermal aggregation is monitored for screening purposes.

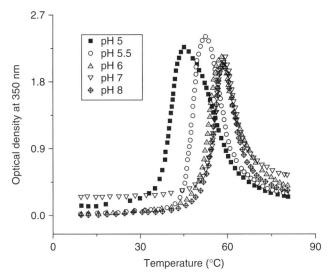

FIGURE 8.8   Aggregation behavior of FGF20. Optical densities at 350 nm (OD_{350}) are recorded as a function of temperature for FGF20 at pH 5–8. *Source:* Adapted from Fan et al. [77].

8.8.2 Monomer Loss Kinetics

Monitoring the time-dependent loss of protein monomeric species can also provide insight into the mechanisms by which aggregation proceeds. In such studies, proteins are incubated over time and the concentration of monomers (after removal of the higher order species using filtration or centrifugation) is determined at different time points employing absorbance measurements, often at 280 nm. The lack of removal of soluble, associated species may, however, limit the accuracy of this approach. The time-dependent monomer concentration data are then used to develop correlations based on the principal monomer loss rate expression:

$$v_M = -d[M]/dt \tag{8.8}$$

where v_M is the monomer loss rate; M, the protein concentration; and t, the time. Monomer loss analyses are much simpler than those of aggregate formation since one has to only deal with homogeneous monomeric protein solutions and does not need to worry about the heterogeneous, multisize distribution of aggregated species. Although used, some argue that definitive conclusions concerning pathways of aggregation should not be drawn based solely on the results from such analyses but that aggregation size and morphology should also be considered [79]. Simultaneous analysis of aggregation growth kinetics is recommended since the presence of soluble aggregates at levels below the limit of detection of most analytical techniques might introduce artifacts in interpretation of kinetic aggregation pathways [68].

8.8.3 Nucleation and Growth

Following the onset of aggregation, the number and size of protein aggregates increase as the native population is depleted. This often results in an exponential growth of aggregates followed by a steady-state plateau in which equilibrium between remaining monomers and the aggregates formed is reached (Fig. 8.9, dashed line).

Many if not most proteins, however, show a characteristic lag phase before the onset of aggregation, during which the protein solution remains clear without the detection of any visual aggregates (Fig. 8.9, solid line). Turbidity measurements may also be unable to detect the presence of any higher molecular weight material. This lag phase presumably reflects the presence of a critical nucleation event [80–84]. Studies on 14 representative proteins involved in a variety of neurodegenerative diseases show that a nucleation-dependent aggregation pathway is involved in the self-assembly of all the examined proteins into amyloid fibrils. In each case, a rate-limiting nucleation event, followed by a fast, autocatalytic growth phase, was observed [84].

In the nucleation phase, serial associations of monomers are usually thermodynamically unfavorable (the intermolecular interactions do not outweigh the entropic contributions). Once the nucleus is formed, however, it serves as perhaps a nonspecified template to which remaining monomeric units can be added, providing a thermodynamically favorable process due to the much greater contact surface area available [85]. Such nucleation-based aggregation mechanisms are, therefore, highly dependent on initial protein concentration where increasing concentrations often result in shortening of the particular lag phase observed.

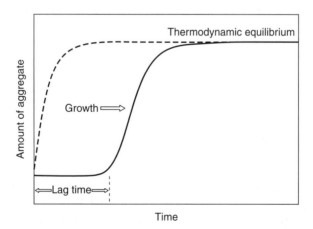

FIGURE 8.9 Experimentally observable formation of aggregates for a nucleation-dependent process above the critical concentration. Aggregate formation is indicated by a solid line. At high concentration, nucleation is so rapid that no lag phase is observable (dashed line). Addition of a nucleus or seed supplants the requirement for nucleation and also results in rapid polymerization. *Source:* Adapted from Jarrett et al. [85].

A classical example is the studies of Hofrichter et al. on deoxyhemoglobin S gelation in which an empirical relationship between the nucleation lag phase (t_d), and initial protein concentration was shown to exist (i.e., t_d is proportional to C_t^{-z}) where C_t is the initial total protein concentration and z is the number of molecules in the nuclei [86,87]. Therefore, employing kinetic turbidity-based measurements supplemented with further mathematical treatments and modeling of the kinetic profiles at the early stages of aggregation, one can estimate the critical nucleus size, an important parameter in nucleation-dependent aggregation often perceived as a barrier above which the growth (i.e., propagation) step starts [88–90].

Figure 8.10 shows the effect of seeding on fibrillogenesis of α-synuclein in which the rate of α-synuclein monomer loss (as measured by A_{280} values on removal of the aggregates using centrifugation) is significantly enhanced as a function of increasing preformed nuclei to the monomeric α-synuclein solution (solid squares are representative of a nonseeded control sample and open squares contain the upper limit of 10% seeded material) [91].

Employing UV-absorption spectroscopy, however, caution should be exercised when interpreting the precise nature of the nucleation phase since turbidity assays may not be sensitive to the presence of aggregates below a threshold size [92] (i.e., critical nucleus concentration).

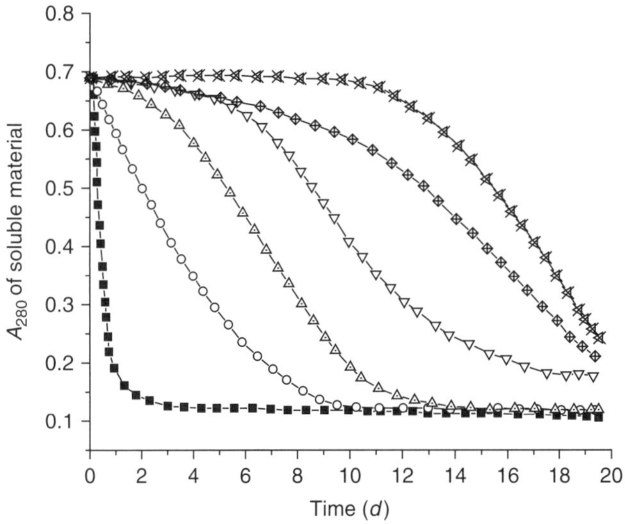

FIGURE 8.10 Seeding of α-synuclein aggregation. Aggregate formation of wild-type α-synuclein at 2 mg/mL as monitored by A_{280} of soluble material following ultracentrifugation. A nonseeded control incubation (✕) is shown along with incubations containing preformed wild-type α-synuclein aggregates as seeds. Seed concentrations from top to bottom in the plot, expressed as a percentage of the soluble α-synuclein amount, are 0.001 (⊕), 0.01 (▽), 0.1 (△), 1 (○), and 10% (■), respectively. *Source:* Adapted from Wood et al. [91].

8.9 UTILITY OF EXTRINSIC DYES TO DETECT PROTEIN AGGREGATION

In addition to intrinsic protein chromophores, a variety of extrinsic chromophores can be used to detect conformationally altered or aggregated proteins. A number of dyes can either covalently or noncovalently interact with proteins in a manner in which they exhibit striking spectroscopic differences in their free and bound states. Extrinsic dyes are often employed in fluorescence spectroscopy but have less frequently been employed in near-UV and visible absorption spectroscopic studies of proteins. CR has been commonly used as a tool for the early detection of amyloidogenesis during amyloid fibril formation in Alzheimer's disease [18,19]. This dye binds with a high selectivity to proteins containing extended intermolecular β-sheet structure, a defining characteristic of amyloid fibrils. Inouye et al. showed that the binding of CR to amyloid fibrils occurs through both ionic and nonionic processes. In the former, the negatively charged sulfonate groups of CR bind to positively charged histidine residues in target proteins, a pH-dependent event. The latter binding was proposed to be due to van der Waals interactions of the dye π system with the protein. Other macromolecules such as RNA polymerase [93], dehydrogenases [94] (e.g., lactic, equine, and yeast alcohol), cellulose [95], elastin [96], chitin [97], and HIV-1 protease [98] also bind CR, making it a frequently effective tool for the study of their solution (aggregation and conformational) behavior.

ThT is another dye commonly used for conformational and aggregation analysis of proteins. As CR, it is especially sensitive to the formation of fibrils. Both the extinction coefficient and the position of the long-wavelength absorption band of ThT depend on solvent polarity [16]. Fibril-bound ThT exhibits a long-wavelength absorption band at $\sim$450 nm, which is significantly redshifted compared to its position in water at $\sim$412 nm. Therefore, it can also be used for the detection of fibril formation as well as perhaps related structures in β-sheet-rich systems.

8.10 SOME PRACTICAL CONSIDERATIONS

8.10.1 Light Scattering Corrections

Some theoretical background and the need for scattering corrections have already been discussed. Corrections can be made either physically (removing aggregates by centrifugation or filtration) or mathematically. Mathematically based analyses include the subtraction of the scattering contribution from the zero-order spectrum (absorbance+light scattering) to obtain true absorbance values. In addition, since OD and the wavelength of incident light (λ) are related according to [99]

$$\ln(OD) = a \ln \lambda + b \tag{8.9}$$

corrections can also be made by fitting the nonabsorbing region of the UV spectrum (320–400) to Equation (8.9) and subtracting it from the zero-order spectrum.

Most currently available spectrophotometric software packages include mathematical algorithms that can be used for correcting light scattering effects. It should also be noted, however, that this procedure only corrects for Rayleigh scattering (i.e., small particles) and not contributions from much larger particles (i.e., which involves Mie and multiple scattering) or the phenomenon of absorption flattening.

8.10.2 Absorption Flattening

As the size of particles become larger, absorption flattening, a phenomenon in which the chromophores within or among particles obscure each other, may occur [100]. This is common when studying proteins at high concentration or in the presence of extensive aggregation in which regions of high local concentrations produce inhomogeneous distributions of the sample, preventing an equal amount of light from reaching each chromophore [42]. Under such conditions, light going through the sample has a lessened probability of encountering the absorbing phase. Care must be taken when analyzing such data since absorption flattening often results in redshifts of the absorption bands and reduced signal intensity. This can be erroneously interpreted as changes in the microenvironment of the chromophore due to protein structural alterations. A simple and common corrective experimental approach is to use short pathlength cuvettes, which results in a more uniform distribution of protein in the light path [101].

8.10.3 Studies of Proteins at High and Low Concentrations

Deviations from the Beer–Lambert law can occur when examining proteins at very high or low concentrations due to the nonlinearity of the Beer–Lambert law at extreme concentrations. Most commercially available spectrophotometers have a wide linear range between 0.05 and 2 absorbance units, although this may vary considerably based on the instrument type and manufacturer as discussed above; it is well established that at high protein concentrations, the presence of aggregation and excessive light scattering signals as well as the phenomenon of absorption flattening can introduce significant artifacts. In addition, at very low protein concentrations (<0.05 A), adsorption of protein to the sides of cuvettes can be problematic since at such low concentrations the ratio of the amount of protein adsorbed to that in solution becomes significant. Since the spectral properties of adsorbed protein can differ significantly from that of native states due to surface-induced conformational alterations [102], great care must also be taken in the interpretation of spectral data under such conditions.

8.11 CONCLUSIONS

Recent advances, particularly the advent of diode-array detectors and applications of high resolution derivative analysis, have renewed interest in the use of absorption spectroscopy to study protein aggregation in conjunction with other techniques. Both major and subtle protein conformational alterations as well as direct detection of aggregation can all be probed by absorption and OD spectroscopy in a single comprehensive measurement conducted over a short period of time. Measurements of protein UV spectra between 190 and 400 nm provide information on secondary (190–220 nm), tertiary (250–300), and aggregation behavior (>320 nm) simultaneously in response to a wide variety of environmental perturbations. Because UV-absorption spectroscopy can measure aspects of secondary, tertiary, and quaternary structure simultaneously, it has the potential to probe the presence of intermediate states that are considered to be aggregation prone. These states are characterized by their extensive secondary structure and minimal tertiary structural interactions [103]. The tertiary structural information obtained from data in the 240- to 300-nm region is especially useful when combined with commonly used secondary structure-sensitive techniques such as CD and FTIR spectroscopy.

Derivative analysis allows highly precise and accurate measurements of both intensity and peak positions of protein chromophores with an effective resolution of the latter approaching 0.01 nm. One significant advantage of the UV-absorption technique is the simultaneous and precise monitoring of the microenvironment of all three aromatic amino acid side chains. Phenylalanine and tyrosine have very low fluorescence quantum yields, and their emission characteristics are relatively insensitive to alterations in their local environments. In contrast, absorption measurements of their properties are quite sensitive.

Information regarding aggregation tendencies as well as detailed descriptions of the underlying mechanisms involved in such events can all be obtained by simply monitoring OD signals at nonabsorbing wavelengths of protein UV spectra. Qualitative and quantitative analysis of the nucleation and growth phases involved in aggregation are possible by studying the shape and often characteristics of the time-dependent turbidity signals and by modeling of such data. Overall, absorption spectroscopy has much to offer in structural analysis of proteins and other macromolecules in the context of their aggregation behavior.

REFERENCES

1. Beaven GH, Holiday ER. Ultraviolet absorption spectra of proteins and amino acids. Adv Protein Chem 1952;7:319–386.
2. Zhang Z, Smith DL, Smith JB. Human β-crystallins modified by backbone cleavage, deamidation and oxidation are prone to associate. Exp Eye Res 2003;77(3): 259–272.
3. Ramachandran LK, Witkop B. Selective cleavage of C-tryptophyl peptide bonds in proteins and peptides. J Am Chem Soc 1959;81:4028–4032.
4. Morrison WW, Frajola WJ. Multiple assay of tryptophan pyrrolase in Drosophila. Ohio J Sci 1968;68(6):285–290.
5. Wetlaufer DB. Ultraviolet spectra of proteins and amino acids. Adv Protein Chem 1962;17:303–390.

6. Balestrieri C, Colonna G, Giovane A, Irace G, Servillo L. Second-derivative spectroscopy of proteins: studies on tyrosyl residues. Anal Biochem 1980;106(1):49–54.

7. Gemmill CL. The effects of iodine on the ultraviolet absorption spectra of thyroglobulin, casein, and insulin. Arch Biochem Biophys 1956;63:192–200.

8. Thompson EOP. Modification of tyrosine during performic acid oxidation. Biochim Biophys Acta 1954;15:440–441.

9. Raven DJ, Earland C, Littler M. Occurrence of dityrosine in Tussah silk fibroin and keratin. Biochim Biophys Acta, Protein Struct 1971;251(1):96–99.

10. LaBella FS, Keeley FW, Vivian S, Thornhill DP. Evidence for dityrosine in elastin. Biochem Biophys Res Commun 1967;26(6):748–753.

11. Waykole P, Heidemann E. Dityrosine in collagen. Connect Tissue Res 1976;4(4):219–222.

12. Harms GS, Pauls SW, Hedstrom JF, Johnson CK. Fluorescence and rotational dynamics of dityrosine. J Fluoresc 1997;7(4):283–292.

13. Rosenheck K, Doty P. The far-ultraviolet absorption spectra of polypeptide and protein solutions and their dependence on conformation. Proc Natl Acad Sci U S A 1961;47:1775–1785.

14. McGlynn SP, Chaudhuri JN, Good M. Possible effect of charge transfer complexation on the dihedral angle of dialkyl disulfides. J Am Chem Soc 1962;84:9–12.

15. Favilla R, Goldoni M, Del Signore F, Di Muro P, Salvato B, Beltramini M. Guanidinium chloride induced unfolding of a hemocyanin subunit from Carcinus aestuarii II. Holo form. Biochim Biophys Acta Protein Struct Mol Enzymol 2002;1597(1):51–59.

16. Vergani L, Grattarola M, Dondero F, Viarengo A. Expression, purification, and characterization of metallothionein-A from rainbow trout. Protein Expr Purif 2003;27(2):338–345.

17. Burke CJ, Sanyal G, Bruner MW, Ryan JA, LaFemina RL, Robbins HL, Zeft AS, Middaugh CR, Cordingley MG. Structural implications of spectroscopic characterization of a putative zinc finger peptide from HIV-1 integrase. J Biol Chem 1992;267(14):9639–9644.

18. Inouye H, Kirschner DA. Alzheimer's β-amyloid: insights into fibril formation and structure from congo red binding. Subcell Biochem 2005;38:203–224. (Alzheimer's disease: cellular and molecular aspects of amyloid β).

19. Inouye H, Kirschner DA. Aβ fibrillogenesis: kinetic parameters for fibril formation from Congo Red binding. J Struct Biol 2000;130(2/3):123–129.

20. Maskevich AA, Stsiapura VI, Kuzmitsky VA, Kuznetsova IM, Povarova OI, Uversky VN, Turoverov KK. Spectral properties of thioflavin T in solvents with different dielectric properties and in a fibril-incorporated form. J Proteome Res 2007;6(4):1392–1401.

21. Luong TN, Kirsch JF. A continuous coupled spectrophotometric assay for tyrosine aminotransferase activity with aromatic and other nonpolar amino acids. Anal Biochem 1997;253(1):46–49.

22. Piersma SR, Visser AJWG, de Vries S, Duine JA. Optical spectroscopy of nicotinoprotein alcohol dehydrogenase from Amycolatopsis methanolica: a comparison with horse liver alcohol dehydrogenase and UDP-galactose epimerase. Biochemistry 1998;37(9):3068–3077.

23. Lucas LH, Ersoy BA, Kueltzo LA, Joshi SB, Brandau DT, Thyagarajapuram N, Peek LJ, Middaugh CR. Probing protein structure and dynamics by second-derivative ultraviolet absorption analysis of cation-π interactions. Protein Sci 2006;15(10):2228–2243.

24. Ichikawa T, Terada H. Estimation of state and amount of phenylalanine residues in proteins by second derivative spectrophotometry. Biochim Biophys Acta Protein Struct 1979;580(1):120–128.

25. Mach H, Volkin DB, Burke CJ, Middaugh CR. Ultraviolet absorption spectroscopy. Methods Mol Biol 1995;40:91–114. Totowa (NJ), USA.

26. Mach H, Sanyal G, Volkin DB, Middaugh CR. Applications of ultraviolet absorption spectroscopy to the analysis of biopharmaceuticals. Therapeutic protein and peptide formulation and delivery, ACS Symposium Series, No. 675.Washington (DC): ACS Publications; 1997. pp. 186–205.

27. Balestrieri C, Colonna G, Giovane A, Irace G, Servillo L. Second-derivative spectroscopy of proteins. A method for the quantitative determination of aromatic amino acids in proteins. Eur J Biochem 1978;90(3):433–440.

28. Servillo L, Colonna G, Balestrieri C, Ragone R, Irace G. Simultaneous determination of tyrosine and tryptophan residues in proteins by second-derivative spectroscopy. Anal Biochem 1982;126(2):251–257.

29. Brandts JF. The thermodynamics of protein denaturation. I. The denaturation of chymotrypsinogen. J Am Chem Soc 1964;86(20):4291–4301.

30. Brandts JF. The thermodynamics of protein denaturation. II. A model of reversible denaturation and interpretations regarding the stability of chymotrypsinogen. J Am Chem Soc 1964;86(20):4302–4314.

31. Hayashi K, Imoto T, Funatsu M. The enzyme-substrate complex in a muramidase-catalyzed reaction. I. Difference spectrum of the complex. J Biochem 1963;54(5):381–387. (Tokyo, Japan).

32. Ray A, Reynolds JA, Polet H, Steinhardt J. Binding of large organic anions and neutral molecules by native bovine serum albumin. Biochemistry 1966;5(8):2606–2616.

33. Donovan JW. Changes in ultraviolet absorption produced by alteration of protein conformation. J Biol Chem 1969;244(8):1961–1967.

34. Chervenka CH. Ultraviolet spectral changes related to the enzymic activity of chymotrypsin. Biochem Biophys Acta 1959;31:85–95.

35. Bailey JE, Beaven GH, Chignell DA, Gratzer WB. Analysis of perturbations in the ultraviolet absorption spectra of proteins and model compounds. Eur J Biochem 1968;7(1):5–14.

36. Kornblatt JA, Kornblatt MJ, Lange R, Mombelli E, Guillemette JG. The individual tyrosines of proteins: their spectra may or may not differ from those in water or other solvents. Biochim Biophys Acta Protein Struct Mol Enzymol 1999;1431(1):238–248.

37. Herskovits T, Laskowski M Jr. Location of chromophoric residues in proteins by solvent perturbation. I. Tyrosyls in serum albumins. J Biol Chem 1962;237:2481–2492.

38. De Young LR, Dill KA, Fink AL. Aggregation and denaturation of apomyoglobin in aqueous urea solutions. Biochemistry 1993;32(15):3877–3886.

39. Stigter D, Dill KA. Theory for protein solubilities. Fluid Phase Equilib 1993; 82:237–249.

40. Fields GB, Alonso DOV, Stigter D, Dill KA. Theory for the aggregation of proteins and copolymers. J Phys Chem 1992;96(10):3974–3981.

41. Fink AL. Protein aggregation: folding aggregates, inclusion bodies and amyloid. Fold Des 1998;3(1): R9–R23.

42. Kueltzo LA, Middaugh CR. Ultraviolet absorption spectroscopy. Biotechnol: Pharm Aspects 2005;3:1–25. (Methods for Structural Analysis of Protein Pharmaceuticals).

43. Lange R, Balny C. UV-visible derivative spectroscopy under high pressure. Biochem Biophys Acta Protein Struct Mol Enzymol 2002;1595(1–2):80–93.

44. Kueltzo LA, Ersoy B, Ralston JP, Middaugh CR. Derivative absorbance spectroscopy and protein phase diagrams as tools for comprehensive protein characterization: a bGCSF case study. J Pharm Sci 2003;92:1805–1820.

45. Fan H, Vitharana SN, Chen T, O'Keefe D, Middaugh CR. Effects of pH and polyanions on the thermal stability of fibroblast growth factor 20. Mol Pharm 2007;4:232–240.

46. Fan H, Kashi RS, Middaugh CR. Conformational lability of two molecular chaperones Hsc70 and GP96: effects of pH and temperature. Arch Biochem Biophys 2006;447:34–45.

47. Fan H, Ralston J, DiBase M, Faulkner E, Middaugh CR. Solution behavior of IFN-β-1a: an empirical phase diagram based approach. J Pharm Sci 2005;94:1893–1911.

48. Fan H, Li H, Zhang M, Middaugh CR. Effects of solutes on empirical phase diagrams of human fibroblast growth factor 1. J Pharm Sci 2007;96:1490–1503.

49. Esfandiary R, Kickhoefer VA, Rome LH, Joshi SB, Middaugh CR. Structural stability of vault particles. J Pharm Sci 2009;98(4):1376–1386.

50. Peek LJ, Brey RN, Middaugh CR. A rapid, three-step process for the preformulation of a recombinant ricin toxin A-chain vaccine. J Pharm Sci 2007;96:44–60.

51. Brandau DT, Joshi SB, Smalter AM, Kim S, Steadman B, Middaugh CR. Stability of the Clostridium botulinum type A neurotoxin complex: an empirical phase diagram based approach. Mol Pharm 2007;4:571–582.

52. Ausar SF, Rexroad J, Frolov VG, Look JL, Konar N, Middaugh CR. Analysis of the thermal and pH stability of human respiratory syncytial virus. Mol Pharm 2005;2:491–499.

53. Ausar SF, Foubert TR, Hudson MH, Vedvick TS, Middaugh CR. Conformational stability and disassembly of Norwalk virus like particles: effect of pH and temperature. J Biol Chem 2006;281:19478–19488.

54. Harn N, Allan C, Oliver C, Middaugh CR. Highly concentrated monoclonal antibodies: direct analysis of structure and stability. J Pharm Sci 2007;96:532–546.

55. Peek LJ, Brandau DT, Jones LS, Joshi SB, Middaugh CR. A systematic approach to stabilizing EBA-175 RII-NG for use as a malaria vaccine. Vaccine 2006;24:5839–5851.

56. Rexroad J, Martin TT, McNeilly D, Godwin S, Middaugh CR. Thermal stability of adenovirus type 2 as a function of pH. J Pharm Sci 2006;95:1469–1479.

57. Rexroad J, Evans RK, Middaugh CR. Effect of pH and ionic strength on the physical stability of adenovirus type 5. J Pharm Sci 2006;95:237–247.

58. Ruponen M, Braun CS, Middaugh CR. Biophysical characterization of polymeric and liposomal gene delivery systems using empirical phase diagrams. J Pharm Sci 2006;95:2101–2114.

59. Thyagrajapuram N, Olsen D, Middaugh CR. The structure stability and complex behavior of recombinant human gelatins. J Pharm Sci 2007;96:3363–3378.

60. Guo J, Harn N, Robbins A, Dougherty R, Middaugh CR. Stability of helix-rich proteins at high concentrations. Biochemistry 2006;45(28):8686–8696.

61. Harn N, Allan C, Oliver C, Middaugh CR. Highly concentrated monoclonal antibody solutions: direct analysis of physical structure and thermal stability. J Pharm Sci 2007;96(3):532–546.

62. Kamerzell TJ, Middaugh CR. The complex inter-relationships between protein flexibility and stability. J Pharm Sci 2008;97(9):3494–3517.

63. Esfandiary R, Hunjan JS, Lushington GH, Joshi SB, Middaugh CR. Temperature dependent 2nd derivative absorbance spectroscopy of aromatic amino acids as a probe of protein dynamics. Protein Sci 2009;18(12):2603–2614.

64. Dwyer JJ, Gittis AG, Karp DA, Lattman EE, Spencer DS, Stites WE, Garcia-Moreno E B. High apparent dielectric constants in the interior of a protein reflect water penetration. Biophys J 2000;79(3):1610–1620.

65. Wang W, Wang YJ, Wang DQ. Dual effects of Tween 80 on protein stability. Int J Pharm 2008;347(1–2):31–38.

66. Adachi K, Asakura T. Nucleation-controlled aggregation of deoxyhemoglobin S. Possible difference in the size of nuclei in different phosphate concentrations. J Biol Chem 1979;254(16):7765–7771.

67. Wegner A, Savko P. Fragmentation of actin filaments. Biochemistry 1982;21(8):1909–1913.

68. Murphy R, Tsai A Misbehaving proteins: protein (mis) folding, aggregation, and stability. New York (NY): Springer Science; 2006.

69. Eberlein GA, Stratton PR, Wang YJ. Stability of rhbFGF as determined by UV spectroscopic measurements of turbidity. PDA J Pharm Sci Technol 1994;48(5):224–230.

70. MacLean DS, Qian Q, Middaugh CR. Stabilization of proteins by low molecular weight multi-ions. J Pharm Sci 2002;91(10):2220–2229.

71. Middaugh CR, Kehoe JM, Prystowsky MB, Gerber-Jenson B, Jenson JC, Litman GW. Molecular basis for the temperature-dependent insolubility of cryoglobulins. IV. Structural studies of the IgM monoclonal cryoglobulin McE. Immunochemistry 1978;15(3):171–187.

72. Kim Y-S, Randolph TW, Seefeldt MB, Carpenter JF. High-pressure studies on protein aggregates and amyloid fibrils. Methods Enzymol 2006;413:237–253. (Amyloid, Prions, and Other Protein Aggregates, Part C).

73. Jones LS, Kaufmann A, Middaugh CR. Silicone oil induced aggregation of proteins. J Pharm Sci 2005;94(4):918–927.

74. Jiang G, Joshi SB, Peek LJ, Brandau DT, Huang CR, Ferriter MS, Woodley WD, Ford BM, Mar KD, Mikszta JA, Hwang CR, Ulrich R, Harvey NG, Middaugh CR, Sullivan VJ. Anthrax vaccine powder formulations for nasal mucosal delivery. J Pharm Sci 2006;95:80–96.

75. Kissmann J, Ausar SF, Foubert TR, Brock J, Switzer MH, Detzi EJ, Vedvick TS, Middaugh CR. Physical stabilization of Norwalk virus-like particles. J Pharm Sci 2008;97(10):4208–4218.

76. Ausar SF, Espina M, Brock J, Thyagarayapuran N, Repetto R, Khandke L, Middaugh CR. High-throughput screening of stabilizers for respiratory syncytial virus: identification of stabilizers and their effects on the conformational thermostability of viral particles. Hum Vaccines 2007;3(3):94–103.

77. Fan H, Vitharana SN, Chen T, O'Keefe D, Middaugh CR. Effects of pH and polyanions on the thermal stability of fibroblast growth factor 20. Mol Pharm 2007;4(2):232–240.

78. Salnikova MS, Joshi SB, Rytting JH, Warny M, Middaugh CR. Physical characterization of clostridium difficile toxins and toxoids: effect of the formaldehyde crosslinking on thermal stability. J Pharm Sci 2008;97(9):3735–3752.

79. Murphy RM. Kinetics of amyloid formation and membrane interaction with amyloidogenic proteins. Biochim Biophys Acta Biomembr 2007;1768(8):1923–1934.

80. Kim Y-S, Cape SP, Chi E, Raffen R, Wilkins-Stevens P, Stevens FJ, Manning MC, Randolph TW, Solomon A, Carpenter JF. Counteracting effects of renal solutes on amyloid fibril formation by immunoglobulin light chains. J Biol Chem 2001;276(2):1626–1633.

81. Hamada D, Dobson CM. A kinetic study of β-lactoglobulin amyloid fibril formation promoted by urea. Protein Sci 2002;11(10):2417–2426.

82. Come JH, Fraser PE, Lansbury PT Jr. A kinetic model for amyloid formation in the prion diseases: importance of seeding. Proc Natl Acad Sci U S A 1993;90(13):5959–5963.

83. Zurdo J, Guijarro JI, Jimenez JL, Saibil HR, Dobson CM. Dependence on solution conditions of aggregation and amyloid formation by an SH3 domain. J Mol Biol 2001;311(2):325–340.

84. Morris AM, Watzky MA, Agar JN, Finke RG. Fitting neurological protein aggregation kinetic data via a 2-step, minimal/"Ockham's razor" model: the Finke-Watzky mechanism of nucleation followed by autocatalytic surface growth. Biochemistry 2008;47(8):2413–2427.

85. Jarrett JT, Lansbury PT Jr. Seeding "one-dimensional crystallization" of amyloid: a pathogenic mechanism in Alzheimer's disease and scrapie? Cell 1993; 73(6):1055–1058.

86. Hofrichter J, Ross PD, Eaton WA. Kinetics and mechanism of deoxyhemoglobin S gelation. New approach to understanding sickle cell disease. Proc Natl Acad Sci U S A 1974;71(12):4864–4868.

87. Hofrichter J, Ross PD, Eaton WA. Supersaturation in sickle cell hemoglobin solutions. Proc Natl Acad Sci U S A 1976;73(9):3035–3039.

88. Cellmer T, Douma R, Huebner A, Prausnitz J, Blanch H. Kinetic studies of protein L aggregation and disaggregation. Biophys Chem 2007;125(2–3):350–359.

89. Kodaka M. Interpretation of concentration-dependence in aggregation kinetics. Biophys Chem 2004;109(2):325–332.

90. Andrews JM, Weiss WF, Roberts CJ IV. Nucleation, growth, and activation energies for seeded and unseeded aggregation of α-chymotrypsinogen A. Biochemistry 2008;47(8):2397–2403.

91. Wood SJ, Wypych J, Steavenson S, Louis J-C, Citron M, Biere AL. α-Synuclein fibrillogenesis is nucleation-dependent. Implications for the pathogenesis of Parkinson's disease. J Biol Chem 1999;274(28):19509–19512.

92. Roberts CJ. Non-native protein aggregation kinetics. Biotechnol Bioeng 2007;98(5):927–938.

93. Woody AYM, Reisbig RR, Woody RW. Spectroscopic studies of Congo Red binding to RNA polymerase. Biochim Biophys Acta Nucleic Acids Protein Synth 1981;655(1):82–88.

94. Edwards RA, Woody RW. Spectroscopic studies of Cibacron Blue and Congo Red bound to dehydrogenases and kinases. Evaluation of dyes as probes of the dinucleotide fold. Biochemistry 1979;18(23):5197–5204.

95. Quenin I, Henrissat B. Precipitation and crystallization of cellulose doped with dyes. Makromol Chem Rapid Commun 1985;6(11):737–741.

96. Tan OT, Faris B, Franzblau C. Aortic elastin fluorescence after in vivo labeling with Congo Red. J Fluoresc 1991;1(2):147–151.

97. Bartnicki-Garcia S, Persson J, Chanzy H. An electron microscope and electron diffraction study of the effect of calcofluor and Congo red on the biosynthesis of chitin in vitro. Arch Biochem Biophys 1994;310(1):6–15.

98. Ojala WH, Ojala CR, Gleason WB. The X-ray crystal structure of the sulfonated azo dye Congo Red, a non-peptidic inhibitor of HIV-1 protease which also binds to reverse transcriptase and amyloid proteins. Antivir Chem Chemother 1995;6(1):25–33.

99. Timasheff SN. Turbidity as a criterion of coagulation. J Colloid Interface Sci 1966;21(5):489–497.

100. Duysens LNM. Flattening of the absorption spectrum of suspensions, as compared to that of solutions. Biochim Biophys Acta 1956;19:1–12.

101. Schneider AS, Harmatz D. An experimental method correcting for absorption flattening and scattering in suspensions of absorbing particles: circular dichroism and absorption spectra of hemoglobin in situ in red blood cells. Biochemistry 1976;15(19):4158–4162.

102. Jones LS, Bam NB, Randolph TW. Surfactant-stabilized protein formulations: a review of protein-surfactant interactions and novel analytical methodologies. Therapeutic protein and peptide formulation and delivery, ACS Symposium Series, No. 675. Washington (DC): ACS Publications;1997. pp. 206–222.

103. Kuwajima K. The molten globule state as a clue for understanding the folding and cooperativity of globular-protein structure. Proteins 1989;6:87–103.

9 Fluorescence Spectroscopy to Characterize Protein Aggregates and Particles

ROBERT A. POOLE, ANDREA HAWE, and WIM JISKOOT

Division of Drug Delivery Technology, Biologics Formulation Group, Leiden University, Leiden, The Netherlands

KEVIN BRAECKMANS

Laboratory of General Biochemistry and Physical Pharmacy, Ghent University, Ghent, Belgium

9.1 INTRODUCTION

Peptides and proteins are susceptible to aggregation [1] and aggregates can have any size ranging from small oligomers to visible particulates. These aggregates can be composed of native or nonnative-like monomers, be ordered or random in structure, and be soluble or insoluble (Chapter 1). Aggregation of proteins and peptides in formulations has to be minimized, not only at release but also for the shelf-life of the product, because aggregation can lead to a loss of activity and aggregates have been implicated as possible triggers of immunological response [2–4].

The stability and lifetime of aggregates depend on the nature of the interactions holding them together (e.g., covalent or noncovalent, hydrophobic, and electrostatic interactions), their degree of order, and extrinsic factors such as temperature, formulation composition, and stress factors. When attempting to study aggregates, it is important to take into account the effect that the technique itself may have on the aggregates or on aggregate formation [5]. Aggregates are also often present only at a very low concentration in the presence of an excess of native monomer, [6] which hampers their detection.

While the characterization of protein aggregates and particulates poses significant analytical challenges, understanding of their nature and the kinetics of their formation is essential for practical applications such as stabilization,

Analysis of Aggregates and Particles in Protein Pharmaceuticals, First Edition.
Edited by Hanns-Christian Mahler, Wim Jiskoot.

TABLE 9.1   Fluorescence-Based Techniques and Their Applications in the Analysis of Protein Aggregates

Technique	Applications
Steady-state fluorescence	Monitoring protein unfolding and aggregation by looking at changes in spectral shape and intensity. The emission spectra of many extrinsic dyes are sensitive to changes in their environment, for example, as a result of interacting with hydrophobic portions of the protein that become exposed on unfolding and formation of aggregates.
Time-resolved fluorescence	Used in combination with steady-state fluorescence to monitor changes in protein structure on aggregation. Resolution of different fluorophore environments is possible.
Fluorescence quenching	Monitoring protein unfolding and changes in accessibility of intrinsic fluorophores, for example, using acrylamide to quench tyrosine and/or tryptophan emission.
Steady-state anisotropy	Anisotropy measurements give a measure of the rotational displacement during the lifetime of the excited state. Anisotropy values are sensitive to the size of the aggregate and to local mobility.
Time-resolved anisotropy	Resolving the origin of changes in anisotropy that have been measured under steady-state conditions.
Fluorescence correlation spectroscopy	Used for determining diffusion coefficients and hence size distributions for a population of aggregates. Fluorescence equivalent of dynamic light scattering (DLS).
Single-particle tracking	Microscope-based technique for determining size distributions of aggregated protein samples.

formulation, and manufacturing of protein pharmaceuticals [1]. There is a need for sensitive techniques to allow detection and structural characterization of even trace amounts of aggregates in often complex therapeutic formulations, which may contain several excipients next to the therapeutic protein.

This chapter focuses on the characterization of protein aggregates using fluorescence-based techniques. Key advantages of using fluorescence-based methods are exquisite sensitivity, nondestructiveness, and the possibility to carry out real-time measurements allowing all stages of aggregate formation to be probed, that is, growth of the aggregate from a single monomer to a large aggregate. In Table 9.1, the most commonly used techniques are listed and their applications are briefly outlined.

9.2 INTRODUCTION TO LUMINESCENCE

Luminescence is the emission of light from a compound or substance occurring from electronically excited states, following absorption of a photon. The process is most easily understood by considering a Jablonski diagram (Fig. 9.1).

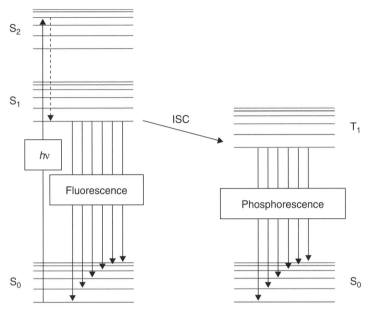

FIGURE 9.1   The simplified Jablonski diagram showing excitation and processes leading to fluorescence and phosphorescence by intersystem crossing (ISC). S_0 is the ground state, S_1 and S_2 are singlet excited states, and T_1 is the triplet excited state. For simplicity, excitation is shown only to one S_2 vibrational state. Upward arrow corresponds to the absorbance of light, and downward arrows depict relaxation pathways.

In Fig. 9.1, the ground state, S_0, the singlet excited states, S_1 and S_2, and the triplet excited state, T_1, for a simple aromatic molecule are depicted. Each electronic state is split into vibrational levels. Following the absorption of a photon of sufficient energy, a valence electron is promoted from the ground state, S_0, to some vibrationally excited singlet state. It then undergoes radiationless decay by vibrational relaxation and internal conversion (e.g., S_2 to S_1) until it reaches the lowest vibrational level of the lowest energy singlet excited state, S_1. From here, a number of deactivation pathways compete: fluorescence, radiationless internal conversion, intersystem crossing to a triplet excited state, or quenching via some energy- or electron-transfer process following interaction with another compound (e.g., a molecule, an ion, or an amino acid residue). Intersystem crossing leading to population of a triplet excited state may lead to phosphorescence. The triplet excited state, T_1, is also subject to deactivation by the processes described for S_1. If the energy gap between T_1 and S_1 is small, thermally activated back intersystem crossing can also compete.

Fluorescence lifetimes are typically of the order of $1-100$ ns and phosphorescence decays may last for several seconds. For a given chromophore, fluorescence and phosphorescence are observed only when they are favored over nonradiative deactivation pathways and quenching by energy or electron transfer. Phosphorescence is seldom observed in solution at ambient temperature since competing deactivation pathways such as reaction with oxygen are usually kinetically dominant. As to our knowledge, phosphorescence has not been applied for studying protein aggregation; this chapter focuses on the application of fluorescence. For the characterization of protein aggregates, either the intrinsic fluorescence of a protein or fluorescent dyes may be used, which can be either used to label the protein of interest or added to the solution.

9.3 INTRINSIC FLUORESCENCE

Most peptides and proteins contain at least one of the naturally fluorescent amino acid residues tryptophan (Trp), tyrosine (Tyr), or phenylalanine (Phe). Thus, they provide a convenient handle to allow fluorescence-based characterization of protein aggregates. They all absorb in the ultraviolet region of the spectrum; absorption maxima for Trp, Tyr, and Phe in water are located at 280 nm ($\varepsilon = 5600$ $M^{-1}/$ cm), 275 nm ($\varepsilon = 1400$ $M^{-1}/$ cm), and 258 nm ($\varepsilon = 200$ $M^{-1}/$ cm), respectively. The emission maximum is at 350 nm for Trp, 304 nm for Tyr, and 282 nm for Phe (quantum yields are 0.13, 0.14, and 0.02, respectively) [7–10].

9.3.1 Phenylalanine

Only few studies of Phe fluorescence in proteins have been reported; it has a much lower quantum yield and extinction coefficient than either Tyr or Trp, and quenching by other amino acids can reduce its fluorescence intensity further [7,10].

9.3.2 Tyrosine

The excited state of Tyr is also susceptible to quenching either by energy transfer to proximate Trp residues or through interactions with the peptide chain. Tyr is, however, a useful probe for proteins that do not contain Trp, in particular, in combination with acrylamide quenching [11].

9.3.3 Tryptophan

Next to the highest quantum yield, Trp has a further advantage over Phe and Tyr in the context of the characterization of protein aggregates: its fluorescence spectrum is strongly dependent on its local environment. Generally, the emission spectrum is blueshifted to shorter wavelengths and becomes more structured with decreasing solvent polarity, for example, when the Trp residues are buried in the hydrophobic core of a protein or protein aggregate [12]. In proteins that contain both Tyr and Trp, an excitation wavelength of 295 nm can be used to selectively excite Trp.

The quantum yield and lifetime of Trp emission are also sensitive to Trp's local environment. The lifetime can vary over the range of about 1–6 ns. Trp fluorescence may be quenched either through interaction with intrinsic quenchers such as amine, carboxylic acid, disulfide, and histidine groups or by the addition of electron-rich species such as iodide and acrylamide [12].

The main disadvantage of using intrinsic fluorophores is that their extinction coefficient and quantum yield are relatively low compared to those of extrinsic dyes; intrinsic quenching often reduces their intensity further, and while this may provide information about the proteins conformation, it can render signal intensities rather low. One clear advantage of using intrinsic fluorescence instead of fluorescent dyes is that they are part of the protein and, thus, do not interfere with the process that is being investigated.

9.4   USE OF DYES (EXTRINSIC FLUORESCENCE)

Dyes may be divided into two categories: those that are covalently linked to the protein and those that interact in a noncovalent way, for example, via a hydrophobic or an electrostatic interaction.

9.4.1   Noncovalent Dyes

Dyes such as ANS, Bis-ANS, Thioflavin T, Congo red, Nile red, and DCVJ have been used for the characterization of protein aggregates [13]. Their fluorescence properties are sensitive to the polarity of their environment (in addition to other factors such as viscosity, temperature, and the presence of hydrogen-bonding interactions). In aqueous medium, these dyes are virtually nonfluorescent. However, in a less polar environment such as in the hydrophobic pockets that may exist on protein aggregates, their spectra are blueshifted and their quantum yield increases significantly [13–15]. In many cases, the dyes interact only weakly with the native monomer, and although there are differences between aggregates, even low concentrations can usually be detected. Even if the dye interacts with the native monomer, which can be the case for hydrophobic proteins or proteins with hydrophobic pockets (e.g., HSA), aggregates can be detected if they are more hydrophobic as compared to the native monomer. Thioflavin T has the added advantage that it has a high selectivity for ordered aggregates such as insulin fibrils that contain a large proportion of β-sheet structure [13]. To understand the photophysical properties of these dyes, it is necessary to add an additional state to our Jablonski diagram (Fig. 9.2).

This additional state is known as a *twisted intramolecular charge-transfer state* (*TICT*). Following excitation, an electron is promoted first to an excited state, S_1(planar), that has geometry that resembles the planar ground state and displays only partial charge transfer. The molecule then undergoes a twist to give the fully charge-separated twisted intramolecular charge-transfer state S_1(twisted) (Fig. 9.3).

Since the TICT state is charge separated, it is stabilized in more polar solvents; thus, the spectra are redshifted [16]. TICT states are also often nonemissive due to rapid nonradiative population of lower energy triplet states, which explains the low quantum yield in polar solvents [17].

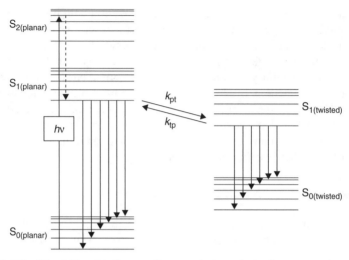

FIGURE 9.2 The Jablonski diagram for a typical extrinsic fluorescent dye, which is able to undergo twisted intramolecular charge transfer (TICT).

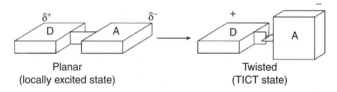

FIGURE 9.3 Schematic of the formation of a TICT state of a fluorescent dye with full charge separation from a planar, partially charge-separated locally excited state [16]. D, donor; A, acceptor. Signs "+" and "−" indicate a charge-separated state. Delta indicates a partial state.

A disadvantage of the use of extrinsic fluorescent dyes is that they may perturb the protein structure and cause or inhibit aggregation. However, in our hands, the influence of dyes on a protein's aggregation state is usually very limited when the dye is added after aggregation has occurred (e.g., by applying heat stress), just before the measurement. The review by Hawe et al. on the use of extrinsic fluorescent dyes for protein characterization provides further background information and application examples [13].

9.4.2 Covalent Dyes

A large number of fluorescent dyes that react to form covalent bonds with the α-amino group of the N-terminus, the ε-amino group of lysine, or the thiol group of cysteine of proteins are commercially available [18].

Labeling protocols are usually provided with the dyes on purchase, and so are not discussed in detail here. However, a number of points are worth mentioning: amine-reactive dyes that form stable amide linkages with proteins are generally preferred; they have the added advantage that by controlling the pH, it is possible to selectively label the α-amino group of the N-terminus rather than the ε-amino group of lysines. It is also important to control the number of labels per protein: the ideal number is dependent on the protein and the intended application, but typically 1–4 labels per protein are best. The number should be high enough to give a signal that is as bright as possible but should be low enough to exclude self-quenching of the dye and structural alternations of the protein. In the context of this chapter, it is important to rule out the possibility that the aggregation behavior of a protein has been influenced by the presence of the label. Given that dyes are typically planar aromatics with low water solubility, this is a real concern and control experiments using unlabeled protein or mixtures of labeled and unlabeled protein should always be performed (see Section 9.12 to see how this point has been addressed in practice).

An interesting possibility with covalent labeling of therapeutic proteins is that it may allow the identification of monomers or their aggregates in body fluids. This could be done either in vitro or perhaps in certain circumstances in vivo (in test animals); with most techniques, it is not possible to distinguish between the protein of interest and the proteins that make up a large proportion of plasma and serum. It has been demonstrated that by using Alexafluor 488-labeled human anti-IgE monoclonal antibody in combination with analytical ultracentrifugation, different aggregation behavior occurs in each of phosphate buffer, human serum, and plasma [19].

Depending on the intended application, it is important to choose an appropriate dye. A useful resource is *The Handbook—A Guide to Fluorescent Probes and Labeling Technologies* [18]. A further point to note is that the fluorescence properties of some dyes, fluorescein being the best-known example, are highly pH sensitive.

9.5 STEADY-STATE FLUORESCENCE

Steady-state fluorescence is the most commonly applied and widely available fluorescence-based technique for the characterization of proteins and their aggregates. By using multiwell plate readers, this technique can also be employed for formulation screening [20,21]. Most studies on protein aggregation look at intrinsic fluorescence in conjunction with extrinsic fluorescent dyes.

In a steady-state fluorescence spectrometer, the sample is illuminated typically by a mercury- or xenon-arc lamp for a period of time much longer than the fluorescence lifetime of the compound being studied. Emission is collected continuously, for example, using a photomultiplier tube as a detector. Steady state refers to the equilibrium, which is reached between the ground- and excited-state populations. Two types of spectra may be recorded: excitation and emission spectra [7]. Fluorescence spectra are usually reported as a plot of intensity versus wavelength. The intensity has arbitrary units because it is dependent on various sample-, experiment-, and instrument-specific factors.

9.5.1 Excitation Spectra

Excitation spectra are obtained by fixing the emission wavelength and varying the excitation wavelengths. For most fluorophores, the shape of their emission spectrum is independent of the excitation wavelength or quantum yield. For dilute samples (absorbance <0.05), excitation and absorption spectra are superimposable. In practice, this is not often observed due to the wavelength-dependent transmission of the excitation monochromator and the properties of the lamp [7,10]. However, it is possible to implement a correction to account for the wavelength-dependent response of the spectrometer being used [10]. It is important to use excitation spectra in combination with absorption and emission spectra to be able to fully understand the fluorescence characteristics of a fluorophore. Comparison between the shapes of absorption and excitation spectra helps to confirm the origin of a fluorescence signal, in particular, for complex systems containing multiple fluorophores, such as proteins.

9.5.2 Emission Spectra

To obtain emission spectra, the sample is excited at a fixed wavelength; the emission monochromator is then scanned to record the variation in intensity as a function of wavelength. The emission spectrum is shifted to longer wavelength as compared to that of the absorption spectrum (Stokes' shift). As mentioned earlier, the excited state decays by radiationless processes (vibrational relaxation and internal conversion) to the lowest energy excited state; it is from this state that fluorescence is usually observed.

Any process that is able to stabilize (or destabilize) the first excited state and thus lower (or raise) its energy leads to a change in Stokes' shift. Protein aggregation may involve partial or full unfolding; this may lead to hydrophobic regions being exposed to the (aqueous) exterior. If a Trp is involved, this will lead to a redshift in the fluorescence emission spectrum as well as a change in the intensity. As mentioned earlier, the spectra of noncovalent extrinsic dyes such as ANS and Nile red are often used to monitor unfolding and aggregation because their spectra and fluorescence quantum yields change considerably depending on whether they are in a hydrophilic or hydrophobic environment.

9.5.3 Experimental Considerations

The form and intensity of emission spectra are sensitive to a number of factors: the concentration of the fluorophore, its extinction coefficient and quantum yield, inner-filter effects, band-pass settings, the uniformity of the light source, and the wavelength-dependent characteristics of the monochromators and the detection system. All these factors may be corrected for, but often this is not done and care must be taken when comparing "uncorrected" data.

For normal right-angle cuvette measurements, it is important that the sample concentration should not be too high. Ideally, the absorbance should be below 0.05: at higher concentrations, much of the excitation light is absorbed at the surface and does not reach the point of observation (inner-filter effect). For compounds with a small Stokes' shift, reabsorption of emitted light may occur, also leading to a loss of intensity. A front-face setup is usually most suitable for concentrated or turbid samples (discussed below).

Emission spectra generally contain components arising from Raman and Rayleigh scattering. Raman scattering is only a problem for samples of low intensity and can be easily identified from the spectrum of the blank solvent. Rayleigh scattering is the scattering of excitation light by particles in solution and is difficult to avoid when characterizing protein aggregates and particulates. The best solution, where possible, is to choose a dye with a large Stokes' shift and use an appropriate cut-on filter between the sample and detector. When only a few large aggregates or particulates are present, the spectrum can appear noisy due to particles diffusing in and out of the observation volume. It is also important to consider whether other fluorescent species or impurities, for example, deriving from excipients in the formulation may be present.

For a detailed discussion, refer to *Principles of Fluorescence Spectroscopy*, 3rd edition [12].

9.5.4 Front-Face Measurements

When solutions of protein aggregates are being characterized, it is not always possible to have an optically "ideal" solution, that is, optically dilute and free of turbidity or particles that scatter the incident light. A useful solution is to use a front-face setup, where the cuvette is rotated at an angle (ideally $34°$ or $56°$—Brewster's angle: an angle at which light of a particular polarization is transmitted perfectly through a surface without reflection) relative to the incident light beam so that interference resulting from reflections are minimized [12,22]. While many spectrometers have the option of orientating the sample at $45°$, this should be avoided since excitation light is reflected directly into the detector.

In front-face measurements, most of the incident light is absorbed near the surface of the sample. A condition that must be fulfilled for front-face measurements is to work at a sufficiently high concentration/optical density where the fluorescence intensity is independent of the fluorophore concentration. To achieve this, the product of the thickness of the cell (centimeter) and the total absorbance of the sample must be at least one.

Limitations of front-face measurements are that reabsorption of emitted light can lead to a reduction in the observed intensity because of the required high fluorophore concentration, in particular, when Stokes' shift is small. Front-face arrangements may not be used for recording excitation spectra since reabsorption depends on the penetration depth of the incident light and is, thus, wavelength dependent. A front-face setup should also not be used for absolute determination of anisotropies.

The versatility of using a front-face setup is illustrated by its common use for studying fluorophores in whole blood. Commercial hematofluorimeters operate using the same principle [23]. Furthermore, it has been used to study protein adsorbed to particles [24].

9.5.5 Fluorescence Plate Reader

An increasingly popular alternative to cuvette-based measurements is to use multiwell fluorescence plate readers. These allow high throughput screening of protein formulations in plates containing up to 1536 wells and require only a few microliters of the sample. Although the same basic principles as in traditional steady-state fluorimeter are valid, there are a number of differences and additional considerations worth mentioning. Excitation and detection are both vertical, which can be a problem especially for formulations containing aggregates as excitation light can be reflected directly into the detector. However, it can also be an advantage since the measurements are less sensitive to the concentration of the sample, that is, in contrast to right-angle measurements where the observation point is usually fixed, in a plate reader the measurement depth can be optimized to give the highest possible signal intensity (note that as a result of the inner-filter effect, the excitation intensity is not uniform across the sample, and for high absorbances, this can greatly reduce the percentage of light that reaches the point of observation). Plate readers are less suitable for highly accurate quantitative measurements but are very useful for qualitative, comparative formulation screening [21].

9.6   TIME-RESOLVED FLUORESCENCE

Fluorescence lifetime measurements often provide more information than steady-state measurements alone; information on different components can be lost in steady-state measurements, where only the intensity-weighted average of the underlying decay process is measured. For example, if an environment-sensitive dye binds to a protein sample that contains monomeric protein and various aggregates, several components may be resolvable by time-resolved measurements, each corresponding to a different binding site. From a steady-state measurement, binding would be apparent only as a change in fluorescent intensity.

The easiest way to understand a fluorescence lifetime measurement is to consider the intensity decay as a function of time for a sample excited with an infinitely short pulse of light. For the simplest fluorophores, the excited state decays according to a first-order rate process to give a plot such as that shown in Fig. 9.4. The lifetime is defined as the *time taken* for the intensity to drop to $1/e$ of its initial value.

In general, the situation is more complicated. For instance, when measuring intrinsic Trp fluorescence, more than one Trp may be present per protein, different

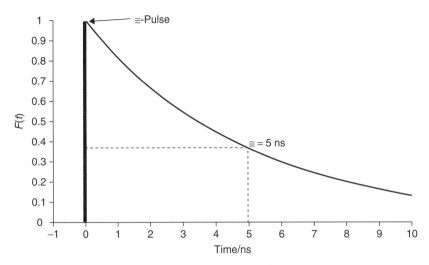

FIGURE 9.4   A schematic plot to show the decay of fluorescence as a function of time.

aggregated species may be present in the sample, or one Trp within a protein may possess a number of different emissive states or conformations. In each of these situations, the resulting decay must be solved as a sum of exponential decays.

$$F(t) = \sum_i \alpha_i e^{\left(\frac{-t}{\tau_i}\right)}$$

There are two techniques that may be used for measuring fluorescence decays: the pulse method and phase-modulation method. In the pulse method, the sample is excited using a short pulse of light (typically of the order of a few hundred picoseconds for a diode laser). The time between the pulse and detection of the first emitted photon is then measured usually using time-correlated single-photon counting. A fluorescence decay such as that shown in Fig. 9.4 is directly obtained by multiple repetition of this process (typically repetition continues until >10,000 counts have been recorded in the detection channel). However, since the excitation pulse is not infinitely short, the measured fluorescence decay is a convolution of the true fluorescence decay of the chromophore and instrument response. To deconvolute these two signals, the instrument response function needs to be measured, usually by either measuring a dilute scattering solution or using a reference dye, for example, N-acetyl-L-tryptophanamide (NATA) with known fluorescence decay.

Alternatively, in the phase-modulation method, the sample is excited by an intensity-modulated source such as a xenon-arc lamp or laser. The excitation is modulated sinusoidally, and as a result, fluorescence is delayed in phase and partially demodulated. By determining the phase difference and modulation ratio, it is possible to calculate the lifetime. For details, the reader is referred to Ref. 12.

9.6.1 Data Treatment

With modern instrumentation, measurement of fluorescence lifetimes is at first glance relatively simple and it is easy to obtain fluorescence decay. However, it is essential to consider factors that may perturb the measurement, such as the appearance of the solution, the presence of fluorescent impurities, or interference from stray or scattered light, which is particularly the case for aggregated samples. Since lifetime decays are usually recorded at a single emission wavelength, it is important to measure steady-state emission spectra both before and after a lifetime measurement to be sure that there has been no change in the spectrum. For example, when monitoring aggregation using extrinsic dyes such as Bis-ANS, the emission maximum can shift by more than 60 nm if aggregation proceeds.

Fitting and interpretation of lifetime decays should also be done with care. The background signal should be subtracted and the above-described deconvolution to obtain the true fluorescence decay is necessary. Most laboratories use commercial software to fit the decays, which is usually a sum of exponentials. However, in particular for more complex system such as aggregate-containing solutions, it can be informative to use lifetime distribution analysis. Thus, the decay is fitted as a series of distinct distributions rather than exact amplitudes and lifetime values [25]. Appropriate statistical analysis of the fit is also essential, that is, residuals, autocorrelations, and χ^2 values should always be reported. For more details, see Ref. 12 and references therein.

9.7 FLUORESCENCE QUENCHING

Quenching is a broad term that may be used to define any process that leads to a reduction in fluorescence intensity following some interaction between two (or more) molecules/residues. Quenching may be divided into two subcategories: static quenching and dynamic (or collisional) quenching. For the characterization of protein aggregates, two main techniques have been widely applied: collisional quenching of Trp by acrylamide or iodide and fluorescent resonance energy-transfer (FRET) experiments between Trp and an extrinsic dye or between two extrinsic dyes. Acrylamide or iodide quenching of Trp is used to gain information on the accessibility of Trp residues for quenching molecules [24,26–29]. Changes in the accessibility of Trp residues within protein aggregates, as compared to the monomeric protein, can reflect structural changes a protein may have undergone on aggregation. The FRET technique allows the determination of distances between pairs of dyes; this is useful for monitoring unfolding of proteins [30]. A requirement for FRET is that there should be an overlap between the emission spectrum of one of the dyes (the donor) and the excitation spectrum of the other (the acceptor). When the two dyes are in close proximity (typically <100 Å), energy transfer from the donor to acceptor can occur; thus, acceptor emission is observed following excitation of the donor. If the distance between the donor and acceptor is too great, no emission is observed. For more details on fluorescence quenching, the interested reader is again referred to Ref. 12.

9.8 STEADY-STATE AND TIME-RESOLVED FLUORESCENCE ANISOTROPY

Anisotropy measurements give a measure of the rotational displacement of a fluorophore during the lifetime of its excited state. The rotational correlation time is a function of size of the rotating species and other factors such as the viscosity of the medium. Thus, changes in anisotropy constitute a useful tool for monitoring aggregation.

All fluorophores possess transition moments for absorption and emission, which are orientated in specific directions. Thus, following excitation with polarized light, the emission is under certain conditions also polarized. The extent of polarization is quantified in terms of the anisotropy, r. In a homogeneous solution, the dipole moments of the molecules are randomly orientated. When excited using polarized light, the population with absorption transition moments orientated along the electric vector of the incident light are preferentially excited. These may then decay by a number of pathways. The most important in the context of this chapter is as a result of rotational diffusion.

An illustration of a typical setup for the measurement of fluorescence anisotropy is shown in Fig. 9.5.

Fluorescence anisotropies are measured using a fluorimeter fitted with excitation and emission polarizers placed in the light path. The sample is illuminated by light that has been passed through the excitation polarizer orientated parallel to the z-axis. The emission is then detected with the emission polarizer orientated first parallel to the excitation polarizer ($I_{\parallel}$) and second perpendicular to the excitation polarizer ($I_{\perp}$). The anisotropy, r, may then be calculated using the

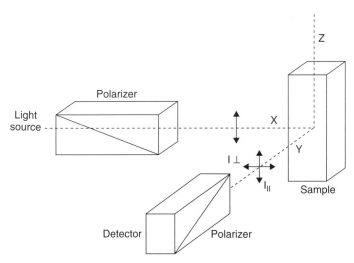

FIGURE 9.5 Illustration of a typical experimental setup for measuring fluorescence anisotropy.

following equation:

$$r = \frac{I_{||} - I_{\perp}}{I_{||} + 2I_{\perp}}$$

If the emission is observed through a monochromator, $I_{||}$ and $I_{\perp}$ cannot be used for the calculations directly as measured since the detection efficiency for vertically and horizontally polarized light is usually not the same. Therefore, it is necessary to correct for this difference using the so-called G-factor. In this case, we use an alternative version of the equation to determine the anisotropy [10]:

$$r = \frac{I_{VV} - GI_{VH}}{I_{VV} + 2GI_{VH}}$$

The G-factor is determinable by using horizontally polarized excitation. From Fig. 9.5, it can be seen that when the excitation polarizer is orientated horizontally, the excited-state distribution is rotated to lie along the observation axis. As a result, both the horizontally and vertically polarized components of the emission are perpendicular to the polarization of the excitation polarizer and, thus, equal and also proportional to $I_{\perp}$. Because of this, any differences between I_{HV} and I_{HH} must be due to differences in the detection system and the G-factor can be calculated as

$$\frac{I_{HV}}{I_{HH}} = G$$

9.8.1   Rotational Diffusion

For a rotating spherical body, for example, a protein monomer or aggregate in solution, the decay of anisotropy following excitation using a pulsed source is monoexponential:

$$r(t) = r_0 e^{-\frac{t}{\theta}}$$

where r_0 is the limiting anisotropy at $t = 0$ and θ is the rotational correlation time of the sphere. The limiting anisotropy r_0 depends on the angle between the excitation and emission dipole of the fluorophore and can range between -0.2 (for perpendicular excitation/emission dipoles) to $+0.4$ (parallel dipoles). A steady-state anisotropy measurement gives us the time-averaged anisotropy and is an average of the anisotropy decay, $r(t)$, over the intensity decay, $I(t)$.

$$r = \frac{\int_0^\infty I(t)r(t)dt}{\int_0^\infty I(t)dt}$$

Thus, an increase in the rotational correlation time corresponds to an increase in the measured steady-state anisotropy. Experimentally, the anisotropy can take any value between the limiting anisotropy r_0 and zero. A value of 0.4 would correspond to an immobilized fluorophore whose excitation and emission electronic dipole moments are parallel. This is nearly true for the membrane probe 1,6-diphenyl-1,3,5-hexatriene (DPH) [12]. For extremely mobile chromophores, that is, when the chromophores' rotational correlation time is much shorter than its fluorescence lifetime, the steady-anisotropy approaches a value of zero.

The simplest way to understand the relationship between rotational correlation times and measured anisotropies is to consider a spherical molecule with a finite emissive lifetime. Immediately following excitation, the anisotropy is at a maximum (or minimum); the measured anisotropy then decays as the sphere rotates. (Note that for a steady-state anisotropy measurement, we observe the time-averaged anisotropy.)

If we now consider a larger sphere with the same fluorescent lifetime as the smaller sphere, the larger sphere rotates more slowly and, thus, the rotational correlation time is larger. The extent to which the molecule rotates by the time the emission decays to zero is less; thus, the measured anisotropy is larger.

This may be described using the Perrin equation:

$$r = \frac{r_0}{1 + \dfrac{\tau}{\theta}}$$

where r is the steady-state anisotropy, r_0 is the anisotropy at $t = 0$, τ is the emissive lifetime, and $\theta(s)$ is the rotational correlation time of the sphere. θ is related to the hydrated volume, V (m3/mol), of the sphere by

$$\theta = \frac{\eta V}{RT}$$

where η is the viscosity (N s/m^2), T is the temperature (K), and $R = 8.31$ J K^{-1}/mol. Thus, in principle, it is possible to estimate the size of a rotating species from the measured anisotropy.

9.8.2 Anisotropy to Characterize Aggregates

From the discussion of the relationship between rotational correlation times and measured anisotropies above, it is clear that anisotropy measurements constitute a useful tool. If the protein undergoes aggregation, the rotational correlation time should increase (if the aggregate is stable) and so should the measured anisotropy.

In practice, the situation is not quite so simple and we must also consider motions of the fluorophore that are independent of the protein. In the case of intrinsic or other covalent fluorophores, this means segmental motion about a bond, that is, rotation of the fluorophore that is independent of the rotation of the protein or aggregate as a whole. With the extrinsic dyes, we must consider the environment of the dye and how strongly it interacts with the protein. Similar to time-resolved fluorescence measurements, the main advantage of using time-resolved anisotropy is that it opens up the possibility of resolving the origins of these contributions. As with all the fluorescence-based techniques described here, anisotropy measurements should be used in combination with other methods to confirm whether the changes observed are due to aggregation, changes in the structure of the native protein, or both. Another advantage of time-resolved anisotropy measurements is that they can be used to prove whether changes in steady-state anisotropy are due to changes in rotational correlation time and not due to changes in emissive lifetime; using steady-state measurements alone, this is not possible.

Another factor to take into account is that for larger proteins and their aggregates, the rotational correlation times can be long, that is, ranging from tens to hundreds of nanoseconds. For example, Lindgren et al. used anisotropy measurements in addition to a number of other fluorescent techniques to investigate aggregation of the protein Transthyretin (TTR): a homotetrameric transport protein with a molecular weight of 55 kDa that has been linked to amyloid diseases including senile systemic amyloidosis and familial amyloidotic poly neuropathy. For native TTR, they obtained different rotational correlation times depending on whether they used ANS or Bis-ANS; they suggest that the difference is, at least in part, due to the shorter fluorescence lifetime of Bis-ANS compared to ANS, which will truncate the measurement. ANS has a longer emissive lifetime and was thus suggested to give more reliable values. For the aggregates (30–50 nm) and fibrils (>100 nm in length), the anisotropy did not decay to zero in the time it took for the dye fluorescence to decay to zero and only limiting values could be reported [31]. One condition that should be fulfilled to carry out feasible anisotropy measurements is that the fluorescence lifetime should be of a similar order to the rotational correlation time. Since most fluorophores have fluorescence lifetimes of only a few nanoseconds, this can pose a problem when studying relatively large aggregates. However, a few fluorophores with longer lifetimes are commercially available, but they must be covalently linked to the protein. Common examples are pyrene derivatives and ruthenium complexes [32–34].

A number of authors have used steady-state and time-resolved anisotropy measurements as tools for the characterization of protein aggregates using intrinsic fluorophores [27,35]; the noncovalent environment-sensitive dyes, such as ANS, Bis-ANS, DCVJ, Nile red, and Thioflavin T, that become highly fluorescent on incorporation into hydrophobic regions of protein aggregates [15,27,31]; or covalent dyes such as pyrene [34]. Further examples are given in the case studies at the end of this chapter [15,34,36].

9.9 FLUORESCENCE CORRELATION SPECTROSCOPY

Fluorescence correlation spectroscopy (FCS) measures fluorescent fluctuations that occur in a small observation volume for a solution kept at thermodynamic equilibrium [37]. A typical setup for an FCS measurement is shown in Fig. 9.6.

The excitation source is usually a laser that is focused through an objective to a diffraction-limited spot. A confocal aperture is used to reject out-of-focus

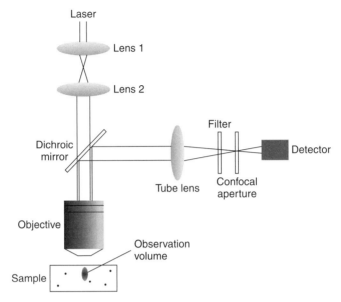

FIGURE 9.6 Experimental setup for carrying out FCS measurements.

light. The concentration of the sample needs to be in a range where only a few molecules (<10) are present in the observation volume at any given time; confocal conditions are necessary to give an adequate signal-to-noise ratio. Furthermore, the sample needs to contain a chromophore that can be excited by the laser light source.

A detector records the fluctuations occurring as fluorescent molecules diffuse in and out of the observation volume. The rate of fluctuations depends on the rates of diffusion, that is, for small molecules that diffuse rapidly, the fluorescence intensity increases and decreases rapidly, whereas for larger molecules that diffuse more slowly, the fluctuations are slower. This is the basic principle that makes FCS of interest for studying solutions containing aggregates. The underlying principle is similar to dynamic light scattering (DLS), with the difference that DLS detects intensity fluctuation of scattered light, whereas FCS detects intensity fluctuations of emitted light.

In FCS fluctuations are recorded using a dedicated correlation board that compares the intensity $F(t)$ to the intensity at a later time $F(t + \tau)$ for a range of delay times τ. This is then reported as a plot of the delay time, τ, versus the function $G(\tau)$. $G(\tau)$ is an autocorrelation function that contains information on the diffusion coefficient and the occupancy of the observation volume. It is defined as the product of the intensity at time t, $F(t)$, and the intensity at a later time point $t + \tau$, $F(t + \tau)$, averaged over a large number of measurements [12,38]:

$$G(\tau) = \frac{\langle F(t)F(t + \tau)\rangle}{\langle F\rangle^2}$$

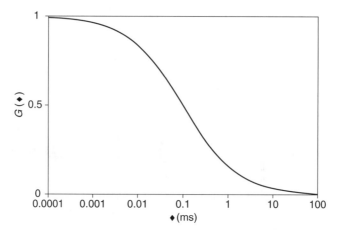

FIGURE 9.7   Simulated autocorrelation function from an FCS measurement.

A simulated autocorrelation is shown in Fig. 9.7.

The inverse of the intensity of the autocorrelation function at $\tau = 0$ gives the average number of molecules being observed ($G(0) = 1/N$). The diffusion coefficient is usually obtained by least-squares fitting of the autocorrelation function. An appropriate fitting function should be chosen based on the expected number of diffusing species (not necessary if the maximum entropy method (MEM) is used since the data is fitted as a continuous distribution of sizes). It is also often necessary to take into account nondiffusive processes that could lead to fluctuations such as chemical reactions, photobleaching, or quenching. For a molecule with a smaller diffusion coefficient, the autocorrelation curve shifts to longer τ.

When a protein undergoes aggregation, there is normally a wide distribution of different aggregate sizes. Thus, while fitting of an autocorrelation for a solution of protein monomer can be done assuming only one diffusing species; aggregated samples often prove more complicated. To overcome this problem, the data may be fitted to a continuous distribution rather than a discrete number of diffusion species. This is done using the MEM (as has been previously mentioned for fitting of lifetime distributions). An example is shown in Fig. 9.8. Distributions of diffusion times can prove informative for comparing aggregate-containing samples. Case study 2 provides another example.

Most FCS studies employ an extrinsic fluorophore (either covalent or noncovalent). Tyr and Trp are generally not seen as suitable chromophores owing to their low quantum yields and photostabilities. The optics used in most microscopes is also not UV transparent. However, it has been demonstrated that the intrinsic Trp fluorescence, excited by a two-photon mechanism, can be used to study the aggregation of Trp-containing proteins by FCS [39]. This approach has two advantages: UV excitation does not need to be used and the requirement for a confocal aperture can be avoided [39].

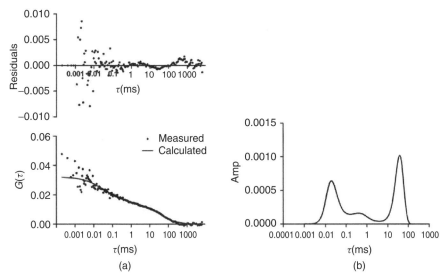

FIGURE 9.8   Analysis of FCS data. (a) MEM analysis of a single autocorrelation function obtained with Nile red in 0.10 µM β-galactosidase solution that was previously heated at 62°C for 5 min. The nonweighted residuals are shown. (b) Distribution of diffusion times (τ) calculated by MEM analysis. *Source:* Adapted from Sutter et al. [15].

9.10   SINGLE-PARTICLE TRACKING

Single-particle tracking (SPT) is an emerging fluorescence microscopy technique in which time-lapse movies are recorded for following the movement of individual fluorescently labeled molecules [40]. The instrument basically itself is an epi-fluorescence microscope setup that is adapted to achieve single-molecule sensitivity. To this end, laser light is used for excitation of the fluorescent molecules in combination with a fast and sensitive CCD camera, such as the electron-multiplying CCD cameras that have single-photon sensitivity. While single molecules are too small to be resolved by a light microscope, they appear as individual diffraction-limited spots in the fluorescence image with a diameter depending on the numerical aperture of the objective lens. For a high quality objective lens, this diameter is approximately 500 nm. The movement of the individual molecules can then be inferred from the movement of the spots of light in the focal plane. Evidently, the concentration of fluorescent molecules should be sufficiently sparse such that the average distance between molecules is substantially larger than the resolution of the microscope. The limited resolution of the light microscope, therefore, imposes an upper limit on the allowed concentration of fluorescent molecules for SPT. Typically, the concentration should be below 1 nM.

From the SPT movies, with suitable image-processing software, it is then possible to calculate with great accuracy the trajectories of individual molecules. Indeed, while the molecules appear in the image as spots of light with a diameter

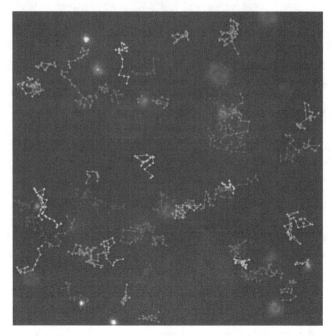

FIGURE 9.9 Fluorescent nanospheres of 200 nm diameter imaged and tracked by SPT. A trajectory starts when the particle moves into the focal plane and ends when it goes out of focus again. The diffusion coefficient (and size) of single particles can be calculated from their trajectories. The field of view is 22.5 μm × 22.5 μm. (*See insert for color representation of the figure.*)

of 500 nm, their position can be determined with an accuracy of typically between 5 and 50 nm by finding the center of the spot. Figure 9.9 shows an example of fluorescent nanospheres diffusing in water that have been tracked. In the case of molecules diffusing in a purely viscous solution, the diffusion coefficient can be readily calculated for each trajectory. The ability to determine the diffusion coefficient (and size) of individual molecules is the most important benefit of SPT, as compared to ensemble averaging techniques, such as FCS where the diffusion coefficient is inferred from the fluctuations of many molecules. SPT, therefore, should be superior in resolving heterogeneous distributions of molecules and molecular aggregates. For this reason, we are currently evaluating the use of SPT for measuring protein aggregates in biological fluids, such as serum or even whole blood. It should be noted that to observe protein aggregates in biological fluids, it is necessary to prelabel the protein with a fluorescent dye.

9.11 IN VIVO AGGREGATE CHARACTERIZATION

The deposition of amyloid fibrils is a characteristic of diseases such as Alzheimer's and Parkinson's. Fibrils, protofibrils, and soluble oligomers are thought to be cytotoxic, and correlation has been found between their accumulation and various disease states. While it is beyond the scope of this chapter, it is worth mentioning that fluorescence-based techniques that may be useful for the characterization of protein aggregates in formulations have also been extensively used in this field. In addition to the methods described earlier, fluorescence microscopy has served an important role [41]. In general, an extrinsic dye or a fluorescent protein such as GFP must be used since ultraviolet light has a very short penetration depth and is also toxic to cells; thus, Tyr and Trp are not suitable. In a number of cases, this problem has been overcome using multiphoton excitation [42]. The most important and widely used techniques include confocal microscopy [43], fluorescence lifetime imaging (FLIM) [44], total internal reflection fluorescence microscopy (TIRFM) [45], fluorescence–resonance energy transfer [46], and fluorescence recovery after photobleaching (FRAP) [47].

9.12   CASE STUDIES

In the following section, selected, illustrative case studies are presented, in which fluorescence-based techniques have been employed to gain more insight into protein aggregation with respect to the underlying kinetics, potential intermediates, or early precursors of aggregation and structure of generated aggregates.

9.12.1   Case Study 1

One challenge in aggregate characterization is the detection of small amounts of large aggregates, which are missed by standard techniques such as size-exclusion HPLC (HP-SEC) [15]. For this purpose, Nile red was used in combination with steady-state fluorescence, time-resolved fluorescence, and FCS to detect nanomolar amounts of heat-induced and denatured aggregates of β-galactosidase, which were too large to be detected by HP-SEC. In steady-state fluorescence, a blueshift of the emission maximum from 660 to 611 nm, accompanied by an increase in fluorescence intensity, was measured for the generated aggregates. Additionally, an increase of the average lifetime of Nile red from 0.4 ns for native β-galactosidase up to 2.5 ns for heat-stressed formulations was observed. It was not possible to estimate the size of the large aggregates by time-resolved anisotropy, because the expected rotational diffusion would have been too slow to be detected by Nile red fluorescence with its average lifetime of longest 2.5 ns. However, an estimation of the hydrodynamic radius of the large aggregates was possible by fluorescence correlation spectroscopy (FCS). For Nile red in buffer or with native β-galactosidase, a fast decay of the correlation function and a diffusion time of about 0.3 ms were measured using a one-component fitting model. This corresponds to a diffusion coefficient $D = 2.9 \times 10^{-6}$ cm^2/s, which is in line with what would be expected given the size of Nile red (318 Da) in aqueous solution. These data further confirm that Nile red did not measurably interact with native β-galactosidase, as already observed in steady-state and time-resolved fluorescence. For a heat-stressed formulation (5 min 62°C), a second diffusion time of 46 ms, corresponding to a diffusion coefficient of $D = 1.8 \times 10^{-8}$ cm^2/s and a hydrodynamic radius of about 130 nm, was measured next to free Nile red. By using a more complex model for fitting the autocorrelation function (MEM, compare section on FCS), it could be shown that the generated aggregates in the formulation exhibited a broad size distribution ranging from 14 to 420 nm, with a major fraction being above 130 nm. In addition, in less stressed formulations (15 min 49°C), traces of these aggregates could be detected by FCS.

9.12.2   Case Study 2

Another approach to visualize small amounts of large aggregates in protein formulations is the use of fluorescence microscopy [36]. Nile red, Congo red, and Thioflavin T were compared for staining immunoglobulin aggregates in the size range from 0.5 µm to several millimeters, of which Nile red offered the most sensitive visualization. Advantages of this technique are the high sensitivity for low levels of aggregates that interact with Nile red, the higher contrast reached as compared to conventional bright field microscopy, and the relative specificity of the dye to protein aggregates. Furthermore, it is possible to use this technique over a wide protein concentration range (in this study 0.7–193 mg/mL without further dilution or concentration steps) and also for turbid solutions.

9.12.3   Case Study 3

An approach to detect early stages of amyloid protein aggregation is to use covalent labeling of α-synuclein variants with pyrene [34]. Pyrene is an environmentally sensitive probe, with an excitation coefficient of about 36,000 M^{-1}/ cm, a long emissive lifetime, exceeding 100 ns, and a pronounced trend to "excimer" (excited-state dimer) formation. The emission spectrum of pyrene exhibits three characteristic bands, from which the ratio of band one and three (I_I/I_{III}) is a measure for the polarity of its direct environment, with a lower ratio corresponding to nonpolar environments (e.g., 0.58 in cyclohexane and 1.95 in DMSO). On aggregation of α-synuclein spiked with pyrene-labeled variants, the aggregation behavior could be monitored by steady-state fluorescence, time-resolved fluorescence, and fluorescence anisotropy. Owing to the long lifetime of pyrene, it was feasible to perform time-resolved anisotropy studies. The fluorescence properties of pyrene underwent characteristic changes during the aggregation process of α-synuclein, with respect to emission intensity, solvent polarity ratio (I_I/I_{III}), excimer intensity, fluorescence lifetime, and anisotropy. These changes reflect the gradual increase of the local hydrophobicity of the probe, induced by the aggregation process and structural changes of the aggregates. Compared to the standard fibrillation assay using the noncovalent dye Thioflavin T, the approach to use pyrene-labeled α-synuclein was more sensitive. Changes in fluorescence intensity and fluorescence anisotropy of pyrene were already monitored in the lag phase of the Thioflavin T assay and have been attributed to protofibrillar oligomeric species.

9.12.4 Case Study 4

Bis-ANS, Nile red, and DCVJ have been used next to a set of spectroscopic and chromatographic techniques to characterize aggregation of a monoclonal antibody (IgG) induced by thermal stress and freeze-thawing [13,48,49]. In steady-state fluorescence, it was shown that all three tested dyes were sensitive to thermally induced changes of the formulations, whereas freeze-thawing did not result in increased dye fluorescence. By light obscuration, it has been shown that freeze-thawing resulted in an increase in subvisible particles in the range of 1–25 μm. Structural changes were monitored within the heat-stressed formulations by circular dichroism and attenuated total reflection Fourier transform infrared spectroscopy, whereas freeze-thawing-induced aggregates were composed of nativelike monomers. However, in steady-state fluorescence, it is not possible to assign the increased dye fluorescence to a particular population, for example, aggregates, particulates, or changed monomers, within the thermally stressed IgG formulation. A combination of extrinsic dyes with separation techniques, such as size-exclusion chromatography (HP-SEC) or asymmetrical flow field-flow fractionation, has been shown to provide further insight into this [15]. For fluorescence detection, the extrinsic fluorescent dye Bis-ANS, which exhibits a good aqueous solubility and a high quantum yield in the presence of hydrophobic aggregates, was added to the mobile phase of the separation system (typically at a concentration of about 1 μM). It is also possible to add the dye directly to the sample and perform the separation with a normal mobile phase. In both approaches, fluorescence detection was performed at an excitation of 385 nm and an emission of 488 nm. By combining HP-SEC and AF4 with online dye detection, an increase in Bis-ANS fluorescence was observed not only for the aggregate fraction but also for the heat-stressed monomer. It was possible to simultaneously detect heat-induced aggregation and structural changes of the monomer and the aggregated IgG. Dyes are also available that can be used to analyze surfactant-containing formulations, [50], which is of practical value as many protein formulations contain a polysorbate (e.g., Tween 20 or Tween 80) as excipient.

9.13 SUMMARY AND CONCLUSIONS

Fluorescence-based characterization of protein aggregates covers far more than simply measuring an emission spectrum. Used in combination, fluorescence methods provide a versatile and highly sensitive way of gaining information about the characteristics of aggregates. They can provide valuable information on the characteristics of protein aggregates, including protein conformation and aggregate size over a wide size range. Moreover, they also open the possibility to detect early-stage aggregates: species that are missed by most other techniques due to their transient nature and low concentration.

REFERENCES

1. Roberts CJ. Non-native protein aggregation kinetics. Biotechnol Bioeng 2007; 98:927–938.

2. Hermeling S, Crommelin DJ, Schellekens H, Jiskoot W. Structure-immunogenicity relationships of therapeutic proteins. Pharm Res 2004;21:897–903.

3. Schellekens H. Bioequivalence and the immunogenicity of biopharmaceuticals. Nat Rev Drug Discov 2002;1:457–462.

4. Rosenberg AS. Effects of protein aggregates: an immunologic perspective. AAPS J 2006;8:E501–E507.

5. Philo JS. Is any measurement method optimal for all aggregate sizes and types?. AAPS J 2006;8:E564–E571.

6. Hawe A, Friess W, Sutter M, Jiskoot W. Online fluorescent dye detection method for the characterization of immunoglobulin G aggregation by size exclusion chromatography and asymmetrical flow field flow fractionation. Anal Biochem 2008;378:115–122.

7. Jiskoot W, Crommelin DJA. Methods for structural analysis of protein pharmaceuticals. New York: AAPS Press; 2005.

8. Demchenko AP. Ultraviolet spectroscopy of proteins. Berlin, London: Springer; 1986.

9. Eftink MR. Fluorescence techniques for studying protein structure. Methods Biochem Anal 1991;35:127–205.

10. Lakowicz JR. Principles of fluorescence spectroscopy. 2nd ed. New York, London: Kluwer Academic/Plenum; 1999.

11. Nielsen L, Frokjaer S, Brange J, Uversky VN, Fink AL. Probing the mechanism of insulin fibril formation with insulin mutants. Biochemistry 2001;40:8397–8409.

12. Lakowicz JR. Principles of fluorescence spectroscopy. 3rd ed. New York: Springer; 2006.

13. Hawe A, Sutter M, Jiskoot W. Extrinsic fluorescent dyes as tools for protein characterization. Pharm Res 2008;25:1487–1499.

14. Neporent BS, Bakhshiev NG. On the role of the universal and specific molecular interactions in the solvent effect on the electronic spectra of molecules. Opt Spektrosk 1960;8:777–786.

15. Sutter M, Oliveira S, Sanders NN, Lucas B, van Hoek A, Hink MA, Visser AJWG, De Smedt SC, Hennink WE, Jiskoot W. Sensitive spectroscopic detection of large and denatured protein aggregates in solution by use of the fluorescent dye Nile red. J Fluoresc 2007;17:181–192.

16. Rettig W. Photophysical and photochemical switches based on twisted intramolecular charge-transfer (TICT) states. Appl Phys B-Photophys Laser Chem 1988;45:145–149.

17. Das K, Sarkar N, Nath D, Bhattacharyya K. Nonradiative pathways of anilinonaphthalene sulfonates - twisted intramolecular charge-transfer versus intersystem crossing. Spectrochim Acta A Mol Biomol Spectrosc 1992;48:1701–1705.

18. Haugland RP, Spence MTZ. The handbook: a guide to fluorescent probes and labeling technologies. 10th ed. Carlsbad, CA, USA: Invitrogen. 2005.

19. Demeule B, Shire SJ, Liu J. A therapeutic antibody and its antigen form different complexes in serum than in phosphate-buffered saline: a study by analytical ultracentrifugation. Anal Biochem 2009;388:279–287.

20. Capelle MA, Gurny R, Arvinte T. A high throughput protein formulation platform: case study of salmon calcitonin. Pharm Res 2009;26:118–128.

21. Capelle MA, Gurny R, Arvinte T. High throughput screening of protein formulation stability: practical considerations. Eur J Pharm Biopharm 2007;65:131–148.

22. Eisinger J, Flores J. Front-face fluorometry of liquid samples. Anal Biochem 1979;94:15–21.

23. Eisinger J, Flores J. Front-face fluorometry of liquid samples. Anal Biochem 1979;94:15–21.

24. Bee JS, Chiu D, Sawicki S, Stevenson JL, Chatterjee K, Freund E, Carpenter JF, Randolph TW. Monoclonal antibody interactions with micro- and nanoparticles: adsorption, aggregation, and accelerated stress studies. J Pharm Sci 2009;98:3218–3238.

25. Alcala JR, Gratton E, Prendergast FG. Interpretation of fluorescence decays in proteins using continuous lifetime distributions. Biophys J 1987;51:925–936.

26. Rezaei-Ghaleh N, Ramshini H, Ebrahim-Habibi A, Moosavi-Movahedi AA, Nemat-Gorgani M. Thermal aggregation of alpha-chymotrypsin: role of hydrophobic and electrostatic interactions. Biophys Chem 2008;132:23–32.

27. Dusa A, Kaylor J, Edridge S, Bodner N, Hong DP, Fink AL. Characterization of oligomers during alpha-synuclein aggregation using intrinsic tryptophan fluorescence. Biochemistry 2006;45:2752–2760.

28. Sharma VK, Kalonia DS. Temperature- and pH-induced multiple partially unfolded states of recombinant human interferon-alpha2a: possible implications in protein stability. Pharm Res 2003;20:1721–1729.

29. Ribeiro MM, Franquelim HG, Castanho MA, Veiga AS. Molecular interaction studies of peptides using steady-state fluorescence intensity. Static (de)quenching revisited. J Pept Sci 2008;14:401–406.

30. Heyduk T. Measuring protein conformational changes by FRET/LRET. Curr Opin Biotechnol 2002;13:292–296.

31. Lindgren M, Sorgjerd K, Hammarstrom P. Detection and characterization of aggregates, prefibrillar amyloidogenic oligomers, and protofibrils using fluorescence spectroscopy. Biophys J 2005;88:4200–4212.

32. Terpetschnig E, Szmacinski H, Malak H, Lakowicz JR. Metal-ligand complexes as a new class of long-lived fluorophores for protein hydrodynamics. Biophys J 1995;68:342–350.

33. Sakamoto T, Mahara A, Munaka T, Yamagata K, Iwase R, Yamaoka T, Murakami A. Time-resolved luminescence anisotropy-based detection of immunoglobulin G using long-lifetime Ru(II) complex-labeled protein A. Anal Biochem 2004;329:142–144.

34. Thirunavukkuarasu S, Jares-Erijman EA, Jovin TM. Multiparametric fluorescence detection of early stages in the amyloid protein aggregation of pyrene-labeled alpha-synuclein. J Mol Biol 2008;378:1064–1073.

35. Eftink M. Quenching-resolved emission anisotropy studies with single and multitryptophan-containing proteins. Biophys J 1983;43:323–334.

36. Demeule B, Gurny R, Arvinte T. Detection and characterization of protein aggregates by fluorescence microscopy. Int J Pharm 2007;329:37–45.

37. Ghosh R, Sharma S, Chattopadhyay K. Effect of arginine on protein aggregation studied by fluorescence correlation spectroscopy and other biophysical methods. Biochemistry 2009;48:1135–1143.

38. Krichevsky O, Bonnet G. Fluorescence correlation spectroscopy: the technique and its applications. Rep Prog Phys 2002;65:251–297.

39. Sahoo B, Balaji J, Nag S, Kumar S, Maitia S. Protein aggregation probed by two-photon fluorescence correlation spectroscopy of native tryptophan. J Chem Phys 2008;129:075103.

40. Remaut K. Nucleic acid delivery: where material sciences and bio-sciences meet. Mater Sci Eng 2007;58:117–161.

41. Munishkina LA, Fink AL. Fluorescence as a method to reveal structures and membrane-interactions of amyloidogenic proteins. Biochim Biophys Acta 2007;1768:1862–1885.

42. Helmchen F, Denk W. Deep tissue two-photon microscopy. Nat Methods 2005;2:932–940.

43. Schmidt ML, Robinson KA, Lee VM, Trojanowski JQ. Chemical and immunological heterogeneity of fibrillar amyloid in plaques of Alzheimer's disease and Down's syndrome brains revealed by confocal microscopy. Am J Pathol 1995;147:503–515.

44. Koh CJ, Lee M. Fluorescence lifetime imaging microscopy of amyloid aggregates. Bull Korean Chem Soc 2006;27:477–478.

45. Yamaguchi K, Takahashi S, Kawai T, Naiki H, Goto Y. Seeding-dependent propagation and maturation of amyloid fibril conformation. J Mol Biol 2005;352:952–960.

46. Nizzari M, Venezia V, Bianchini P, Caorsi V, Diaspro A, Repetto E, Thellung S, Corsaro A, Carlo P, Schettini G, Florio T, Russo C. Amyloid precursor protein and Presenilin 1 interaction studied by FRET in human H4 cells. Ann N Y Acad Sci 2007;1096:249–257.

47. Luheshi LM, Dobson CM. Bridging the gap: from protein misfolding to protein misfolding diseases. FEBS Lett 2009;583:2581–2586.

48. Hawe A, Friess W, Sutter M, Jiskoot W. Online fluorescent dye detection method for the characterization of immunoglobulin G aggregation by size exclusion chromatography and asymmetrical flow field flow fractionation. Anal Biochem 2008;378:115–122.

49. Hawe A, Kasper JC, Friess W, Jiskoot W. Structural properties of monoclonal antibody aggregates induced by freeze-thawing and thermal stress. Eur J Pharm Sci 2009;38:79–87.

50. Hawe A, Filipe V, Jiskoot W. Fluorescent molecular rotors as dyes to characterize polysorbate-containing IgG formulations. Pharm Res 2010;27:314–326.

10 Infrared Spectroscopy to Characterize Protein Aggregates

MARCO VAN DE WEERT and LENE JØRGENSEN

Department of Pharmaceutics and Analytical Chemistry,
University of Copenhagen, Copenhagen, Denmark

10.1 INTRODUCTION

Infrared (IR) spectroscopy is the field of spectroscopy that deals with vibrational motions in multiatomic molecules. Even at 0K, the atoms in a molecule are in motion (zero-point vibration), resulting in movements that can be described as harmonic oscillations. The energy required to excite these oscillations depends on the atoms, type of chemical bond (including hydrogen bonds), and change in bond angles involved in the oscillation. Thus, IR spectroscopy allows the analysis of molecular structure, including the presence and absence of various functional groups as well as the configuration and morphology of the compound. Combined with the ability to measure samples in any physical state, this has made IR spectroscopy one of the most common analytical methods in organic chemistry and material science.

In particular, in the last two decades, IR spectroscopy has also been widely used to study the structure of proteins in various environments. Protein secondary structure is defined by bond angles and hydrogen-bonding characteristics of the amide backbone. Thus, it can be expected that the exact position of the absorbance band of the amide backbone depends on protein conformation. Decades of research, starting in the early 1950s, has indeed shown a correlation between IR spectra and protein conformation. This chapter discusses how IR spectroscopy can be used to characterize protein structure, with an extended discussion on protein aggregates, and also takes a look at the characterization of particulates containing protein. The instrumentation and sampling methods are also discussed. For an in-depth discussion on IR spectroscopy, the interested

Analysis of Aggregates and Particles in Protein Pharmaceuticals, First Edition.
Edited by Hanns-Christian Mahler, Wim Jiskoot.
© 2012 John Wiley & Sons, Inc., Published 2012 by John Wiley & Sons, Inc.

reader is referred to various textbooks; the multivolume *Handbook of Vibrational Spectroscopy* [1] is perhaps the most comprehensive textbook available.

10.2   INFRARED SPECTROSCOPY—THE BASICS

10.2.1   Vibrations and IR Absorption

Vibrational motions in molecules can be described as the periodic motion of an atom or multiple atoms about an equilibrium position. For example, in the simple diatomic molecule carbon monoxide (CO), the distance between the carbon and oxide atom is not fixed but oscillates (vibrates) around an average (equilibrium) distance. The energy required for this vibrational motion can be described in good approximation by the harmonic oscillator as derived for two masses (the atoms) connected by a spring (the bond) and is given in Equation 10.1. The actual energy values required for the vibrational motions in molecules mostly lie within the IR region of the electromagnetic spectrum (1–100 μm):

$$f = \frac{1}{2\pi}\sqrt{\frac{k}{\mu}} \quad \text{with } \mu = \frac{m_1 \cdot m_2}{m_1 + m_2} \tag{10.1}$$

where f is the vibration frequency, k the bond strength, and μ the reduced mass of the two atom masses, m_1 and m_2.

Equation 10.1 shows that the oscillation frequency depends on both the molecular masses of the atoms as well as the bond strength. Thus, diatomic molecules have highly unique absorption bands that reflect these differences. For large molecules, the IR spectrum generally contains a number of absorption bands that are specific for various functional groups, for example, amide bonds and methyl groups, as well as absorption bands that are caused by vibrational motions of larger parts of the molecule. The presence and absence of absorption bands in the IR spectrum can then be used to derive the presence (and absence) of certain functional groups, as well as other characteristics of the molecule, including configuration and physical state (e.g., cis–trans and para–meta–ortho isomers, crystallinity, and protein conformation).

In principle, there are $3N - 6$ fundamental vibrational modes for a molecule ($3N - 5$ for a linear molecule). Figure 10.1 shows three of the four fundamental vibrations of carbon dioxide (CO_2) as well as the rotation of the molecule. The bending vibration is actually doubly degenerated, but only one is shown in the figure. Of these fundamental vibrations, only the two bending vibrations and the asymmetric stretching vibration result in a change in dipole moment. The symmetric stretching vibration does not alter the dipole moment. However, to interact with IR radiation, there must be an oscillating dipole that changes in magnitude. Hence, this fourth vibrational mode cannot be excited by IR radiation. The rotational motion is excited in connection with simultaneous excitation of a vibrational motion. At room temperature, the rotational motion is not at its ground

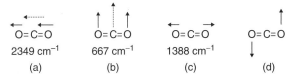

FIGURE 10.1 Rotational–vibrational motions in CO_2. Asymmetric stretching vibration, bending vibration 1 (in plane of paper), symmetric stretching vibration, and rotation. Bending vibration 2 (out of plane of paper) is not shown, as it is identical in energy to bending vibration 1. The solid arrows indicate the direction of the movement of the oxygen atoms compared to the stationary carbon atom. The dashed arrows indicate the change in dipole moment. The numbers indicate the required excitation energy for the vibration. Note that the symmetric stretch ($1388 \ cm^{-1}$) is not observed in IR spectra.

state energy, and excitation of the rotational–vibrational motion can, thus, occur with higher and lower energy than that of the vibrational motion alone.

The extinction coefficient of the absorption bands depends on the change in magnitude of the oscillating dipole moment. Thus, C=C vibrations will yield (much) less intense absorption bands than that by C=O vibrations. The relative intensities of absorption bands in the IR spectrum can, therefore, be used to estimate the relative amounts of specific functional groups in an unknown molecule.

The combination of vibrational and rotational excitation modes can be observed in Fig. 10.2a for the spectrum of water vapor (also containing CO_2). Note that the scale of the x-axis is given in wavenumber, which is the reciprocal value of the wavelength. About 3800 and $1600 \ cm^{-1}$ are the absorption bands of the O–H stretch and H–O–H bending vibration of water, respectively. The absorption bands consist of a large number of very sharp bands, divided by a clearly visible gap. It is the center of this "gap" that corresponds to the energy required to excite the vibrational motion (quantum number v excited from 0 to 1). However, since all quantum numbers must change on excitation, we only see the absorption bands for those vibrational transitions in which the rotational quantum number (J) also changes.[1] At room temperature, a molecule populates many different rotational states, hence the observation of sharp bands both above (higher energy, the so-called P branch) and below (lower energy, the R branch) the vibrational excitation.

In this same spectrum, the absorption band of the CO_2 asymmetric stretch vibration can be observed about $2300 \ cm^{-1}$. Here, the absorbance peak appears to consist of two bands, but these two lobes are actually the P and R branch for the rotational motions of CO_2. However, for CO_2, the energy difference between the rotational motions is much smaller, which means that the individual bands are too close together to be able to be resolved using the applied resolution settings for the spectra shown in Fig. 10.2.

---

[1]There are many exceptions to this rule. For example, methane gas does show a transition $\Delta J = 0$, known as the Q branch.

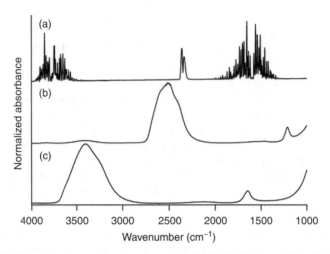

FIGURE 10.2   IR spectra of water vapor (a), liquid D_2O (b), and liquid H_2O (c).

The IR absorption bands of solid and liquid samples are very broad. However, the freedom of rotation in liquids and solids is much lower than that in gases, and the peak broadening is thus not due to simultaneous excitation of a vibrational mode and the various rotational motions. Rather, it is due, among others, to the uncertainty principle, Doppler broadening, and collisions (especially in the liquid state). Moreover, intra- and, particularly, intermolecular interactions may cause further band broadening [2].

Figure 10.2 also shows the IR spectra of liquid water (c) and deuterated water (b). In liquid water, the spectrum is significantly different from that of water vapor. Owing to intermolecular interactions, mainly the formation of hydrogen bonds, the absorption wavenumber shifts to lower values (corresponding to lower energies), and the relative extinction coefficients of the two vibrational movements (O–H stretch and H–O–H bend) changes. The spectrum of deuterated water shows that significant band shifts may occur on using isotope-labeled compounds, as can be derived from Equation 10.1. That is, Equation 10.1 shows that on inclusion of a heavier isotope of an atom, the reduced mass increases, which, in turn, reduces the vibration frequency (k remains almost the same on isotope exchange).

10.2.2   Measuring IR Spectra (of Protein Samples)

Unlike most other optical spectroscopy methods, current IR instrumentation does not use a dispersive system to scan through the wavelength range. Rather, an interferometer, which involves the so-called beam splitter and a movable mirror, is used to simultaneously send all wavelengths from the IR source through the sample. It is beyond the scope of this chapter to discuss the interferometer and mathematics involved to obtain the IR spectrum in detail, and the interested reader is referred to textbooks (cf. [1]). However, a short discussion on some aspects is required to understand some of the peculiarities of the method as well as the typical settings used for measuring protein-containing samples.

First, the interferometer-based IR spectrometers yield much faster scanning over a large wavelength range as well as a better signal-to-noise ratio than any dispersive systems, but do require various mathematical "tricks" to transform the so-called interferogram into an IR spectrum. The latter involves a Fourier transformation and, hence, the common reference to Fourier transform infrared (FTIR) spectroscopy.

The Fourier transform in IR spectrometers includes the use of a weighting function, called an *apodization function*. Unfortunately, there are no literature reports that discuss the effect of the various possible apodization functions on protein structural analysis. Although different apodization functions do have different effects on the band shape [3], these effects are generally relatively small. Nonetheless, it is recommended to stick to one apodization function, in particular, the more conservative functions, such as the triangular or (medium) Norton–Beer function. In some software packages, the choice of apodization function may be slightly hidden, and within the (protein analysis) literature, the applied function is almost never indicated.

The resolution (R) of an FTIR spectrum solely depends on the maximum distance (X) the movable mirror in the interferometer is allowed to travel:

$$R = \frac{1}{X} \tag{10.2}$$

This is in contrast to dispersive spectrometers, in which slits are used to alter the resolution. In the dispersive spectrometers, increasing the resolution (e.g., from 4 to 2 cm^{-1}) requires smaller slit widths, which decreases the signal-to-noise ratio. Thus, longer scan times per wavelength are required to obtain the same signal-to-noise ratio. In FTIR spectrometers, increasing the resolution means scanning to a larger maximum distance X, thus always increasing the time required for one scan. However, the signal-to-noise ratio of a single scan is (almost) independent on the resolution setting.

A suitable resolution for most protein-containing samples is 4 cm^{-1}, although various investigators use a resolution of 2 cm^{-1}. The latter is a more appropriate setting if water vapor is a significant concern for protein structural analysis (see below). Moreover, better resolutions are also required if the observed spectral changes are close to the resolution setting. In such cases, a reanalysis with higher resolution is needed to confirm that the observed change is real.

The highly digitized nature of FTIR means that the resolution of a spectrum can be directly observed in the data density. That is, the distance between data points on the wavenumber axis is about the same[2] as the resolution setting. However, the *apparent* resolution may be increased in FTIR instruments by applying the so-called zero filling. The latter method adds 'zeroes' to the interferogram beyond

[2]In practice, slightly smaller.

the maximum distance X. These zeroes are taken into account in the wavenumber calculations, resulting in a smoother spectrum. It is of importance to realize that zero filling also increases the data density of a spectrum, doubling the number of data points for each level of zero filling. While resolution settings are easily accessible, the zero filling is sometimes hidden deep in the software settings and hardly ever reported in the literature. This can generate problems in comparing spectra, as well as in repeating the methodology of others.

Further peculiarities of FTIR spectroscopy are related to the data presentation. First, as previously noted, the x-axis scale is often given in cm^{-1} or the wavenumber ($\bar{\nu}$) scale. The wavenumber is simply the reciprocal value of the wavenumber and thus corresponds to an energy value. In general, the scale (left-to-right) goes from high energy to low energy, for the mid-IR region corresponding to 4000–400 cm^{-1}. A second peculiarity is the still common use of percent transmission ($\%T$) as the y-scale. Many databases for organic compounds use this scale, despite the fact that absorption spectra are much easier and more appropriate to compare. We strongly recommend using absorbance for the y-scale.

A final note should go to the detectors that may be used. The two most common types are the DTGS (deuterated triglycine sulfate) and MCT (mercury cadmium tellurium) detectors. The DTGS is usually the standard detector in an IR instrument, owing to its robustness and relatively low cost. The MCT is much more sensitive and allows faster scanning, but is also more expensive, requires cooling with liquid nitrogen, and its response is not linear at high absorbances. Thus, for measurements with high absorbance samples, such as for protein solutions, the DTGS is best suited. For kinetics and samples with low absorbance, the MCT detector is a better choice. Failure to maintain proper cooling of the MCT detector may yield spectral distortions, which are not always immediately recognizable in the spectrum.

10.2.3   Sampling Methods for Solid Materials

The versatility of IR spectroscopy is in part due to the many different types of sampling methods that have been developed. Only the most relevant sampling methods for solid and liquid (protein-containing) samples are considered here.

For solid samples, such as freeze-dried proteins or dried particulate matter, the most popular method is to disperse the sample of interest into an IR-transparent matrix, usually potassium bromide, and press this mixture into a transparent disk of a few millimeters thickness. The disk is then placed in a holder and measured in transmission mode. As a rule of thumb, a few milligrams (1–2) of the sample homogeneously dispersed into 300 mg (IR spectroscopic grade) KBr, pressed into a 13-mm diameter disk at 4 kN pressure, produces a proper IR absorbance to allow structural analysis of a protein. Problems may arise if the content of protein in the sample is low, since at least 0.2 mg of protein in the disk is required to obtain a useful absorbance signal. Moreover, the nonproteinaceous bulk of the sample may be so large that it is difficult to obtain an IR-transparent KBr disk.

The bulk material may also have a significant signal in the relevant spectral regions of the protein. Unfortunately, it is almost impossible to prevent some level of spectral distortions using this methodology, which makes it very difficult to subtract the contribution of large interfering signals of the bulk material.

It is also of importance that the sample contains a limited amount of water (20% or lower) to prevent the formation of amorphous KBr. The latter makes the disk less transparent and potentially very brittle. Large and/or highly deformable particles in the sample may cause significant scattering, resulting in band broadening and sloping baselines. Some sample milling may, thus, be required to create smaller particles, if possible at all.

It has been reported that the high pressure required to make KBr pellets may cause changes in the secondary structure of a protein [4], although others report those changes to be very minor [5]. Nonetheless, we recommend that the pressure used to create the disks is kept below 4 kN, in particular, if those lower pressures are sufficient to produce transparent pellets.

Yet another common method to measure solid-state spectra is based on diffuse reflectance (often known as *diffuse reflectance infrared Fourier transform*, *DRIFT*). In this method, the sample is physically mixed with an IR-transparent scattering material (often KBr), and the diffusively reflected IR radiation is then analyzed for absorption by the sample. The best spectra are obtained with small particles (<5 μm); thus, some sample milling may be required. Importantly, DRIFT spectra are not the same as transmission spectra, but are the result of reflection, meaning that they only reflect the surface layer of the sample. Moreover, the reflective properties depend on sample properties. The so-called Kubelka–Munk conversion, available in most FTIR software packages, can transform the DRIFT spectrum to a transmission spectrum. However, there are some assumptions in this conversion, and (usually small) spectral differences may still be present, even if the sample is structurally exactly the same as measured in transmission. DRIFT has been used for the analysis of lyophilized protein and shown to give similar results to other sampling methods [6].

A final popular method to analyze solid samples is attenuated total reflectance (ATR), which does not require the use of a matrix material such as KBr. It allows the measurement of anything from powders to large pieces (centimeters or more) of material. In this sampling method, the IR beam is allowed to reflect inside a crystal, usually made of germanium, zinc selenide, or diamond. At the reflection points, an evanescent wave protrudes from the surface of the crystal into the sample compartment, and it is this evanescent wave that may interact with a material in direct contact with (or in close proximity to) the crystal. Any absorption of radiation results in attenuation of the IR beam, which can then be converted to an absorption spectrum. In addition, in this method, the spectrum differs from transmission spectra, partly due to the increasing depth of penetration of the evanescent wave with decreasing wavelength. IR software packages generally contain a correction routine for this wavelength dependency, but these do require knowledge (or at least an educated guess) of the refractive index of the material.

Other spectral deviations may be caused by the so-called anomalous dispersion effect, which is related to differences in the refractive index of a compound within absorption bands [7,8]. The anomalous dispersion may lead to small shifts of peak maxima toward lower energy compared to transmission spectra and is most prominent for strong absorption bands. Correction routines are available, but they are usually not included with common IR software packages.

Since the depth of penetration of the evanescent wave into the sample is usually below 2 μm, depending on the crystal material, incident angle, and sample itself, the user should be aware that only the sample surface is analyzed and that good sample/crystal contact is required. The latter is not always easy to achieve. However, the ATR method does put fewer restraints on the sample in terms of, for example, particle size and water content than the other sampling methods. That is, as long as the material can be pressed into close contact with the crystal, the material can be analyzed.

The appropriate choice of the ATR crystal depends on several factors. The cheapest and most common ATR crystals are made of ZnSe and are relatively large, meaning that a lot of material is required to obtain a good signal, in the order of several hundred milligrams. The angle of incidence, usually 45° or 60°, determines both the total number of reflections (along with ATR geometry) and the depth of penetration, which, in turn, determines the total pathlength. For strongly absorbing samples, one should limit this pathlength, meaning a bigger angle of incidence. Highly crystalline materials may damage the relatively soft and brittle ZnSe crystals, and for such materials, it is recommended to switch to (the more expensive) diamond or germanium crystals. Especially the diamond crystals are usually small, with at most one to three reflections, meaning that they not only use less sample but also are less suited for looking at low absorbing compounds.

10.2.4 Sampling Methods for Liquids and Suspensions

The most common method to analyze liquids is a simple transmission cell, in which the liquid sample is introduced into a small chamber between two inert IR-transparent plates, for aqueous samples usually crystalline calcium fluoride. Owing to the strong absorption of water in the relevant IR region, the pathlength of these cells should be below 10 μm, with 6 μm optimal for protein concentrations up to ~50 mg/mL. At higher protein concentrations, a smaller pathlength may be required to keep the absorbance around 1650 cm^{-1} below ~1.2–1.3. Using smaller pathlengths may thus be necessary for some of the protein pharmaceuticals currently under investigation, such as high concentration monoclonal antibody formulations [9]. Larger pathlengths can often be used for deuterated water, sometimes up to 50–100 μm. Accurate control of the pathlength is often difficult, especially for cells with a pathlength below 10 μm, but it is of importance to keep the variation limited. It takes some experience to find the best way to fill and assemble the cells properly, so new users should prepare for the occasional frustration of having to start all over. If suspensions are to be measured, for example, protein solutions containing visible particles, the particles in those suspensions should either be smaller than the pathlength of the cell or be deformable enough to allow pressing the plates together to the required pathlength. Moreover, crystalline particles, such as those used in some (older) insulin formulations, may damage the CaF_2 windows and should thus be analyzed with caution.

The most viable alternative to transmission measurements is the previously discussed ATR method. Rather than pressing a solid material on the ATR crystal, here a solution or suspension is applied onto the crystal. In addition, for solutions/suspensions, the penetration depth of the evanescent wave is limited to a few micrometers or less, thus potentially resulting in a significant contribution of surface-adsorbed protein. This adsorbed protein may also be difficult to remove, resulting in possible carryover to subsequent samples. For high concentration protein solutions, however, the potential spectral artifacts due to sampling surface-adsorbed protein are very limited [10]. The most important spectral deviations between transmission and ATR spectra appear to be the aforementioned anomalous dispersion effects and wavelength-dependent penetration depth. Ultimately, however, the differences observed within the conformationally sensitive bands usually are very limited. The most significant disadvantage of ATR is that it often requires larger sample volumes than the transmission measurements (depending on the system up to a factor 50) and has a lower signal-to-noise ratio at the same number of scans. Moreover, the total pathlength of the ATR system (approximated as the depth of penetration × number of reflections) at 1650 cm^{-1} must remain below $7-8$ μm to prevent too high absorbance values in this conformationally sensitive spectral region. This means that not all ATR systems can be used for solutions.

The selection of the required sampling method will ultimately depend on the sample itself, as well as the experience of the laboratory doing the experiments. For the majority of cases, the KBr pellet method for solids and a CaF_2 transmission cell with a 6-μm spacer will be sufficient. For some, a longer pathlength liquid transmission cell may prove useful to allow sensitive measurements in D_2O, while in particular, a diamond-based ATR system will increase sample flexibility.

10.3   PROTEIN STRUCTURE AND INFRARED SPECTROSCOPY

10.3.1   Protein Analysis by IR Spectroscopy—The Basics

A typical IR spectrum of a protein is shown in Fig. 10.3. Similar to the spectra of other compounds, the protein spectrum contains a number of absorption bands related to specific functional groups, as well as absorption bands that are the result of vibrations of (large parts of) the protein chain. In order to analyze protein conformation, the only absorption bands of relevance are those originating from the amide groups in the backbone of the protein. After all, it is the bond angles and hydrogen bonding in those amide groups that define protein conformation.

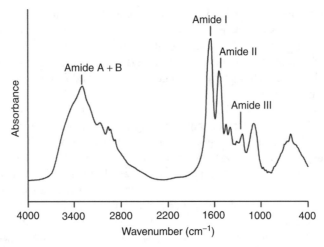

FIGURE 10.3   Solid-state IR spectrum of a protein (lysozyme).

TABLE 10.1   Important Absorption Bands of the Amide Backbone in Proteins

Name	Spectral Region (cm^{-1})	Vibrational Motion
Amide A	∼3500	Fermi resonance of N-H stretch and Amide II overtone
Amide B	∼3100	
Amide I	1700–1600	Mainly C=O stretch
Amide II	1580–1520	N–H bending and C–N stretching combination
Amide III	1340–1210	Complex vibrational motion of several sections of the amide bond including overtones

The characteristics of the most important amide vibration bands are summarized in Table 10.1.

Although all amide-bond-related vibrations contain information on the protein conformation, there are a variety of issues that make the Amide I absorption band (1700–1600 cm^{-1}) most applicable. For example, the Amide A and B bands are hampered by the presence of N–H stretch and O–H stretch vibrations of various amino acid side chains. The Amide III absorption bands (1340–1210 cm^{-1}) are relatively weak and many other compounds absorb strongly in this region. In contrast, the Amide I and, to a lesser extent, the Amide II band (1580–1520 cm^{-1}) are found in a region where few other absorption bands are found. For most proteins, the absorption bands of amino acid side chains in the Amide I and II regions are limited and, hence, of limited significance for the structural analysis. Finally, decades of experience have shown the Amide I band to be more sensitive to protein conformational differences than the Amide II band.

The Amide I band has one notable disadvantage compared to the Amide II and III bands, which is the strong absorption band of the H$-$O$-$H bending vibration of water within the same region. The molar absorption coefficient of the latter vibration is about a factor 15$-$20 lower than that of the amide C=O stretching vibration, but because of the large excess of water, even at high protein concentrations (e.g., 50 mg/mL), the Amide I signal only constitutes a few percent of the total signal observed about 1650 cm^{-1}. In the early days of IR analysis of protein structure, this problem was overcome by using D_2O, since D_2O does not absorb strongly in the Amide I region (Fig. 10.2). However, proper analysis of protein structure does require full hydrogen$-$deuterium exchange, which, in turn, often requires long-term incubation and sometimes even partial unfolding during the exchange process. It may also alter the properties of proteins (cf. [11]) and is thus not always a viable option. Fortunately, improved understanding and better equipment (including the short-pathlength cells) has now allowed the analysis of proteins in H_2O. Although concentrations as low as 5 mg/mL have been used, it is advised to use higher concentrations whenever possible.

Subtracting the contribution of water is mostly based on the water overtone vibration band about 2100 cm^{-1} (Fig. 10.2). Since very few other compounds absorb in this spectral region, a flat baseline indicates the full removal of the contribution of water. An additional check of proper subtraction is the Amide I/II intensity ratio. In transmission measurements, this ratio is generally about 1.5:1$-$2:1. For ATR measurements, the ratio is smaller, about 1.2:1 (before any ATR corrections) [10].

Proper subtraction of the water contribution does require that the water structure in the sample is similar to that in the reference, since the water absorption band is sensitive to water structure. Large variations in temperature ($>1°C$) or large differences in salt content between the sample and reference may cause significant changes in water structure, which, in turn, may affect the accurate analysis of protein conformation due to poor subtraction of the water contribution.

If other compounds are present that absorb in the Amide I region, it is best to subtract their contribution after subtracting the water contribution, rather than attempting to subtract both at the same time[3]; small differences in concentration between the sample and control may ultimately have a large influence on the final spectrum and affect the conformation analysis. One such interfering substance is water vapor (Fig. 10.2). In most properly purged instruments and using proper procedures, the water vapor contribution can be reduced to almost zero. While this may be sufficient for most applications, conformational analysis, in particular using second-derivative spectra (see below), may be significantly affected by almost invisible contributions. Thus, this contribution often needs to be subtracted from the spectrum before further analysis and preferably as the last subtraction routine. In our experience, it is most convenient to use the region around 3650 cm^{-1} to subtract water vapor contributions, although the region just above 1700 cm^{-1} may also be suitable.

[3]Note that proper subtraction may not always be possible, since interactions between analyte and matrix may alter the spectrum of the matrix.

10.3.2 Extracting Structural Information from Infrared Spectra

Analysis of model peptides with a well-known single conformation has shown that different conformations give a specific absorption band in the Amide I region (cf. [12]). Various attempts at calculating the expected absorption bands of several conformational elements have been made, with reasonable correlation to the observed spectra (cf. [13–17]). These theoretical calculations show that the band positions are not static but may change according to length/size as well as possible distortions of the conformational segment. This means that the assignment of band positions to specific conformations is prone to errors, yet at the same time may yield a deeper insight into protein secondary and tertiary structure [13]. Table 10.2 summarizes the spectral ranges in the Amide I band in which typical secondary structural elements may be found. There is significant overlap between certain structural elements, while some band assignments are still rather uncertain, in particular those for turns and the 3_{10} helix. This uncertainty needs to be taken into account when using IR spectroscopy to quantitatively determine protein secondary structure or when assigning spectral changes to specific conformational changes.

Most proteins contain multiple conformational elements and thus exhibit a very broad and often seemingly featureless absorption band (Fig. 10.3) [18]. As the individual absorption bands of the conformational elements are by nature also broad, increasing the spectral resolution generally does not improve the ability to observe the individual bands and thus is a futile exercise. Rather, mathematical methods have been developed to extract this information. Common methods include curve fitting, Fourier self-deconvolution (FSD),

TABLE 10.2 Typical Positions of Absorption Bands of Specific Secondary Structural Elements

	Spectral Region (in cm^{-1})	
Structure	In H_2O	In D_2O
α-Helix	1650–1658	1648–1657
3_{10} Helix[a]	1662–1666	1640, 1664?
β-Sheet (all types)	1620–1640	1615–1638
	1680–1695[b]	1670–1695[b]
Intermolecular β-sheet	1620–1630	1615–1625
	1690–1700[b]	1680–1690[b]
Turn[c]	1662–1686	1653–1691
Unordered	1640–1650	1639–1650

[a]Assignment of this structural element is still difficult as few proteins contain a significant amount of 3_{10} helix to allow unequivocal assignment.
[b]For parallel β-sheets, the high energy component has very low intensity compared to antiparallel β-sheets.
[c]Assignment of turn structures is hampered by the existence of many different types of turn structures, usually in relatively small amounts.

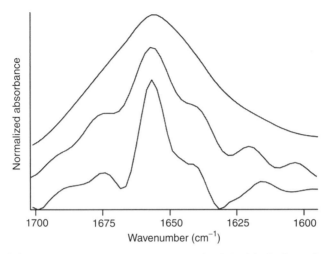

FIGURE 10.4 From top to bottom: The unresolved Amide I absorption band and resolution-enhanced spectra of the same band (Fourier self-deconvolution and inverted second derivative). The protein is lysozyme, a mixed α/β-protein ($\sim$40/10%).

second-derivative analysis, combinations of the former three methods [19], as well as various pattern-recognition methods [20]. Figure 10.4 shows a typical Amide I spectrum of a protein and the underlying absorption bands as determined by the FSD and second derivative.

Curve fitting is an iterative procedure in which a number of curves are used to reconstruct the (sometimes resolution-enhanced) spectrum. Unfortunately, the procedure is operator biased, and it is easy to find a wide range of different approaches to curve-fit protein spectra in the literature. Important input parameters are the number of bands, (initial) band position, width, height and shape, and any baseline. The number of bands, band positions, and height may be based on the second-derivative spectrum (see also below), although this method usually does not resolve all underlying absorption bands, or based on the known spectral ranges of secondary structural elements (Table 10.2). Bandwidth is often allowed to vary, but there will be upper and lower limits that need to be accepted by the operator. Band shapes in solutions can usually be approximated best by a mixture of Lorentzian and Gaussian band shapes, adding the level of mixing of these two as yet another fitting parameter. However, with each additional parameter that is allowed to vary, the possibility increases of having multiple solutions that yield a proper fit. The goodness of fit can be evaluated using the χ^2 value (should be small) or low and random residuals.

The results of curve fitting are curves at certain wavenumbers with known shape and area. These curves can then be assigned to certain structural elements and the relative areas used to determine the relative percentage of this structural element. Several studies have shown a reasonable agreement between the calculated secondary structure in FTIR and in X-ray crystallography (cf. [21]), but this is not always the case. Typical issues with curve fitting are proper assignment to specific structural elements, using sufficient curves, and the unproven assumption that the extinction coefficients of all secondary structural elements are equal. Finally, significant contribution of side-chain absorptions may occur [22] and correction for side-chain absorptions adds yet another (group of) fitting parameters. It is, therefore, common to see considerable differences in calculated secondary structural content and band assignments for the same protein.

A more objective method of curve fitting is based on neural networks (or pattern recognition), in which a database of known protein spectra, with their associated secondary structural content, is used to fit the spectrum of the sample. The only parameter to be fitted is the relative proportion of each of the reference spectra needed to properly fit the sample spectrum. The secondary structure is then calculated based on the linear combination of the known secondary structures of these reference proteins. This procedure can only be used if the sample protein and reference proteins are expected to contain similar structural elements. Moreover, it does not show whether any peak shifts have occurred without a concomitant significant change in secondary structural content.

The FSD and second-derivative analysis are two methods that mathematically decrease the bandwidth of IR absorption bands. In the FSD, a math function is applied to the interferogram, which on Fourier transformation to the spectrum results in narrower absorption bands. The choice of proper deconvolution parameters is not always easy, and significant distortion of the band shape is possible if improper parameters are chosen. After deconvolution, this new spectrum can be subjected to curve fitting. Owing to the better resolution of bands, the fitting process is usually much faster and the algorithm more likely capable of finding a global minimum. However, this does not necessary equal a more accurate result in terms of secondary structural content.

Second-derivative analysis detects subtle changes in the band shape, thus increasing the apparent resolution. In addition, here parameter choice can be tricky, in particular when trying to mimic results of others. Most investigators use the so-called second-order Savitzky–Golay derivative algorithm. In the latter procedure, a function is fitted to the spectrum within a small spectral window. The second derivative of that function is then determined for the midpoint of the spectral window, the window displaced by one point, and the procedure repeated. Of crucial importance is choosing the right spectral window. A very small spectral window will overemphasize very sharp bands, such as those from water vapor. A very large spectral window smoothes out all underlying spectral features. In general, using a spectral window that covers about $15-25$ cm^{-1} is reasonable for the Amide I band. Note, however, that the input parameter of the Savitzky–Golay function is the number of data points, while resolution and zero filling (see below) determine the data spacing. Thus, the operator needs to know this data spacing to determine the number of data points to use in the Savitzky–Golay routine. Second-derivative analysis is well suited to identify the presence of underlying absorption bands in the Amide I spectrum, and relative band intensities often fit well with the secondary structure content. However, relative band intensities are unreliable if bandwidths differ. For example, intermolecular β-sheets often have a more narrow bandwidth than other structural elements, while in the analysis of lyophilized proteins, several structural elements may show broadening. However, no systematic studies have been performed on this aspect.

A final and very common method in analysis of protein pharmaceuticals is spectral comparison. In most cases, the formulation scientist is not interested in detailed knowledge on secondary structural content, but rather in *changes* of secondary structural content. One approach is to overlay two area-normalized resolution-enhanced spectra and compare the two by eye. This "eyeballing" of the data is obviously subjective, but quite suitable to detect those spectral regions where changes in band positions or intensity have occurred. If a more objective numerical value is required, it is possible to determine the area overlap between the area-normalized sample and reference spectrum [10,23]. There is some level of subjectivity in the baseline correction that is often needed to properly normalize the data, which should be taken into account when comparing with results of others.

The choice of methodology to use in the analysis of protein FTIR spectra will, of course, depend on the required detail. If one merely wants to see if structural changes have occurred, the area-overlap method is very suitable. However, it should be remembered that the area overlap itself does not directly reflect the magnitude in structural change. For example, complete transition from α-helix to random coil involves a small shift in wavenumber (<10 cm^{-1} in H_2O), and the absorption bands of these two structural elements show major overlap. In contrast, a full transition from α-helix to intermolecular β-sheet involves a much larger shift in wavenumber (30 cm^{-1} or more), and those absorption bands will not overlap. Hence, the area overlap will be much smaller in the latter case, despite the magnitude of the structural change being the same. This also means that the sensitivity of detecting changes will depend on the nature of the structural change.

Much more detailed information can be obtained using the various fitting procedures, and there will be a much lower difference in sensitivity toward changes than discussed for the area-overlap method. However, as noted earlier, they include either an operator bias (curve fitting) or a possible database bias (neural networks).

10.4 PROTEIN AGGREGATION

In the case of FTIR spectroscopy, covalent intermolecular bonds in proteins (usually) cannot be identified, due to the complexity of protein IR spectra and the minor changes expected on the formation of one covalent bond. Moreover, deviations from the native secondary structure observed by FTIR do not necessarily imply the formation of any protein associates. However, in many, but certainly not all, cases, noncovalent aggregation is considered to be connected to the formation of intermolecular β-sheets, which yield a rather specific signal in the Amide I band (Table 10.2). Intermolecular β-sheet formation is generally the rule for thermally induced protein aggregation but is also frequently observed for surface-/interface-induced protein aggregation (cf. [24,25]). In a number of cases, noncovalent aggregation has been observed for monoclonal antibodies subjected to freeze-thawing [26] and shaking/stirring stress [27] without any evidence for the formation of intermolecular β-sheets.

Figure 10.5 shows a typical example of the formation of intermolecular β-sheets, in this case the (second-derivative) FTIR spectrum of heat-aggregated lysozyme. Native lysozyme contains a significant amount of α-helix (1656 cm^{-1}), as well as some β-sheet (1641/1690 cm^{-1}). In contrast, the heat-aggregated lysozyme has apparently lost most of its α-helical structure as well as its β-sheet, at the expense of a conformational element that yields two absorption bands around 1624 and 1698 cm^{-1}. The large apparent splitting of these two bands, as well as the observation of the same signal in model peptides forming an extended network of β-sheets, suggests that these new bands are due to the formation of an intermolecular network of β-sheets. The presence of the high energy peak (1698 cm^{-1}) indicates that this network contains a significant amount of antiparallel β-sheets, since parallel β-sheets generally do not yield a high energy absorption band [14,15,28]. Moreover, a recent study by Zandomeneghi et al. shows that β-sheets in native proteins generally have a different signal from the intermolecular β-sheets in amyloid fibrils [29]. Combined with a range of other studies on aggregated proteins (cf. [30–37]), it has now been well established that noncovalent protein aggregates involving intermolecular β-sheets can be detected by a sharp band around 1620–1630 cm^{-1} (in water), in particular when this band is absent in the native protein spectrum. This band can often already be observed in the unresolved

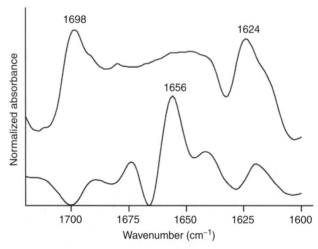

FIGURE 10.5 Inverted second-derivative IR spectrum of (top) dried heat-aggregated lysozyme and (bottom) native lysozyme in solution.

spectrum. The exact position of the intermolecular β-sheet absorption band is variable due to differences in type of β-sheets (parallel vs antiparallel) and also size and shape (e.g., kinked or flat) of the β-sheet. Unfortunately, little high resolution structural data on protein secondary structure within aggregates is currently available, which makes it difficult to make any solid correlations.

It should be noted here that some investigators have linked the presence of two absorption bands around 1615 and 1700 cm^{-1} in some lyophilized protein samples to intermolecular β-sheets (cf. [38]). Since the samples containing these bands yield aggregates on rehydration, this assignment appears very reasonable. However, van de Weert et al. noted similar bands with even higher intensities in three commercially available dry proteins, but none of these proteins were aggregated on rehydration [10]. This apparent contradiction has not been resolved yet and illustrates the uncertainties involved in band assignments in FTIR spectroscopy of proteins.

Although many proteins may show an almost complete change in secondary structure to β-sheets (and their associated turns) in aggregates caused under stresses such as heating, other proteins may retain a significant amount of native-like structure. That is, only part of the protein denatures and forms the intermolecular β-sheet structure, whereas the rest of the protein chain retains its normal fold. An example is shown in Fig. 10.6, where the inverted second-derivative IR spectra of native and fully aggregated α-amylase are shown. The aggregate spectra not only contain the distinctive intermolecular β-sheet bands around 1618 and 1693 cm^{-1} but also show a significant amount of residual α-helical structure. Thus, the presence of absorption bands that are also present in the native structure does not necessarily mean that the sample contains a mixture of native and aggregated protein.

An additional interesting observation shown in Fig. 10.6 is the different relative intensities of the bands at 1618 and 1693 cm^{-1} in the two aggregate spectra. This difference may appear small, but was found to be reproducible and directly correlated with the solubility of the aggregate (personal communication Dr. Søren Nymand Olsen). It is as yet unknown how this macroscopic property would alter the relative intensities of the two intermolecular β-sheet absorption bands, and whether this correlation also holds for other proteins.

10.5 PARTICLES AND INFRARED SPECTROSCOPY

The observation of particulate material in protein solutions is common and may be caused by the formation of insoluble aggregates. However, proteins may precipitate as native or denatured species, while other compounds may (also) be present in the precipitate. In this respect, IR spectroscopy can be very useful, as it can be directly applied on the precipitated material, either still hydrated or dried, after isolation using, for example, centrifugation. One may even use IR microscopy (discussed in Chapter 12) to analyze different parts of the precipitated material. Scattering is generally limited even for large particles (>2 μm),

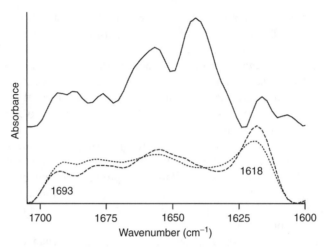

FIGURE 10.6   Inverted second-derivative spectra of α-amylase in its native state (solid line), and fully aggregated from a solution containing 5 mM NaCl (dashed line) and 160 mM NaCl (dotted line). α-Amylase is a mixed α/β protein (26/24%). This data was kindly provided by Dr. Søren Nymand Olsen.

in particular when ATR is used as the sampling technique. Since essentially all organic compounds yield a specific IR spectrum, IR spectroscopy often helps to identify the precipitated material or at the least gives an indication of the presence of proteins or other organic compounds in the precipitate. Depending on the complexity of the spectrum, it may even be possible to identify these organic compounds, in particular if reference spectra of the possible components are available.

When the precipitate is found to contain protein, the secondary structure of the protein can be determined using IR spectroscopy using the various methods discussed above. Problems may occur if the precipitate contains significant amounts of materials that also absorb in the Amide I region. It may not always be possible to subtract the contribution of such (possibly unknown) material. Note that this includes the presence of relatively large amounts of water (equal weight to protein, or more). The water spectrum may be altered to such an extent by being in a solid or solidlike matrix that there is no proper reference spectrum to subtract this contribution. In such cases, it may be more appropriate to rehydrate the precipitated material and perform the analysis in aqueous solution or suspension.

The usefulness of IR spectroscopy in characterizing protein structure in particulate materials has been shown best by various studies on proteins entrapped in particular drug-delivery systems (cf. [39–46]). Obviously, the protein has been deliberately entrapped into the particulate material in these drug-delivery systems, but in essence, the analytical principle is the same for any undesired and unknown particulate material. For example, Van de Weert et al. used IR spectroscopy to identify an unknown precipitate left after full degradation of a semisolid polyorthoester matrix containing a model protein [47]. The precipitate was identified as mainly consisting of protein, and the spectrum indicated that the protein contained a significant amount of intermolecular β-sheets. Similarly, a precipitate after shaking and/or stirring antibody formulations has been analyzed by FTIR, and in this case, the protein was found not to contain significant amounts of intermolecular β-sheets [27].

10.6 SUMMARY: ADVANTAGES AND DISADVANTAGES OF IR SPECTROSCOPIC ANALYSIS OF PROTEINS, PROTEIN AGGREGATES, AND PARTICULATE MATERIAL

The main advantage of IR spectroscopy over other methods is the ability to measure IR spectra in both liquid and dried state. Even highly opaque samples and/or complex samples can often be analyzed. As long as potential interfering absorptions of the matrix can be subtracted, these samples can then also be subjected to conformational analysis of proteins present in the sample. Moreover, if an unknown sample is analyzed, IR spectroscopy will allow a reasonable indication as to the organic materials present in that sample. Thus, a precipitate in a protein sample can be analyzed (after separation) and characterized.

The analysis of protein-containing samples can be used to determine protein secondary structure, even though its quantitative application is hampered by uncertainty as well as the many steps involved in extracting the information. Qualitatively, the appearance of an absorption band in the region 1620–1630 cm^{-1}, in particular when absent in the native protein spectrum, is indicative of protein aggregation through the formation of intermolecular β-sheets.

A disadvantage of FTIR is its inability to analyze low protein concentrations (<5 mg/mL in water), although at the same time it allows the analysis of very high concentrations (cf. [36,37]), which is not possible with many other techniques. Moreover, the IR spectrum of a protein sample will be a global average and cannot distinguish between changes in the whole population or the existence of two different populations. In conclusion, IR spectroscopy cannot stand on its own in characterizing or identifying protein aggregation, but is a powerful tool in combination with other methods described in this book. It is unique in its ability to identify the formation of (usually noncovalent) protein aggregates containing intermolecular β-sheets in any physical state.

REFERENCES

1. Chalmers JM, Griffiths PR. Handbook of vibrational spectroscopy. Chichester: John Wiley & Sons Ltd.; 2001.
2. Painter PC, Pehlert GJ, Hu Y, Coleman MM. Infrared band broadening and interactions in polar systems. Macromology 1999;32:2055–2057.
3. Hendra PJ, Birembaut F. How FTIR works II. Int J Vib Spec 2002;6(2):3. [www.ijvs.com].

4. Chan HK, Ongpipattanakul B, Au-Jeung J. Aggregation of rhDNase occurred during the compression of KBr pellets used for FTIR spectroscopy. Pharm Res 1996;13:238–242.

5. Meyer JD, Manning MC, Carpenter JF. Effects of potassium bromide disk formation on the infrared spectra of dried model proteins. J Pharm Sci 2004;93:496–506.

6. Souillac PO, Middaugh CR, Rytting JH. Investigation of protein/carbohydrate interactions in the dried state. 2. Diffuse reflectance studies. Int J Pharm 2002;235:207–218.

7. Goormaghtigh E, Raussens V, Ruysschaert J-M. Attenuated total reflection infrared spectroscopy of proteins and lipids in biological membranes. Biochim Biophys Acta 1999;1422:105–185.

8. Jackson M, Mantsch HH. Artifacts associated with the determination of protein secondary structure by ATR-IR spectroscopy. Appl Spectrosc 1992;46:699–701.

9. Harn N, Allan C, Oliver C, Middaugh CR. Highly concentrated monoclonal antibody solutions: direct analysis of physical structure and thermal stability. J Pharm Sci 2007;96:532–546.

10. van de Weert M, Haris PI, Hennink WE, Crommelin DJA. Fourier transform infrared spectrometric analysis of protein conformation: effect of sampling method and stress factors. Anal Biochem 2001;297:160–169.

11. Dennison SR, Hauss T, Dante S, Brandenburg K, Harris F, Phoenix DA. Deuteration can affect the conformational behaviour of amphiphilic α-helical structures. Biophys Chem 2006;119:115–120.

12. Goormaghtigh E, Cabiaux V, Ruysschaert JM. Determination of soluble and membrane protein structure by Fourier transform infrared spectroscopy. I. Assignments and model compounds. Subcell Biochem 1994;23:329–362.

13. Brauner JW, Flach CR, Mendelsohn R. A quantitative reconstruction of the amide I contour in the IR spectra of globular proteins: from structure to spectrum. J Am Chem Soc 2005;127:100–109.

14. Chirgadze YN, Nevskaya NA. Infrared spectra and resonance interaction of amide-I vibration of the antiparallel-chain pleated sheet. Biopolymers 1976;15:607–625.

15. Chirgadze YN, Nevskaya NA. Infrared spectra and resonance interaction of amide-I vibration of the parallel-chain pleated sheet. Biopolymers 1976;15:627–636.

16. Ganim Z, Chung HS, Smith AW, Deflores LP, Jones KC, Tokmakoff A. Amide I two-dimensional infrared spectroscopy of proteins. Acc Chem Res 2008;41:432–441.

17. Nevskaya NA, Chirgadze YN. Infrared spectra and resonance interactions of amide-I and II vibrations of α-helix. Biopolymers 1976;15:637–648.

18. Goormaghtigh E, Cabiaux V, Ruysschaert JM. Determination of soluble and membrane protein structure by Fourier transform infrared spectroscopy. III. Secondary structures. Subcell Biochem 1994;23:405–450.

19. Jackson M, Mantsch HH. The use and misuse of FTIR spectroscopy in the determination of protein structure. Crit Rev Biochem Mol Biol 1995;30:95–120.

20. Hering JA, Innocent PR, Haris PI. Towards developing a protein infrared spectra databank (PISD) for proteomics research. Proteomics 2004;4:2310–2319.

21. Byler DM, Susi H. Examination of the secondary structure of proteins by deconvolved FTIR spectra. Biopolymers 1986;25:469–487.

22. Goormaghtigh E, Cabiaux V, Ruysschaert JM. Determination of soluble and membrane protein structure by Fourier transform infrared spectroscopy. II. Experimental aspects, side chain structure, and H/D exchange. Subcell Biochem 1994;23:363–403.

23. Kendrick BS, Dong A, Allison SD, Manning MC, Carpenter JF. Quantitation of the area of overlap between second-derivative amide I infrared spectra to determine the structural similarity of a protein in different states. J Pharm Sci 1996;85:155–158.

24. Husband FA, Garrood MJ, Mackie AR, Burnett GR, Wilde PJ. Adsorbed protein secondary and tertiary structures by circular dichroism and infrared spectroscopy with refractive index matched emulsions. J Agric Food Chem 2001;49:859–866.

25. van de Weert M, Hoechstetter J, Hennink WE, Crommelin DJA. The effect of a water/organic solvent interface on the structural stability of lysozyme. J Control Release 2000;68:351–359.

26. Hawe A, Kasper JC, Friess W, Jiskoot W. Structural properties of monoclonal antibody aggregates induced by freeze-thawing and thermal stress. Eur J Pharm Sci 2009;38:79–87.

27. Kiese S, Pappenberger A, Friess W, Mahler H-C. Shaken, not stirred: mechanical stress testing of an IgG1 antibody. J Pharm Sci 2008;97:4347–4366.

28. Cerf E, Sarroukh R, Tamamizu-Kato S, Breydo L, Derclaye S, Dufrêne Y, Narayanaswami V, Goormaghtigh E, Ruysschaert J-M, Raussens V. Antiparallel β-sheet-a signature of the oligomeric amyloid-beta peptide. Biochem J 2009;421:415–423.

29. Zandomeneghi G, Krebs MRH, McCammon MG, Fändrich M. FTIR reveals structural differences between native β-sheet proteins and amyloid fibrils. Protein Sci 2004;13:3314–3321.

30. Allain A-F, Paquin P, Subirade M. Relationships between conformation of β-lactoglobulin in solution and gel states as revealed by attenuated total reflection Fourier transform infrared spectroscopy. Int J Biol Macromol 2006;26:337–344.

31. Benseny-Cases N, Cócera M, Cladera J. Conversion of non-fibrillar β-sheet oligomers into amyloid fibrils in Alzheimer's disease amyloid peptide aggregation. Biochem Biophys Res Commun 2007;361:916–921.

32. Dzwolak W, Ravindra R, Lendermann J, Winter R. Aggregation of bovine insulin probed by DSC/PPC calorimetry and FTIR spectroscopy. Biochemistry 2003;42:11347–11355.

33. Dzwolak W, Muraki T, Kato M, Taniguchi Y. Chain-length dependence of α-helix to β-sheet transition in polylysine: model of protein aggregation studied by temperature-tuned FTIR spectroscopy. Biopolymers 2004;73:463–469.

34. Lefévre T, Arseneault K, Pézolet M. Study of protein aggregation using two-dimensional correlation infrared spectroscopy and spectral simulations. Biopolymers 2004;73:705–715.

35. Paquet M-J, Laviolette M, Pézolet M, Auger M. Two-dimensional infrared correlation spectroscopy study of the aggregation of cytochrome c in the presence of dimyristoylphosphatidylglycerol. Biophys J 2001;81:305–312.

36. Matheus S, Friess W, Mahler H-C. FTIR and nDSC as analytical tools for high-concentration protein formulations. Pharm Res 2006;23:1350–1363.

37. Matheus S, Mahler H-C, Friess W. A critical evaluation of $T_{m(FTIR)}$ measurements of high-concentration IgG$_1$ antibody formulations as a formulation development tool. Pharm Res 2006;23:1617–1627.

38. Allison SD, Dong A, Carpenter JF. Counteracting effects of thiocyanate and sucrose on chymotrypsinogen secondary structure and aggregation during freezing, drying, and rehydration. Biophys J 1996;71:2022–2032.

39. Carrasquillo KG, Costantino HR, Cordero RA, Hsu CC, Griebenow K. On the structural preservation of recombinant human growth hormone in a dried film of a synthetic biodegradable polymer. J Pharm Sci 1999;88:166–173.

40. Castellanos IJ, Cruz G, Crespo R, Griebenow K. Encapsulation-induced aggregation and loss in activity of γ-chymotrypsin and their prevention. J Control Release 2002;81:307–319.

41. Fu K, Griebenow K, Hsieh L, Klibanov AM, Langer R. FTIR characterization of the secondary structure of proteins encapsulated within PLGA microspheres. J Control Release 1999;58:357–366.

42. Griebenow K, Castellanos IJ, Carrasquillo KG. Application of FTIR spectroscopy to probe and improve protein structure in sustained release devices. Int J Vib Spec 1999;3(5):2.

43. Sarmento B, Ferreira DC, Jorgensen L, van de Weert M. Probing insulin's secondary structure after entrapment into alginate/chitosan nanoparticles. Eur J Pharm Biopharm 2007;65:10–17.

44. van de Weert M, van 't Hof R, van der Weerd J, Heeren RMA, Posthuma G, Hennink WE, Crommelin DJA. Lysozyme distribution and conformation in a biodegradable polymer matrix as determined by FTIR techniques. J Control Release 2000;68:31–40.

45. Yang T-H, Dong A, Meyer J, Johnson OL, Cleland JL, Carpenter JF. Use of infrared spectroscopy to assess secondary structure of human growth hormone within biodegradable microspheres. J Pharm Sci 1999;88:161–165.

46. van de Weert M, van Dijkhuizen-Radersma R, Bezemer JM, Hennink WE, Crommelin DJA. Reversible aggregation of lysozyme in a biodegradable amphiphilic multiblock copolymer. Eur J Pharm Biopharm 2002;54:89–93.

47. van de Weert M, van Steenbergen MJ, Cleland JL, Heller J, Hennink WE, Crommelin DJA. Semisolid, self-catalyzed poly(ortho ester)s as controlled-release systems: protein release and protein stability issues. J Pharm Sci 2002;91:1065–1074.

11 Raman Microscopy for Characterization of Particles

STEFAN FISCHER

Late-Stage Pharmaceutical and Processing Development, Pharmaceutical
and Device Development, Pharma Technical Development Biologics
Europe, F. Hoffmann-La Roche Ltd, Basel, Switzerland

OLIVER VALET and MARKUS LANKERS

rap.Id Particle Systems GmbH, Berlin, Germany

11.1 INTRODUCTION

Particulate contamination in parenteral products, in particular protein pharmaceuticals, is an important issue for the pharmaceutical industry. Significant research has been performed with respect to particle detection in parenterals. There is a particular emphasis on visible particle inspection. These methods are described elsewhere (Chapter 6) and are beyond the scope of this section. Historically, drivers for visible inspection were to mitigate the risk of blocking blood vessels by particulates [1–3]. Consequently, parenteral drug products had to, and continue to, comply with compendial/regulatory requirements for particulate contamination. According to the United States Pharmacopoeia (USP) XXIV [4], parenteral drugs have to be "essentially free from visible particles." Therefore, parenteral drug products are subject of a 100% control by means of visible inspection during manufacturing. Various particulate contaminants such as glass, metal, rubber, starch, zinc oxide, carbon black, cellulose fibers, and fragments [5,6] have been described. It seems, however, that particulate contamination can never be completely eliminated. M.J. Groves states, "...whatever the process, the solution passes through, and no matter how undesirable the particles are, some are inevitably going to be present" [5]. To reduce particulate contamination, analytics for particle identification came into play. Groves said that Garvan and Gunner claimed to have found carbon black, whiting, and other materials while filtering injection solutions [2,7,8] "...although identification procedures were not always given" [5]. Groves considered the evidence "flimsy" because the

Analysis of Aggregates and Particles in Protein Pharmaceuticals, First Edition.
Edited by Hanns-Christian Mahler, Wim Jiskoot.

process for cleaning filters before collection and microscopic examinations was not described [5]. Groves' conclusions emphasize the importance of efficient sample preparation before any identification analysis as well as sound reasoning linking particles to their source.

Several microscopic techniques such as scanning electron microscopy (SEM) and infrared (IR) microscopy (Chapter 12) as well as Raman microscopy have been applied for particle detection [9,10]. This chapter predominantly discusses Raman microscopy and its application for particle identification. For the general physics background on Raman scattering and spectroscopy, the reader is referred to Refs. 11 and 12. Nevertheless, the general principles of Raman spectroscopy are briefly described.

In Raman spectroscopy, the molecule is illuminated by a monochromatic source of light (i.e., a laser beam). Photons of the incident radiation with their given frequency raise the potential energy of the molecule to a virtual state (i.e., an excited electronic state), an energetic state above the ground electronic state. Almost immediately, the molecule returns to its energetic ground state by emission of a photon of the same energy as incident photon. This common phenomenon is called *Rayleigh scattering* and belongs to a class of elastic scattering. The term *elastic scattering* is based on the fact that the energies of incident and emitted photons are identical. In addition to the common phenomenon of Rayleigh scattering, the molecule's energetic state may drop to a first excited energetic/vibrational state. This process is accompanied by emitting a photon of different energy. This effect is called *inelastic scattering* since the energies of incident and scattered photons are different. This process of inelastic scattering is known as *Stokes–Raman scattering*. In summary, the Raman effect is a light scattering effect and is caused by transitions between two vibrational states of energies. This vibrational information is specific to chemical bonds, functional groups, and molecule symmetry, which provides an unique fingerprint spectrum of molecules. Consequently, the Raman effect can be used, for example, for identity testing of substances as it is performed, for example, by means of FTIR (Fourier transform infrared spectroscopy). In this chapter, the use of Raman spectroscopy is elucidated with respect to particle identification in parenterals. More precisely, Raman spectroscopy in combination with a microscope, namely, Raman microscopy, is described.

In terms of application, Raman spectroscopy provides significant practical benefits to the pharmaceutical industry because it is user friendly, requires minimal sample handling, and provides unique spectra of various analytes, for example, contaminants, packaging materials, excipients, active agents, etc. Scientists working with Raman quickly recognized the advantages and opportunities it could provide the pharmaceutical industry. A review by Cutmore and Skett gives a good overview [13]. Although interference from samples' fluorescence may hamper acquiring Raman spectra, applications such as drug and polymorph screening have been studied employing Raman techniques.

Regarding particle identification, the aforementioned technologies—in their classical setup—may only analyze a couple of particles without a significant statistical base. Automating such technologies would enable the detection of a greater amount of particles and thereby provide a sound statistical base [14]. Several approaches have been taken to develop automated analytical technologies for airborne particles. Triggered mass spectrometry was applied by Prather et al. [15–17] to analyze the chemical composition of single particles. Hill et al. [18,19] developed a laser fluorescence technique to distinguish between biotic and abiotic particles. However, these techniques are not applicable to particles in liquid matrices. For this reason, particles could be separated by filtration and analyzed on a filter membrane. Automated SEM/energy dispersive using X-ray (EDX) [20,21] systems are available for particle analysis but provide data only on the elemental composition of a sample. Although this data may be helpful, elemental composition information is likely not enough for the characterization and discrimination of organic materials. This is due to the fact that various highly differing organic molecules are equal in respect to their elemental formula. Moreover, the elemental composition does not elucidate unique molecular properties that provide a fingerprint in vibrational–rotational spectroscopic methods. Unique fingerprint spectra increase the likelihood of reliable material identification. The combination of Raman microscopy and image analysis adds morphological information (i.e., shape and size of the particles) [22,23] creating yet another dimension of information.

11.2 STRENGTHS AND WEAKNESSES OF DIFFERENT METHODS FOR PARTICLE IDENTIFICATION

Raman microscopy allows for easy sample measurement. Ideally, it can be performed without destroying the sample, using a noninvasive and inexpensive sample preparation technique. Samples can be placed directly on the microscope stage. The risk of sample destruction and other limitations are discussed later. In contrast to IR measurements, water causes only a slight distortion to the spectrum due to its weak Raman scattering. Consequently, water-containing samples, for example, biological samples, living cells, or liquid protein formulations can also normally be investigated using Raman spectroscopy. The resolution of Raman spectroscopy corresponds to the laser wavelength, which is typically below 1 µm. Specialized Raman techniques such as tip-enhanced Raman spectroscopy (TERS) enable the analysis of particles as small as 100 nm. IR microscopy can typically investigate particles down to 10 µm and larger [24].

Both Raman and IR spectra provide a similar vibrational molecular fingerprint, making both techniques applicable for unknown particle identification. In addition, both vibrational techniques are easy to use and do not require specifically trained staff. It should be noted that molecules have chemical bonds and functional groups that may give stronger signals in Raman as compared to IR and vice versa. Therefore, IR and Raman can be considered complementary vibrational techniques.

Raman spectroscopy has a major disadvantage compared to IR with regard to sample heating using intensive laser radiation. If the sample's absorption bands overlap with the excitation wavelength of the laser, it can lead to the destruction of the sample. Suitable strategies have to be applied to balance the risk of sample destruction and obtaining reasonable spectra with good signal-to-noise (S/N) ratio, for example, by starting the measurements with rather low exposure times. This is especially important in applications for particle identification, where only few particles can be analyzed and no back-up sample is available. For particle identification in parenterals, the analyst may face the situation of having to analyze few visible particles in a single glass vial.

The most important disadvantage of Raman spectroscopy is its interference with fluorescence, which, in many cases, prevents the generation of Raman spectra. Fluorescence, because of its higher quantum efficiency, competes with the Raman effect and may mask its vibrational information. This situation may also arise if the particle contains a very small amount of fluorescent compound.

SEM is often applied especially because of its very high resolution. Since its inception decades ago, SEM has evolved from a simple analytical tool, with a resolution of about 50 nm, to a computer-assisted tool with a very high resolution. For a general introduction to SEM, the interested reader is referred to Ref. 25. Modern SEM setups allow to obtain images of a sample's surface with a resolution down to 2 nm and smaller (depending on the instrumental setup). Besides their high resolution, SEM micrographs found their way to many applications especially because of their large depth of field. More precisely, characteristic three-dimensional micrographs allow to map and describe the surface structure of a sample. The magnification range can be adjusted from $\times 10$ to $\times 50,000$. The magnification depends on the sample and appropriate sample preparation, but as a rule of thumb, SEM enables magnifications more than 100 times larger than that by a light microscope.

SEM combines imaging capabilities, structure analysis, and elemental analysis [25]. In terms of particle identification, the elemental analysis is not of great use for organic substances, as the detection of carbon will neither allow for the identification nor to link the particle to its source. For inorganic substances, however, SEM techniques can be of great use for particle identification. A major weakness of SEM is that it requires sputtering conductive coatings on a sample surface for sample preparation, which can alter or even destroy a sample [25]. This makes SEM prone to artifacts. In addition, the sputtering process is rather time consumptive.

Destructive sample preparation can be overcome by the use of an environmental scanning electron microscope (ESEM) [26,27]. In this instance, the untreated sample can be analyzed in a chamber with a reduced vacuum. Humid, wet samples as well as nonconducting samples can be investigated without further coating of the sample.

In summary, Raman spectroscopy and SEM are not competing but complementary techniques that give vibrational and elemental information on the particle. However, the combination is quite difficult because the Raman light objective must be mounted in close proximity to the vacuum part right above the sample. This setup is not easy to handle, and therefore, one supplier has already stopped manufacturing this equipment. The advantages of elemental and structural spectroscopic methods have led to breakthrough developments and the creation of a combination instrument with both laser-induced breakdown spectroscopy (LIBS) and Raman spectroscopy.

LIBS (metal.ID, rap.ID Particle Systems GmbH, Berlin, Germany) analyses detect the elemental composition of particles ranging from 10 μm and larger. The same area is then measured automatically with both technologies without any sample movement. The instrument has unparalleled advantages owing to the combination of an optical microscope (ambient air), easy sample transfer as well as real image.

11.3 EXPERIMENTAL SETUP OF RAMAN MICROSCOPY

11.3.1 General Setup and Requirements

First, we start with some considerations about sample volume and sensitivity. In a micro-Raman setup, a laser beam is focused onto the sample, enabling the measurement of extremely small sample volumes. The spot size is influenced by several optical factors. The focus of the Raman spectroscopic probe can theoretically be minimized to an area with a lateral diameter of about 250 nm (half of the laser wavelength of 532 nm). Focus depth depends on the confocality of the setup and is for a ×100 objective about 2 μm. With all these assumptions, a sampling volume of 0.75 $μm^3$ or in chemical measures just reaching down to the level of picomol can be measured. Therefore, virtually any object can be measured by means of Raman microscopy.

Owing to the minimal focus and particle size, the particle must remain still and perfectly aligned to the laser beam at the time of spectroscopy. Otherwise, the signal is lost or incorrect particles or areas are accidentally measured. One significant advantage of Raman spectroscopy is that, in principle, the wavelength of the laser can be selected freely. Several laser detector systems are available with a typical wavelength from 532 up to 1064 nm. A shorter wavelength has faster integration time and lower energy intensity compared to that of longer wavelengths.

The laser power in a 532-nm system is typically selectable from 10 down to 1 mW. The unit that determines the throughput of the optical system is typically counts/second. Many factors influence the sensitivity of a micro-Raman system including numerical aperture of the objective, transmission of the spectrometer, beam profile of the laser, sensitivity of the charge, and coupled device detector system.

Particle measurements can be performed in situ or on particle isolation. Both approaches are discussed in the following sections.

11.3.2 In Situ Measurements

Root-cause investigations of visible particle findings can be beneficial when measuring particles in situ within a closed container, for example, a prefilled syringe

[28]. In situ approaches mitigate the risk of particle contamination during sample preparation and all further steps required for retrieving a Raman spectrum. Measurements analyzed with this approach demand that the particle remains still and in a fixed position. For example, if the particle is adjacent to the inner wall of the container, then proper alignment with the laser focus can be ensured. In addition, in situ approaches require further prerequisites: the container wall, consisting of, for example, glass, also gives a Raman signal that has to be manually subtracted from the particles' signal using several mathematical operations. Such operations require very skilled operators and are quite time consuming. Finally, there is another prerequisite for in situ measurements that is briefly discussed. In the example of a particle attached to the inner wall of a syringe, the in situ approach may be only applicable if the particle is foreign (extrinsic), that is, is not a part of the matrix (i.e., formulation) or active itself. Otherwise, the Raman signals from the particle likely compete with signals from the solution. This effect may be even more prominent if a strong Raman scatterer is in solution. Consequently, in situ particle identification may be feasible, but standard procedure consists of particle isolation, which is discussed in the following section.

11.3.3   Particle Isolation

To isolate particles of interest from the solution, a filtration step is the method of choice. Filtration is also necessary if automated or statistically relevant investigations are planned with the samples. Several precautions have to be considered for successful filtration [29].

First, the filtration equipment as well as the filter itself should be clean and free of any particulate contamination. However, it is important to understand that a zero level of particulate contamination is highly unlikely. Therefore, to account for false-positive results, a blank measurement is highly recommended. The blank measurement provides information on the level of inherent particle contamination in the process before sampling and ensures that those low particle levels can be put into perspective for the real sample measurement. It is also beneficial to use special metal-coated filter membranes prepared in a clean room with a minimized level of contaminants (Fig. 11.1). The metal coating alone does not provide a Raman signal, whereas the organic filter membrane material, for example, polycarbonate, would provide a background signal. To minimize matrix effects, a special washing step may be required. For drug formulations, it may be mandatory to wash away excipients. However, this may bear the risk of particle redissolution. This can be balanced by analyzing the filter before and after washing.

Usually particle-free water (e.g., water for injection (WFI)) is used to wash the buffer salts and other excipients off.

A risk associated with washing is to obtain false-positive results resulting from the belief that contaminants have been washed away, which, however, dried on the filter instead. Once dried up, the salts from the buffers or other crystals may not necessarily redissolve again or redissolve quickly enough. The same is true for the active ingredient itself. Hence, filtration implies a risk of creating protein particles in protein samples.

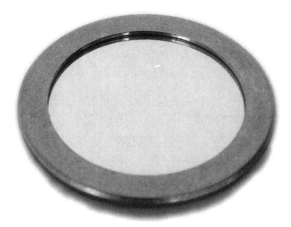

FIGURE 11.1   Filter membrane technology. The synthetic polycarbonate membrane is coated with a 100-nm gold layer and set in aluminum. Available pore sizes range from 0.2 to 8 μm (filtr.AID, rap.ID Particle Systems GmbH).

Part of the sample preparation is, of course, to determine the ideal amount of sample needed. If an imaging system is overloaded with particles, it can only count a mass of particles but cannot distinguish individual particles. In addition, the pores may be blocked and after a certain sample volume the filtration simply stops. Overall, particle filtration should be a standardized process with careful considerations for risks, especially regarding false-positive results. However, specific samples may require case-to-case adaptations.

11.3.4   General Setup of a Micro-Raman System

Figure 11.2 shows the general setup of a micro-Raman system. The $x-$, $y-$, z-positioning system in combination with the objective and video camera systems focuses on the particles and provides sharp and crisp dark-field images of the filter surface. The imaging and acquisition systems are able to see a laser light source, aligned with the image, to generate vibrational spectra using a spectrometer detection system.

The computer system automates the entire process and combines the imaging analysis data with the data from the integrated chemometrical identification [30].

11.3.5   Particle Detection Through Imaging Analysis

Once isolated on the filter membrane, the particles have to be visualized with a microscope. Several factors have to be considered to visualize the particles on the membrane. Important factors are the stability and technology of illumination. The metalized filter surface allows for a good contrast between recovered particles

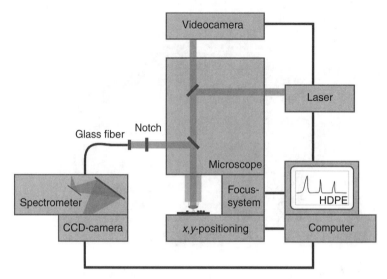

FIGURE 11.2   General setup of a micro-Raman system.

and the filter membrane using a dark-field illumination technique. Consequently, the smooth background appears black and the particles appear bright.

To detect particles in the nanometer range, a high level of optical magnification power is necessary. The single-particle explorer device (rap.ID Particle Systems GmbH) covers a measurement range from 500 nm to 150 µm. Representative microscopic images are shown in Fig. 11.3. Using a ×100 objective and a 2 MP digital camera one pixel represents a size of 110 nm.

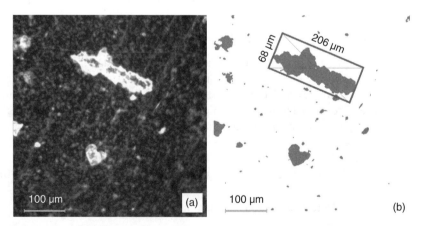

FIGURE 11.3   (a) Microscopic images of a membrane with white particles. (b) This image represents the same microscopic membrane as (a) after image recognition. Microscopic images of the membrane are represented as white particles in (a) and the same picture after image recognition in (b).

A stable acquisition of the image is necessary for fully automated particle recognition through an automatic image analysis system. The imaging system automatically takes up to 600 individual images (fields of view) from the membrane until the entire effective filtration area is evaluated by the system. The automated focusing feature provides sharpness in the images without user interaction.

The image is binarized and the particles are recognized (Fig. 11.3). The automated thresholding algorithm determines the grayscale threshold, making the result free of subjective judgment and therefore reproducible and easy to validate [22,31,32]. Particles overlapping multiple fields of view are stitched by a special algorithm to determine their real size easily reaching the millimeter level.

Analogous to the method of membrane evaluation described in the USP 788 [4], microscopic images of the entire membrane surface covered with particles are automatically recorded and evaluated.

Using this procedure, the position, length, and width of particles are determined down to the submicrometer. The entire particle-loaded area is scanned, a montage is obtained (Fig. 11.4), and particles overlapping multiple fields are combined and stitched to a single large particle with an integrated merging algorithm.

After image analysis, the coordinates (center of gravity and orientation) of all particles in the scanned area are obtained. The locations are determined and stored for subsequent automated integrated Raman spectroscopy.

Selection criteria for spectroscopy are set before or during the measurement. Particles meeting certain size criteria are chosen automatically for the analysis. Shape parameters, such as elongation or rectangularity, can also be used to preselect particles for fully automated analysis and to determine the automated Raman microprobe measurement of the particles. The movement of the membrane is controlled, and the motorized stage works in 50-nm steps. This is necessary to align the laser for the Raman analysis with an accuracy of 200 nm, enabling the

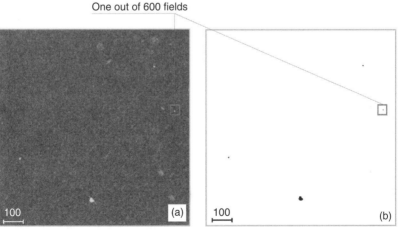

FIGURE 11.4   Montage of 600 individual fields of view (FOV), obtained within 7 min by the instrument.

automated spectroscopy of 500-nm particles such as single bacteria. The device carries out Raman spectroscopic examinations on the selected particles.

The resulting spectra are automatically matched to the pharmaceutical and customer-specific database created with Raman chemical fingerprints of material samples. The system also recognizes mixed composition materials, such as rubber stoppers or dyed polymers, due to their characteristic chemical fingerprint. A report is automatically created providing the size, shape, and best-matched Raman identification and spectrum quality for each individual particle in the form of hypertext protocol.

The analysis of thousands of particles helps users to locate major sources of contamination in various manufacturing processes. Over time, the ability to compare analytical results assists in detecting trends and implementing appropriate quality management. Routine use of the method contributes to ongoing supervision and optimization of production processes.

11.3.6   Reference Databases and Chemometry

This chapter discussed prerequisites for the general setup, sample preparation, and imaging analysis. This section focuses on reference databases. At the very end of the workflow, particle identification can only be as reliable as the reference spectra are. Generally, database spectra should show an excellent S/N ratio, at least 20. The better the database spectra and the clearer the distinctive features of the Raman fingerprint measurements are, the better the chemometrical recognition will work. Once an S/N value of 20 or better is obtained, the spectra can be put directly into the reference library. Therefore, time should be invested into obtaining excellent high quality spectra. High quality spectra provide better material retrieval through the chemometrical database search process.

The regular background level from fluorescence or elastic scattered light should be removed. This operation, called *detrending*, is usually automated within the spectroscopic software of the system. Software optimization could smooth spectra to remove the noise level.

In practical terms, the intrinsic particle sources (such as excipients) are well known regarding their quality, lot, etc. Moreover, they are available in sufficient amounts, either as highly pure powder or as liquid substances. This facilitates the generation of reference spectra, as they can be measured directly without any further sample preparation. The material sample is transferred into the system on a metalized surface or a stainless steel plate. Then, usually with an integration time of 30 s, Raman spectra with a suitable S/N ratio are obtained. The active pharmaceutical ingredient may present a special challenge with regard to reference spectra. Proteins, for example, are relatively weak Raman scatterers. They may be either in a dried or liquid state with at least a minimum matrix, for example, a buffer salt system. Besides having the protein solely in a buffer system, entire protein formulations, that is, including excipients, may be analyzed. For the latter case, the protein in a formulation may be ideally separated from the matrix because of the reasons described earlier. In principle, there are two major strategies to obtain protein reference spectra: (i) the measurement of protein in liquid and (ii) creating protein particles by stress and subsequent analysis of single particles. Approach (i) involves measuring a droplet of a protein solution in a low concentration buffer system. A sufficiently high protein concentration may turn the matrix signals (e.g., a histidine buffer) to negligible levels. The advantage of this strategy is that the protein can be measured in its native state. This may not be necessarily guaranteed by approach (ii), where the protein is stressed to obtain protein particles. To create protein particles, approaches such as heat denaturation or mechanical shaking may be applied. Consequently, the particles may be separated and collected on a filter as described earlier. The advantage is that such strategies try to mimic protein particles as a consequence of protein destabilization. However, the analyst should be aware of the fact that heat denaturation does not necessarily mimic the situation in a liquid formulation within a vial or syringe at real-time storage conditions. Therefore, one should handle such references with care. Raman spectroscopy provides structural information on proteins and their aggregates [33]. Slightly differing spectra may be obtained from a protein depending on the stress applied and the resulting conformational changes in the protein. For more information, we refer to an article by Wen [24] discussing a comprehensive review of Raman analysis on protein pharmaceuticals.

Extrinsic sources of particulate matter such as glass from syringes, cellulose fibers from various wipers, or sheets of paper are also measured and stored in the reference library [34–36] (Fig. 11.5). Samples with the size of a match head are directly measured, and the resulting Raman spectra are stored in the reference library. Sample material should be cross referenced according to its macroscopic appearance, for example, color and further by the material sample's use in the process. For example, plastic material is mainly made up of polypropylene and characterized by a color used for a tray in the filling line. The database entry could be "polypropylene—blue—filling line." In any case, a consistent strategy should be applied for naming reference spectra. More precisely, a material class is not necessarily linked to a particular particle source, especially in ubiquitous materials such as cellulose. The label "wiper" for respective reference spectrum may likely match many particle findings for most cellulose-based materials. The link to the particle source wiper may thus be misleading. However, this should also be considered vice versa. The analyst does not often have detailed information on the material class of a particles' source. The wiper may not be consisting of 100% cellulose; therefore, the label "cellulose" may be misleading as well.

If spectra have a high enough S/N ratio, several filters such as detrending and smoothing can be applied to prepare the spectra for automated identification using the chemometry function of an automated database search. "Pearsons" algorithm [37] can be used to retrieve a particle by comparing its spectrum with the spectra in the library database. Two individual factors influence the quality of the database match. One factor is the position of the peak and the other is the area under the peak. If both factors share strong similarities, a number from 500 to 1000 is calculated. This number describes the quality of the match and,

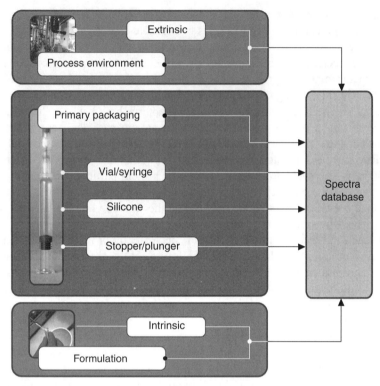

FIGURE 11.5   Sources of particulate contamination used for the setup of a spectral database.

depending on the algorithm, a value of 1000 would mean the spectra are identical. Numbers between 700 and 1000 are matches with a suitable quality. If the S/N ratio is above 20 and the match is below 700, this implies that the substance of interest is not located in the library. Consequently, this is not a match and the particle of interest is not identified.

Identification of a single particle would take about 60 s with traditional Raman methods. Therefore, it would take a total of 16 h to measure 1000 particles. Filters and statistics are usually applied to further improve and accelerate automated analysis and to find the predominant particle source. One could, for example, identify the largest 200 particles in an automated run with a measurement time of approximately 3 h.

11.4   USE OF RAMAN SPECTROSCOPY IN PARENTERALS

11.4.1   Optimization of Manufacturing Processes

Raman microscopy may be used for particle identification in the manufacturing process. Continuous use of this method may provide a historical database of particulate contaminants over time and enable the creation of a historical particle profile spanning several manufacturing batches.

Automated Raman microscopy provides information on which materials have been detected (e.g., cellulose, polypropylene, etc.) and also adds quantitative information (size, number, etc.). Sampling at different stages of the process helps to identify critical process steps/sources of interest. Deviations from historical profiles may be easily detected and troubleshooting exercises can be foreseen. The expandable customer library pinpoints the particle source location in the manufacturing process much easier, because it continually includes material from potential contamination sources [38].

11.4.2 Formulation Development and Stability Studies

During drug formulation development/screening studies, the drug product is manufactured, filled into primary packaging, and typically exposed to real-time and accelerated stress conditions for the sake of stability studies. The stability profile is analyzed during predetermined time points with various analytical endpoints and is compared to initial values (time point zero). Parenteral drugs, in particular, must be analyzed for visible particles as outlined in the introduction. In the event that visible particles are present in the formulation, the scientist is immediately interested in the particle source. The discussion of extrinsic versus intrinsic particles (Fig. 11.5) addresses whether the appearance of particulates is due to formulation instability at a defined stress condition and a certain time point or to other factors, for example, manufacturing or primary packaging.

For biotech parenterals, discrimination of protein particles from other sources is especially important. A major task for biotech formulations is to prevent the protein from precipitation or aggregation. Figure 11.6 illustrates Raman analysis on visible particles that appeared during the reconstitution of a lyophilized monoclonal antibody formulation. These vials were taken out of a climate chamber after storage for several months to analyze the stability profile. Raman microscopy analysis provides the formulation scientist with the following information: the visible particles are fiberlike (Fig. 11.6a), and their Raman spectrum (Fig. 11.6b) matches a cellulose-derived source (Fig. 11.6c) and differs significantly from the reference spectrum of the active, monoclonal antibody as shown in the normalized overlay (Fig. 11.7). The information acquired by the analysis answers the question of extrinsic particle contamination and confirms that the appearance of visible particles is not due to protein precipitation/aggregation. Such a conclusion, in formulation screening studies, may already be the desired outcome.

However, the issue of "how one would spot the source of contamination" is a significant issue that must be discussed. First, it is necessary to be aware of the overall workflow and manufacturing process. Lyophilized vials also undergo a 100% visible inspection on manufacture, but in already lyophilized state, thus making an inspection of particulates in solution challenging. There could be various sources responsible for this particulate contamination: it is possible that cellulose could have been a contaminant located in the primary packaging and

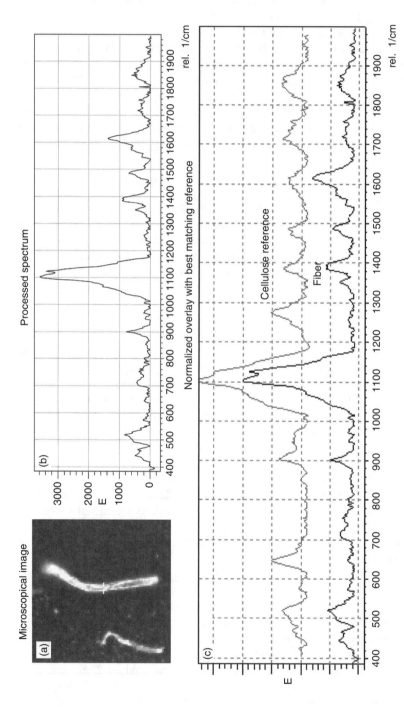

FIGURE 11.6 Raman microscopical analysis of visible particles observed on reconstitution of a lyophilized monoclonal antibody formulation. (a) Microscopical image: particles are fiberlike (note that only a representative fiber is shown). (b) Processed spectrum obtained from the fiber. (c) Normalized overlay of the fiber spectrum with the best matching reference, which was found to be cellulose-based material.

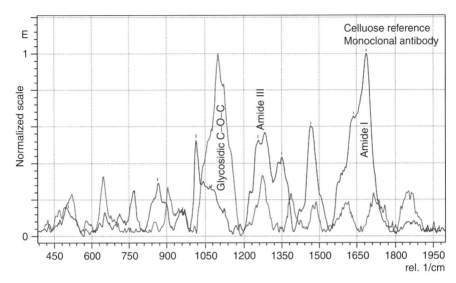

FIGURE 11.7   Overlay of a Raman spectrum of cellulose and a monoclonal antibody. The cellulose spectrum comprises the typical C–O–C–ether band; the monoclonal spectrum exhibits the typical Amide III and Amide I band. *(See insert for color representation of the figure.)*

some fibers were not washed away during the vial washing procedure, cellulose could derive from wipers or clothes used in the sterile facility, or finally the vial could have been contaminated during the reconstitution procedure. To pinpoint the contamination source, it is important to understand possible contaminants in the overall workflow as described in the previous section. Ideally, as outlined in Section 11.3.6, such possible contaminants would all be part of the reference database.

Overall, Raman microscopy can be a powerful tool for particle identification in formulation development and stability studies. It may facilitate the discrimination between extrinsic and intrinsic particles. Spotting the actual source can still be a challenge, especially for ubiquitous materials that can be derived from various sources in the overall process. The likelihood of success can be increased by a sound reference database pertaining to materials and process steps. This includes manufacturing processes as well as the primary packaging per se, which is discussed in the following section.

11.4.3   Optimization of Primary Packaging

Another application example is the detection of particulate matter in the primary packaging material. This is crucial in terms of minimization of visible rejects and finally the production of high quality parenterals. As shown in Fig. 11.5, typical examples are glass particles, silicon oil, and material from the closure.

It should be noted that, from a primary packaging perspective, particles leached from primary packaging and foreign particles in primary packaging are of interest.

The release of particles from a surface is dependent on several surface characteristics, such as smoothness, electrical charge, and the geometry of a primary packaging material. These characteristics influence the cleaning characteristics of each material as well as the cleanliness of testing procedures. A major prerequisite for such testing is reliable extraction methods for extracting particles from a material, container, or device. A validated procedure facilitates cleanliness levels control and ensures cleanliness levels comparison, over time, in differing production facilities.

Sample handling differs from simple filtration of, for example, a liquid parenteral formulation because it requires a reliable release of particles from the surface and subsequent sampling, for example, on a filter. Above all, this is mostly an incubation step, for example, in WFI allowing for subsequent filter analysis. Blank measurements and other sample preparation precautions (as described earlier) are necessary.

It is important to mention that particles may also appear due to interaction between the formulation and primary packaging material. Formulation screenings and stability studies should thus be carried out in representative packaging material.

Overall, Raman microscopy can be used for optimization and troubleshooting with respect to primary packaging.

11.5   SUMMARY

In summary, Raman spectroscopy/microscopy is a powerful tool used to help identifying particles in parenterals. As outlined above, Raman microscopy is capable of analyzing aqueous samples that contrast requirements for, say, FTIR instrumentation. In addition, the analyst receives additional information on particle shape, as simply assessed by microscopical analysis. This may not necessarily reflect the origin of a particle, but may provide useful hints. The Raman spectrum is based on molecular vibrational fingerprints that have similar features as IR spectra, whereas methods such as SEM-EDX provide only the elemental composition while neglecting unique molecular properties. It is important to note that both particle visualization and Raman analysis can be run in a fully automated manner.

In Situ measurements have been described for liquid formulations in different containers without further sample preparation [28], for example, foreign particles adsorbed to the inner wall of a prefilled syringe. Sample preparation is both time consuming and risks particle contamination; hence, in situ measurements can be very useful. However, in situ measurements are definitively not a routine procedure and require highly trained operators, especially for data processing (i.e., subtraction of matrix spectra). Consequently, standard procedures include isolating the particle from the liquid by means of filtration on a suitable filter. The sample preparation has to be handled with care due to particle contamination risks, matrix effects, and general artifacts obtained during workflow preparation. Unfortunately, Raman analysis also risks sample destruction through laser excitation. A high laser intensity or exposure time may be necessary during the measurement itself to obtain spectra with a sufficient S/N ratio.

Rayleigh scattering and interference from sample fluorescence is also a significant disadvantage to the method.

A key element for successful particle identification is the quality of reference spectra. The user should invest sufficient time to generate high quality spectra with a good S/N ratio. Consistent naming standards should be applied for reference spectra. Naming is important for foreign particle sources where sometimes the exact composition is unknown.

However, even with perfect reference databases, the likelihood of success depends on other factors as well, for example, the Raman intensity of the material of interest (strong vs poor Raman scatterers). Therefore, in many situations, the analyst may require case-to-case adaptations of the overall analysis workflow. This encompasses sample preparation, overcoming matrix effects and general strategies to obtain reasonable spectra both of analyte and reference.

Raman microscopy may be a powerful tool used to interpret particulate contamination sources in parenteral formulations. Such analysis may be used in manufacturing processes, formulation screening/stability studies, and primary packaging.

REFERENCES

1. Bruening E.J. Origin and significance of intra-arterial foreign body emboli in lungs of children. Virchows Arch 1955;327:460–479.
2. Garvan J. M, Gunner B.W. The harmful effects of particles in intravenous fluids Med J 1964;2:1.
3. Vonglahn W.C, Hall J.W The reaction produced in the pulmonary arteries by emboli of cotton fibers. Am J Pathol 1949;25(4):575–595.
4. USP. USP/NF General Chapter <788>. Particulate matter in injections. Rockville (MD): United States Pharmacopeial Convention; 2008.
5. Groves M.J. Parenteral products: the preparation and quality control of products for injection. London: William Heinemann Medical Books Ltd; 1978.
6. Godding E.W. Foreign matter in solutions for injections. Pharm J 1945;154:124.
7. Garvan J.M, Gunner B.W. Intravenous fluids: a solution containing such particles must not be used. Med J Aust 1963;50(2):140–145.
8. Garvan J.M, Gunner B.W. Particulate contamination of intravenous fluids. *Br J Clin Pract* 1971;25:119.
9. Lankers M. Visual inspection of parenterals—do you remember the reasons? In: Twelfth Arden House European Conference; London. 2007:
10. Knapp J.Z. Origin, result and measurement of USP "essentially free" inspection for visible contaminating particles. PDA J Pharm Sci Technol 2000;54(3):218–232.

11. Chalmers J.M, Griffiths P.R. Handbook of vibrational spectroscopy. New York: John Wiley & Sons; 2002.

12. Smith E, Dent G. Modern Raman spectroscopy: a practical approach. Hoboken, NJ, USA. Wiley & Sons; 2005.

13. Cutmore E.A, Skett P.W. Application of Fourier transform Raman spectroscopy to a range of compounds of pharmaceutical interest. Spectrochim Acta A Mol Spectrosc 1993;49(5–6):809–818.

14. Lewans M. Fingerprinting particles automatically. CleanRooms Magazine 2001;9–10.

15. Gard E, Mayer J.E, Morrical B.D, Dienes T, Fergenson D.P, Prather K.A. Real-time analysis of individual atmospheric aerosol particles: design and performance of a portable ATOFMS. Anal Chem 1997;69(20):4083–4091.

16. Whiteaker J.R, Prather K.A. Detection of pesticide residues on individual particles. Anal Chem 2003;75(1):49–56.

17. Silva P.J, Prather K.A. Interpretation of mass spectra from organic compounds in aerosol time-of-flight mass spectrometry. Anal Chem 2000;72(15):3553–3562.

18. Nachmann P, Chen G, Pinnick R.G, Hill S.C, Chang R.K, Mayo M.W and Fernandez G.L. Conditional-sampling spectrograph detection system for fluorescence measurements of individual airborne biological particles. Appl Opt 1996; 35(7):1069–1076.

19. Pinnick R.G, Hill S.C, Nachmann P, Videen G, Chen G, Chang R.K. Aerosol fluorescence spectrum analyzer for rapid measurment of single micrometer-sized airborne biological particles. Aerosol Sci Technol 1998; 28(2):95–104.

20. Kelly J.F, Lee R.J, Lentz S. Automated characterization of fine particulates Scan Electron Microsc 1980;1:3111.

21. Lee R.J, Kelly J.F. Applications of SEM-based automated images analysis. In: Wittry D.B, editor. Microbeam analysis. San Francisco: San Francisco Press; 1980.

22. Niemann M, Valet O. Development of an integrated measurement system for foreign particles testing in OINDP based on IPAC-RS recommendations. Respir Drug Deliv Eur 2005;1:181–184.

23. Blanchard J, Coleman J, Crim C, Dabreu-Hayling C, Fries L, Ghaderi R, Haeberlin B, Malcolmson R, Mittelman S, Nagoa L, Saracovan I, Shtohryn L, Snodgrass-pilla C, Sundahi M, Wolff R. Best practices for managing quality and safety of foreign particles in orally inhaled and nasal drug products, and an evaluation of clinical relevance. Pharm Res 2007;24(3): 471–479.

24. Wen Z. Raman spectroscopy of protein pharmaceuticals. J Pharm Sci 2007;96(11):2861–2878.

25. Goldstein J, Newbury D, Joy D, Lyman C, Echlin P, Lifshin E, Sawyer L, Michael J. Scanning electron microscopy and X-ray microanalysis. 3rd ed. New York: Kluwer Academic/Plenum Publishers; 2003.

26. Manero J.M, Gil F,J, Padros E, Planell J.A. Applications of environmental scanning electron microscopy (ESEM) in biomaterials field. Microsc Res Tech 2003;61(5):469–480.

27. Danilatos G.D. Bibliography of environmental scanning electron microscopy. Microsc Res Tech 1993;25(5–6):529–534.

28. Cao X.L, Wen Z.Q, Vance A, Torraca G. Raman microscopic applications in the biopharmaceutical industry: in situ identification of foreign particulates inside glass containers with aqueous formulated solutions. Appl Spectrosc 2009;63(7):830–834.

29. Valet O. Made to measure. CleanRoom Technol 2002.

30. Lankers M. Determining particle composition: consider the path to the source. PennWell: Cleanrooms; 2002;11–12.

31. Valet O, Niemann M. Qualification of the liquid particle explorer system for foreign particles counting and identification in a dry powder inhaler product based on IPAC-RS recommendations. Respir Drug Deliv 2006;3:761–764.

32. Valet O, Hess U. Method for foreign particles counting and identification in a cellulose containing suspension of a nasal spray formulation. Respir Drug Deliv Eur 2007;1:325–328.

33. Li C.H, Li T Application of vibrational spectroscopy to the structural characterization of monoclonal antibody and its aggregate Curr Pharm Biotechnol 2009;10(4):391–399.

34. Hayashi T. Relationship between the compositions of rubber closures and occurences of particulate matter in parenteral solutions. Yakuzaigaku 1980;40:68–73.

35. Dolcher, D, Material and process environment related particles from elastomeric closures. In: Proceedings of P.D.A. International Conference on Particle Detection, Metrology and Control; 1990; Washington, DC. pp. 103–132.

36. Dolcher D. Particles on rubber closures 1991. pp. 246–247.

37. Pearson K. Notes on the history of correlation. Biometrika 1920;13(1):25–45.

38. Valet O, Lankers M. Measurement and identification of foreign particles in a QbD environment - streamlining with efficient analytical methods. Respir Drug Deliv 2008;3:723–726.

12 Microscopic Methods for Particle Characterization in Protein Pharmaceuticals

PATRICK GARIDEL

Pharmaceutical Development, Process Science/Biopharmaceuticals, Boehringer Ingelheim Pharma GmbH & Co. KG, Biberach an der Riss, Germany

ANDREA HERRE and WERNER KLICHE

Biopharmaceuticals, Quality Control and Materials Testing, Boehringer Ingelheim Pharma GmbH & Co. KG, Biberach an der Riss, Germany

12.1 INTRODUCTION

Proteins have the tendency to form aggregates. This depends on the protein stability properties, protein solution conditions, and various stresses that a protein may encounter, for example, during its manufacturing (Chapter 1). In addition, small changes in the three-dimensional structure or amino acid modifications (e.g., oxidation) are possible causes for the formation of protein aggregates [1]. Protein aggregates can cover an extremely broad size range, starting in the range of a few nanometers up to particles of a few millimeters. Thus, a particle size range of more than six orders of magnitude is covered, and none of the actually available techniques is able to correctly analyze samples containing this multitude of particle sizes. Especially techniques for the subvisible particle range are scarce.

The term *particle* is used as a generic term including nonproteinaceous particles (e.g., glass particle, metal particle, and silicone oil droplet) as well as proteinaceous particles (aggregates and associates) [2]. As protein aggregates can become large enough and thus become accessible to different microscopic techniques, it is obvious that one could try employing microscopy to get more insights into the formation of protein aggregates. Moreover, the progresses in the improvement of the resolution, as well as the development of new techniques,

Analysis of Aggregates and Particles in Protein Pharmaceuticals, First Edition.
Edited by Hanns-Christian Mahler, Wim Jiskoot.
© 2012 John Wiley & Sons, Inc., Published 2012 by John Wiley & Sons, Inc.

allow the investigation of very small particles in the range of a few nanometers (Table 12.1).

There are a number of techniques to detect, characterize, and quantify protein aggregates, but all these methods have some technical limitations as described by Garidel and Kebbel [2] and other chapters in this book.

The easiest way to detect visible protein aggregates is visual inspection of the protein solution, as described in Chapter 6. This enables the analysis of protein particles down to 0.1 mm under optimal conditions. In certain cases, a magnifying glass is necessary. For the visualization of smaller aggregates/particles, other techniques are available. The most prominent method is the classical light microscope. Depending on the light and wavelength used as well as technical components (e.g., filters and detector components), currently available light microscopes differ a lot in resolution (for more details, see Ref. 3).

Using light with a wavelength of 400–600 nm, the theoretical resolution is 0.2 µm. This is the so-called Abbe limit, which was described at the end of the nineteenth century by the optic laws presented by Ernst Abbe [4]. The resolution of 0.2 µm is obtained using a wavelength of 550 nm with an aperture of 1.4 [5]. Different variants of light microscopic methods are applied for the analysis of particles in biopharmaceuticals: static light microscopy (LM, manual or automated) and, more recently, dynamic LM (microflow imaging; see Chapter 7).

For smaller particles, several electron microscopic techniques are used [6].

Another high resolution technique is atomic force microscopy (AFM) that allows the resolution of a few nanometers, depending on the sample analyzed.

All these techniques rely on the visualization of the investigated particles. The identification of the particles is based on "experience" or data bases. In general, no information on the chemical nature of the particle is obtained, with the exception of SEM-EDX (scanning electron microscopy combined with energy dispersive X-ray analysis). However, there are techniques available with lower resolution that may allow the chemical identification of particles. Among these methods are, for example, Fourier transform infrared (FTIR) or Raman microscopy (for more details, see Chapter 11).

A major challenge using microscopic techniques is the isolation and preparation of the particle(s) of interest, because one has to show that the particle isolation protocol has no impact on the nature of the particle and that the analyzed sample aliquot is representative for the whole sample. The latter is especially important when precise and accurate particle numbers per sample are to be obtained. For most microscopic techniques, the information that can be obtained regarding the number of particles is very limited. A technique (microscopic flow imaging) overcomes this problem for the characterization and quantification of particles larger than 2 µm (Chapter 7).

In this chapter, we describe the application of selected microscopic techniques: LM, electron microscopy (EM), AFM, flow imaging techniques (Chapter 7), and

TABLE 12.1 Overview of Selected Microscopic Techniques

Technique	Particle Size Range	Advantages	Disadvantages[a]	Applicability for Protein Pharmaceuticals
Visual inspection	~150 μm to cm	No cost investment Easy to perform Detection of foreign and protein particles (training of analyst needed) Fast Nondestructive	Subjective method Very limited quantitative information Limited qualitative information	100% visual inspection (drug product) Release and stability testing Troubleshooting
LM	~0.2 μm to cm	Detection of foreign and protein particles (training of analyst needed), protein particles by staining with protein-specific dyes Easy to perform Low cost investment Quantitative method for subvisible particles (EP)	Subjective method with respect to the characterization of particles, which depends on user/reference samples/data base Time consuming for particle counting	Routine release and stability testing Trouble shooting
Automated light microscopy	~2.5 μm to cm	Automated morphometric analysis High reproducibility Qualitative (particle size classes) and quantitative method (number per class)	Higher costs than manual microscopy	For example, routine water monitoring Routine release and stability testing Troubleshooting

(continued)

TABLE 12.1 *(continued)*

Technique	Particle Size Range	Advantages	Disadvantages[a]	Applicability for Protein Pharmaceuticals
Electron microscopy (General)	~0.1–1 nm to cm	Detection of foreign and protein particles (protein particles by staining with protein-specific dyes); High resolution; Detailed information on Topography (surface characteristics); Morphology (size, shape)	High costs for investment and maintenance; Low sample throughput; May require complex sample preparation; Time consuming; Not quantitative (particle number)	Troubleshooting; Characterization
Transmission electron microscopy (TEM)	~0.1 nm to cm	Thin samples	Possible sample damage due to beam impact	Troubleshooting
Reflection electron microscopy (REM)	Nanometer to millimeter	Massive samples	Costly equipment; Surface analysis	Troubleshooting
Scanning electron microscopy (SEM)	~1 nm to cm	Three-dimensional structure of the sample ("topographic images")	Costly equipment; Coating of the sample with several nanometers of conductive material needed, which might disturb the delicate sample structure, and the sample appear to be "smoothed"	

Method	Resolution/Range	Properties	Limitations	Application
		Qualitative sample identification	Costly equipment	Troubleshooting
		Relative quantitative elemental information (particles 1 μm in diameter and 1 μm in depth)		
		Images of a few millimeters can be investigated with a depth of field on the order of millimeters		
Scanning transmission electron microscopy (STEM)	~0.1 nm to cm	Form atomic resolution images	Costly equipment	Troubleshooting
		Using dark-field microscopy allows high contrast imaging of biological samples without requiring a staining		
Atomic force microscopy AFM	~0.1 nm to 100 μm	High resolution	High costs for investment and maintenance	Troubleshooting
		Detailed information on Topography (surface characteristics)	Low sample throughput	Characterization
			Time consuming	

(continued)

TABLE 12.1 (*continued*)

Technique	Particle Size Range	Advantages	Disadvantages[a]	Applicability for Protein Pharmaceuticals
		Morphology (size and shape)	Can "only" image a maximum height on the order of micrometers and a maximum scanning area of about 150 × 150 μm	
			Cannot normally measure steep walls or overhangs	
		True three dimensional	Not quantitative (particle number)	
		No need for sample manipulation		
		Applicability under ambient air conditions manipulation surface profile		
		Possibility to investigate samples under fully hydrated conditions		
Flow imaging techniques	~ 2 to 400 μm	(Automated) analysis of the particle size and shape	Particle detection limit > 2 μm	Troubleshooting
		Quantitative method (particle number and size)	Generation of extremely large amounts of data, which may pose a challenge for data evaluation	
		No sample preparation necessary		

Fourier transform infrared (FTIR) microscopy	~25 μm to cm	Identification of single particles	High costs for investment and maintenance	Troubleshooting
		Identification of subcomponents of "mixed" particles	Low sample throughput	Characterization
		Protein particles: characterization of secondary structure	Time consuming	
			Not quantitative (particle number)	
			Establishment of spectra library necessary for the identification of particles	

[a]For each method described, the preparation of the particles is challenging and bears the risk to lose particles or to contaminate the sample with particles from the environment or equipment. Additionally, selecting a representative sample volume may be challenging for any microscopic method, especially with increasing magnification and thus decreasing sample aliquot per analysis.

infrared (IR) microscopy for the investigation of particles with a focus on protein particles. Note that Raman microscopy is discussed in Chapter 11.

12.2 LIGHT MICROSCOPY (LM)

The basic physical principles of LM are known since ages with the studies of Christiaan Huygens, Robert Hooke, Antoni van Leeuwenhoek, Michel Ferdinand d'Albert d'Ailly, just to name a few protagonists of the seventeenth century [6]. For an introduction, refer to Refs 3, 5, and 6.

Although it is an "old" technique, LM is still successfully used for the characterization of biological samples such as tissues, cells, and protein assemblies [7–11], also in combination with, for example, polarized light [12]. The methods are often used in medical research for the identification of pathological relevant protein aggregates, for example, in Alzheimer disease (A-β peptides, τ-protein), spongiform encephalopathies (prions), and Parkinson disease (α-synuclein). By applying LM, information on particle size and overall particle morphology (shape, surface roughness, compactness, color, and transparency) can be obtained.

The resolution of LM is in the tenth of micrometer range (theoretical resolution 0.2 µm). Although the resolution is low, the advantage of the method is the low cost investment of the equipment as well as the ease of use. A droplet (a few microliter) of the sample containing the particles may be placed on a microscopic glass and directly investigated. In this case, the handling is limited. However, a challenging issue can be to assure isolating a representative aliquot of the sample, especially in case that only few particles are present in a large volume of sample. A possibility for particle separation may be isolation via filtration. Generally, one has to make sure that the collection of the sample will have no impact on the sample quality. Besides particle loss due to adsorption to pipette tips or vials, potential contamination with non-sample related particles has to be avoided (e.g., by working under laminar airflow conditions). For protein pharmaceuticals, both generation and disassembly of proteinaceous particles may occur during sample preparation. The sample amount required depends on the amount of particles per volume and how easily these particles can be suspended and be collected via filtration.

Figure 12.1 shows an example of particles that were formed in a protein formulation after stirring the solution for 4 h at room temperature. The experimental stress conditions are described elsewhere [13]. In Fig. 12.1a, it is shown that a number of particles in the size range of a few micrometers have been formed. The shape and size of the particles widely differ. In an accelerated shaking stress test of a protein formulation in a siliconized syringe, LM showed the appearance of spherical particles (Fig. 12.1b), which were likely to be silicone emulsified in the aqueous solution [14]. On the basis of the morphology of the investigated particles, the authors were able to discriminate silicone oil particles from protein particles.

The European Pharmacopeia describes how to quantify the amount of subvisible particles using a microscope [15]. In brief, a binocular microscope is used

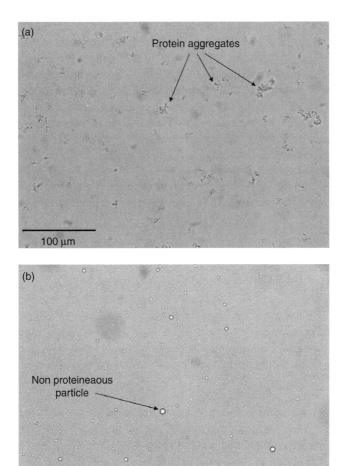

FIGURE 12.1 (a) Protein particles, formed by stirring a liquid protein formulation for 4 h at room temperature in a 2 R vial, as observed by light microscopy. (b) Light microscope investigation of a sample filled in a siliconized syringe under accelerated shaking stress stability conditions.

and a filtration stage using membrane filters for the collection of the particles. The microscope is equipped with a calibrated ocular micrometer enabling the determination of the size of particles investigated by microscopy. Furthermore, the microscope is equipped with two illumination systems, one of which illuminates the sample from the top and the other one from the side at an angle of 10–20°. According to the European Pharmacopeia, the magnification is set to 100 ± 10. For the determination of the particle size, a linear scale is used with scale division of 10 μm.

Using LM, the characterization of the observed particles generally depends on the training of the user, reference samples, and/or a data base, especially for the morphological classification of the particles. For particle counting as described in the pharmacopeial microscopic methods, another limitation is that the particle sizing process with the use of a circular diameter graticule is carried out "by transforming mentally the image of each particle into a circle and comparing it to the 10- and 25-μm graticule reference circles" [15]. This procedure is rather difficult and imprecise for irregular-shaped particles. Additionally, it is time consuming. For this reason, the pharmacopeial methods allow partial filter counting and determination of total filter count by calculation. However, in doing so, only a small aliquot may be analyzed, raising the question on the representativeness of the aliquot for the whole sample.

For protein pharmaceuticals, another drawback can be that protein particles that may have only limited visible contrast are not or only partially detected. The methodological limitations of the pharmacopeial methods may be partially overcome by two techniques: (i) automated microscopy with image analysis and (ii) the application of staining techniques using dyes.

In automated microscopy, a microscope with a motorized stage automatically scans a sample deposited on a filter taking various picture frames per filter. All picture frames are then combined to a single picture covering the whole filter area (Fig. 12.2). This picture is analyzed with imaging software differentiating filter background from particles by setting a grayscale threshold value that is intermediate between the filter background grayscale and the particle grayscales. Identified particles can be classified by the imaging software according, for example, to their size or shape. Thus, particle sizing is no longer user dependent, and as the method is automated, less user-time is required for the analysis. As a consequence, larger filter areas corresponding to larger sample volumes can be analyzed, increasing the representativeness of the analyzed sample aliquot and consequently the accuracy and precision of the particle counting results. Simultaneously, particles can be photodocumented for potential later analysis by the imaging software. However, the method cannot be fully automated as, for example, threshold setting has to be done manually. Additionally, the elimination of potentially overlapping particles or of particles that may have been segmented by the imaging software also has to be conducted manually to guarantee precise and accurate particle quantification. Segmented particles may be of special concern when analyzing protein particles combining low and high contrast areas within one particle as the imaging software may not be able to distinguish low contrast areas from filter background, thus segmenting the particle during image analysis artificially into two or more particles.

With the aim to increase the detectability of low contrast protein aggregates, fluorescence microscopy may be applied together with dyes that selectively bind to proteins. Demeule et al. [16] presented a study for the detection and characterization of protein aggregates by fluorescence microscopy (in this book) using the hydrophobic dye Nile Red and comparing their results with protein aggregate staining using Congo Red and Thioflavin T. They found that Nile Red staining is a valuable option for the detection of protein aggregates (Chapter 9). The advantage of this approach is its high detection sensitivity [17].

FIGURE 12.2   Picture of filter surface composed of various picture frames taken by auto-mated scanning of the filter surface. (Picture was provided by Carl Zeiss MicroImaging GmbH.)

Li et al. [18] also addressed this issue using a commercially available staining kit, using a dye that selectively binds to proteinaceous samples. They concluded that by using such an approach for the detection of insoluble aggregates (i) particles are easier observed because of the staining and (ii) the staining method is selective for protein aggregates and thus avoids interferences from most other nonprotein particles.

A 0.22-μm filter membrane is used for the assay to filter the solution containing the protein aggregates. First, the filter has to be washed, thus making sure that no contamination occurs. The filtered particles are then stained for 5 min (according to the manufacturer's protocol using a defined staining concentration) on the membrane. The filter is again washed to remove the staining solution and air dried. The washing step has to be performed with care to avoid loss of particles. These steps should be performed under a laminar flow hood to avoid contaminations. The filter with the stained particles is transferred to the microscope (sample has to be covered to avoid external contamination) and then investigated. Figure 12.3 shows an example of staining protein aggregates using this kit. As can be seen, some particles were stained, which are of proteinaceous nature. These particles that are stained may be protein aggregates or nonproteinaceous particles on which protein is adsorbed. In the last case, one option is to strongly wash the particles with, for example, detergent solutions to remove the adsorbed protein. However, the success of such a procedure depends on the nature of the particles. For instance, particles were also observed that were not

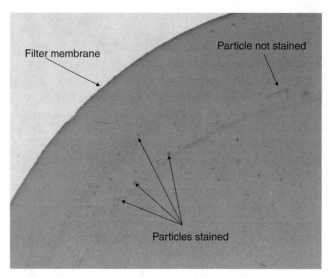

FIGURE 12.3 Identification of protein aggregates by means of a protein-specific staining procedure (see text) using light microscopy.

stained. In the presented case, these particles were cleaning paper as used in the laboratory. The assay is quite time consuming and external contaminations are difficult to avoid. Therefore, this method can be used for troubleshooting purposes, but not as a routine detection method.

12.3 ELECTRON MICROSCOPY (EM)

Compared to LM, where the illumination is performed using visible light, EMs use a beam of highly energetic electrons to examine objects on a nanometer scale and thus create a highly magnified image. The magnifications obtained with EM are much higher than those obtained with light microscopes, reaching magnifications of up to two million times for EM compared to the lower magnification of maximum 2000 times for LM. The information derived from EM investigations of a biological sample are as follows [6]:

1. Topography, that is, the surface characteristics of the sample and its texture. On the basis of this information, one can derive additional sample properties such as the hardness of the sample, its reflectivity, etc.
2. Morphology, that is, the shape and particle size of the sample.
3. Composition, that is, the chemical elements the analyzed sample is composed of and their relative amounts.

There are different types of EM techniques [6]. They can be distinguished on the nature and chemical composition of the investigated samples. One criterion is the geometry and physical and chemical properties of the sample. For massive samples, one can measure the signals that are reflected from the sample surface according to reflection geometry (reflection EM). If the sample is thin enough, transmission is feasible (transmission EM). Another differentiation criterion is based on the used instrument type, depending on whether the image is generated by means of a system configured on the physical principle of LM or based on a rastering approach as used in classical television (raster EM).

The four large EM families are described in the following sections.

12.3.1   Transmission Electron Microscopy (TEM)

As described above, transmission electron microscopy (TEM) functions by applying a high voltage electron beam to the sample and thus creating an image of the sample. The electron source is an electron gun (tungsten cathode), from which the electrons are emitted, and the electron beam is accelerated by an anode (40–400 keV). The beam is focused by electrostatic and electromagnetic lenses and transmitted through the sample that is partly transparent to electrons and partly scatters the electrons.

When the electrons emerge from the sample, the electrons have interacted with the sample, and as a consequence, the electron beam carries information about the sample structure that is magnified by the objective lens system of the microscope. The spatial variation in this information (the "image") is viewed by projecting the magnified electron image onto a fluorescent viewing screen. The images can be recorded using a charge-coupled device camera. The TEM resolution is limited primarily by spherical aberration [5]. However, with the development of new devices, it was possible to partially overcome spherical aberration to increase resolution. The highest image resolution using TEM lies in the Angstrom range at magnifications above 50 million times. Such high resolutions are especially obtained in material sciences [6].

12.3.2   Reflection Electron Microscopy (REM)

In reflection electron microscopy (REM), an electron beam is incident on a sample surface, but instead of using the transmission (TEM) or secondary electrons (SEM), the reflected beam of elastically scattered electrons is detected. The advantages, limitations, and applications of these techniques have been summarized by Egerton [19].

12.3.3   Scanning Electron Microscopy (SEM)

In TEM (see above), the electrons of the high voltage beam carry the information for generating the image of the sample. This is different for SEM, namely, the electron beam is not at any time carrying the complete image of the specimen, but the image is produced by probing the sample with a focused electron beam that is scanned across a rectangular area of the sample (raster scanning technique). At each point on the specimen, the incident electron beam loses some energy, and that lost energy is converted into other energy forms, such as heat, emission of low energy secondary electrons, backscattered electrons, light emission (cathode luminescence), or characteristic X-ray emission. These different physical principles of the interaction of the primary electron beam with the sample are used for sample characterization [19].

The display of the SEM maps the varying intensity of any of these signals into the image in a position corresponding to the position of the beam on the sample when the signal was generated. The normal operating SEM mode is the use of a secondary electron detector for generating the image.

The image resolution of SEM is, in general, about an order of magnitude lower than that of a TEM. However, because the SEM image relies on surface processes rather than transmission, it is able to image bulk samples up to several centimeters in size (depending on instrument design) and has a much greater depth of view and so can produce images that are a good representation of the three-dimensional structure of the sample [6] (Fig. 12.4).

SEM has certain popularity in life-science applications among the different EM techniques, because it allows the generation of three-dimensional-like images (topographic images) of the sample surface. This three-dimensional-like image appearance is due to the large depth of field of the scanning EM as well as to the shadow relief effect of the secondary and backscattered electron contrast. This is clearly shown in Fig. 12.4b.

SEM also allows the generation of sample information with regard to its composition. The characteristic X-rays are emitted as a result of the primary electron beam bombardment of the sample. The analysis of the characteristic X-radiation emitted from samples allows qualitative sample identification as well as quantitative elemental information from regions of a sample nominally 1 μm in diameter and 1 μm in depth under normal operating conditions (for more details, see Ref. 20).

With a conventional electron source, the lateral resolution is ~10–50 nm and the depth resolution 10–1000 nm (backscattered electrons) or 1–10 nm (secondary electrons).

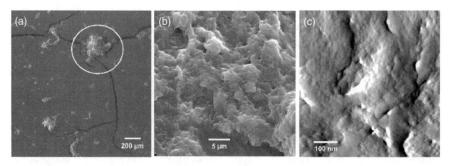

FIGURE 12.4 Scanning electron microscopic (SEM) investigation of protein aggregates (a) and (b) SEM images at different magnification. (c) Atomic force microscopic (AFM) investigation of the protein aggregate in the noncontact mode.

12.3.4 Scanning Transmission Electron Microscopy (STEM)

The scanning transmission electron microscopy (STEM) rasters a focused incident probe (incident electron beam) across a thin sample to facilitate the detection of electrons scattered through the sample. Thus, the high resolution as obtained in TEM is also possible in STEM. The focusing action (and aberrations) occurs before the electrons hit the specimen in the STEM, but afterward in the TEM [20].

EM systems involve both high investment costs and high costs for maintenance.

Furthermore, depending on the type of EM experiment performed, there is a more or less complex sample preparation involving, for example, chemical fixation, cryo fixation, sample dehydration, embedding, sectioning, staining, freeze fracturing, and freeze etching [6,20,21]. Such preparations are especially necessary for the investigation of biological samples such as protein–protein or protein–membrane complexes or cells. Such samples are, in general, mechanically fragile and must be stabilized by fixation, are too thick to be investigated, lack electron contrast (staining is necessary), or are hydrated (dehydration necessary). All these preparations may lead to artifacts and sample damage. Therefore, various techniques are applied to investigate a sample to be able to recognize possible artifacts induced by the sample manipulation and preparation [22–27].

However, the first challenge is sample isolation (see Section 12.2).

For most EM techniques, the samples are viewed in vacuum, with the exception of environmental SEM (ESEM) allowing the analysis of hydrated samples. ESEM is a special adaptation of SEM, with the main differences being the lower vacuum in the sample chamber and the accordingly modified detector [19], resulting in a lower resolution compared with other EM techniques.

When operating a SEM experiment, one usually has conductive or semiconductive samples. However, for biological samples, which are nonconductive, the sample has to be prepared and coated with a thin layer (several nanometers) of conductive material (e.g., gold) to be investigated by SEM. This coating has the potential to disturb the delicate sample structure, and the sample appears to be "smoothed."

However, all these limitations are known and can be handled by appropriate experimental protocols [6,19]. EM offers a unique chance to investigate samples at extremely high resolution. Therefore, EM investigations are highly used, especially when combined with new image analysis capabilities [28–32]. A number of applications for biological samples and in medical research (e.g., medical devices, implants) are available [33–35].

A SEM image of protein aggregates with sizes in the range between 50 and 200 μm are shown in Fig. 12.4a, and 12.4a magnification of the large aggregate (marked by a circle in Fig. 12.4a) is represented in Fig. 12.4b, showing a cloudlike structure. Such a structure is often observed for thermally induced protein denaturation and the formation of aggregates. Figure 12.4c shows the same sample as investigated by AFM (see discussion below).

12.4 ATOMIC FORCE MICROSCOPY (AFM)

AFM is a follow-up microscope based on the scanning tunneling microscope, which was developed about 20 years ago [36]. AFM, or scanning force microscopy, is a very high resolution type of scanning probe microscopy allowing lateral resolutions in the nanometer range (for biological samples).

The information is gathered by "feeling" the surface with a mechanical probe, such as the needle of a record player "feeling" the record [37].

Thus, the AFM consists of a cantilever (mechanical probe) with a sharp tip (probe with a radius of curvature on the order of nanometers) at its end that is used to scan the sample surface. When the tip is brought into proximity of a sample surface, various forces between the tip and the sample lead to a deflection of the cantilever according to Hooke's law. In general, the cantilever deflection is measured using a laser spot reflected from the top surface of the cantilever into an array of photodiodes. The cantilever is now scanned over the sample. The measured height deflection is measured and the information converted into a false-colored image.

The AFM can be operated in a number of modes, depending on the application and sample nature. In general, possible imaging modes are divided into static (also called *contact*) modes and a variety of dynamic (or *noncontact*) modes where the cantilever is vibrated [21,36,38,39].

In the static mode operation, the static tip deflection is used as a feedback signal. Because the measurement of a static signal is prone to noise and drift, low stiffness cantilevers are used to boost the deflection signal. However, close to the surface of the sample, attractive forces can be quite strong, causing the tip to "snap-in" to the surface. Thus, static mode AFM is almost always done in contact where the overall force is repulsive. Consequently, this technique is typically called *contact mode*. In the contact mode, the force between the tip and surface is kept constant during scanning by maintaining a constant deflection [40].

Using the constant-height mode, the spatial variation of the cantilever deflection (deflection mode) can be used directly to generate the topographic data set because the height of the scanner is fixed as it scans.

In the dynamic mode, the cantilever is externally oscillated at or close to its fundamental resonance frequency. The oscillation amplitude, phase, and resonance frequency are modified by tip–sample interaction forces; these changes in oscillation with respect to the external reference oscillation provide information about the sample's characteristics. Schemes for dynamic mode operation include frequency modulation and the more common amplitude modulation [36,40]. In frequency modulation, changes in the oscillation frequency provide information about tip–sample interactions.

Operating using amplitude modulation, changes in the oscillation amplitude or phase provide the feedback signal for imaging. In amplitude modulation, changes in the phase of oscillation can be used to discriminate between different types of materials on the surface. Amplitude modulation can be operated either in the noncontact or in the intermittent contact regime [36]. In ambient conditions, most samples develop a liquid meniscus layer. Because of this, a major hurdle for the noncontact dynamic mode in ambient conditions is keeping the probe tip close enough to the sample for short-range forces to become detectable while preventing the tip from sticking to the surface. This can have an impact on the sample imaging procedure. Dynamic contact mode (also called *intermittent contact* or *tapping mode*) was developed to bypass this problem. In dynamic contact mode, the cantilever is oscillated such that the separation distance between the cantilever tip and sample surface is modulated [21].

Biological samples are often investigated using the noncontact mode, because the impact of the AFM tip with the soft biological sample is minimized.

The lateral resolution is in the nanometer range and the height resolution in the lower nanometer to Angstrom range.

Compared to EM, which provides in most cases a two-dimensional projection or a two-dimensional image of a sample, AFM provides a true three-dimensional surface profile. Furthermore, there is no need for sample manipulation for AFM as it is necessary for SEM (coating required for biological sample). A further advantage of AFM is the applicability under ambient air conditions and the possibility to investigate samples under fully hydrated conditions [36].

In principle, AFM can provide higher resolution than that by SEM.

A major drawback of AFM is the fact that the method is time consuming; thus, it is a tool not for routine analysis, although in chip-development AFM is used as a quality indicating method.

A further disadvantage of AFM compared with SEM is the image size, which is under investigation. Using SEM, images of a few millimeters can be investigated with a depth of field on the order of millimeters. Depending on the scanner used, AFM can only image a maximum height in the order of micrometers and a maximum scanning area of around 150×150 μm. One has also to consider that the nature of AFM probes normally does not allow to measure steep walls or overhangs.

However, AFM is used for the investigation of a number of biological samples from biological membranes up to single proteins [41–45].

San Paulo and García [46] imaged single antibodies using AFM and were able to demonstrate the Y-shape of these proteins (see also Ref. 47).

Maco et al. [48] have recently shown the structure of the nuclear pore complex by using AFM combined with information from EM.

Figure 12.4 shows a protein aggregate sample investigated by SEM (Fig. 12.4b) and AFM (Fig. 12.4c). AFM allows a much higher resolution at the cost of viewing just a small part of the sample. Two (dried) protein aggregates of sizes between 10 and 30 μm are shown in Fig. 12.5. Figure 12.5a represents the height mode, whereas the deflection mode is shown in Fig. 12.5b. Using the deflection mode, the three-dimensional aspect of the sample is slightly lost; the sample looks flattened. However, more details of the surface are observed.

The mechanism of how larger protein aggregates are formed can be estimated based on the results shown in Fig. 12.6a–c (a: height, b: amplitude, and c: phase

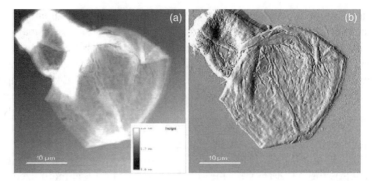

FIGURE 12.5 Atomic force microscopic (AFM) investigation of protein particles in the contact mode under ambient air conditions: (a) height mode and (b) deflection mode.

mode). The large protein aggregate of ~600 nm is composed of smaller units of a size of ~50–100 nm. Another example is shown in Fig. 12.6d–f (d: height, e: amplitude, and f: phase mode), where again the protein particle seems to consist of subunits of similar size. Thus, it may be that first a certain protein aggregate population of about 50–100 nm is formed and these particles associate to form much larger aggregates.

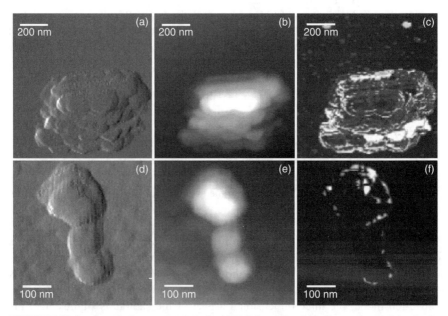

FIGURE 12.6 Atomic force microscopic (AFM) investigation of protein particles in the noncontact mode at room temperature: (a, e) height mode, (b, d) amplitude mode, and (c, f) phase mode for two examples (a–c and d–f).

12.5 EMERGING MICROSCOPIC TECHNOLOGIES

The described techniques EM or AFM allow the investigation of protein aggregates at extremely high resolution. Because these methods are time consuming, just a selected amount of aggregates can be analyzed. Quantification of the particles in a solution is not practicable with these methods.

Since a few years, new approaches were developed for the quantification of particles in solution, however, with a drawback in size resolution. Most of these approaches are based on flow microscopy.

For the characterization of particles, the first parameter to identify is the size. However, this is not enough to fully characterize particles. Therefore, particles are better characterized using a number of morphological parameters such as equivalent circle diameter (ECD, diameter of a circle with equivalent area to particle), circularity (ratio between the circumference of circle of equivalent area and the actual perimeter of the particle; the more spherical a particle is, the closer the circularity is to 1), convexity (ratio between the actual particle area and actual particle perimeter), Feret diameter (the measured distance between theoretical parallel lines that are drawn tangent to the particle profile and perpendicular to the ocular scale), aspect ratio according to Feret (ratio between the maximum Feret diameter and the minimum Feret diameter), brightness, etc. For each of these parameters, a statistical distribution is calculated and combined in scatter diagrams.

Therefore, controlled sample orientation is used because random orientation reduces the information contained in the gathered data. Consistency of orientation is important for statistically significant size and shape measurement.

Two systems discussed in this chapter, Sysmex FPIA-3000 (Malvern) and the Micro-Flow Imaging™ system (Brightwell Technologies), differ in their setup.

Sysmex FPIA-3000 from Malvern [49] is an instrument for flow particle image analysis of size and shape. The system is an automated analysis of the particle size as well as the shape of the particle. According to the manufacturer's information, the smallest particles that can be detected are in the range of 1 μm. Particles up to 40–80 μm can be detected, depending on the setup. The standard required sample volume is 5 mL, however, can be reduced to 1 mL. Measuring time is within minutes, excluding data analysis [49].

A sample is passed through a measurement sample cell where images of the particles are captured using stroboscopic illumination and a CCD camera. The heart of Sysmex FPIA-3000 is the sheath-flow cell, which allows the sample flow to produce an ideal particle presentation for imaging. The sample is injected between two hydrodynamic sheath flows. Thus, the sample and particles within the sample are retained at plane focus, with particles separated. Owing to the fact that the sample is sandwiched by the sheath liquid, the particles are aligned within the flow with their major axes in the direction of the flow. As sheath liquid aqueous solutions, as well as methanol, ethanol, isopropyl alcohol, or a 25% ethylene glycol solution can be used. However, one has to test whether these liquids will have an impact on the analyzed sample. The sheath liquid is consumed during the experiment. According to the manufacturer, about 120 mL is used per sample. Komabayashi and Spoingberg [50] recently presented a study for the analysis of mineral oxides using this method (for more details, see referred study).

The Micro-Flow Imaging System works without the need of a sheath liquid. The setup is illustrated in Chapter 7. The sample is filled in a small capillary. Bright-field images are captured in successive frames as s continuous sample stream passes through a flow cell positioned in the field of view of a custom magnification system with a well-characterized and extended depth of field. A focusing routine that directly measures or is traceable to measurements on a reference bead population ensures consistent flow-cell placement [51]. The images are analyzed in real time by the image analysis software. The images are analyzed to compile a full database about the morphological characteristics of the particles such as size, shape, or transparency. On the basis of statistical data evaluation and classification algorithms, these different parameters can be plotted and analyzed. Using a Micro-Flow Imaging System DPA4100, the particles that can be investigated are between about 1 and 400 μm. The focus depth is 400 μm and the field of view 1760 × 1400 μm. The analysis rate is 200 μL/min and the used sample volume 500 μL.

Figure 12.7a shows a representative image obtained with Micro-Flow Imaging System for a stressed protein sample. The analysis of the images shows various particle morphologies (Fig. 12.7b). The spherical particles are silicone droplets [52], whereas the other particles are probably protein aggregates.

All these systems rely on reference samples that are stored in a data base and on which the analyzed particles are compared and thus "identified."

As mentioned earlier, the size is just one parameter for the characterization of particles; other parameters are necessary to better discriminate particles. Figure 12.8 shows two particles of similar dimension, however, of completely different shape. These particles can be discriminated using morphological particle parameters.

The presented flow microscopy systems are also used for the determination of the particle concentration in a sample. This is exemplarily shown in Fig. 12.9, where the particles are size clustered and the number of each class plotted. Recently, Huang et al. [53] presented a comparative study using a flow microscopy system and the classical light obscuration method. They found some differences between the methods and explained this by the fact that the presence of nonspherical particles as well as particles that possess a refractive index similar to the solvent appear to be detected by the flow microscopy system, but not by the light obscuration system. Thus, the particle concentration detected by the flow microscopy system was higher in their study.

Using such systems, especially when viscous solutions are investigated, one has to make sure that the system is free of air bubbles; otherwise, these "particles" will also be counted.

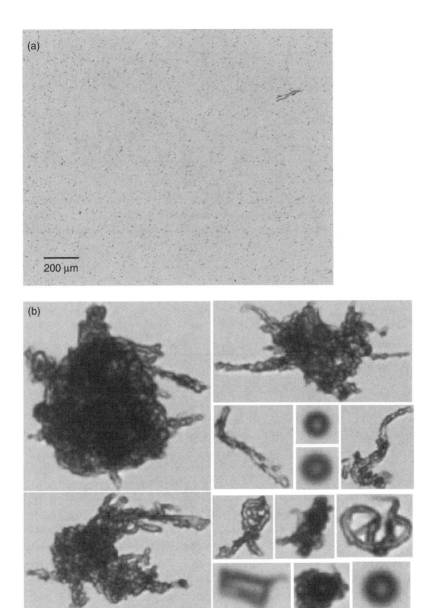

FIGURE 12.7   (a) A representative image captured during a microflow imaging exper-iment. Image dimension $= 1757 \times 1406 \times 100 \ \mu m$ (corresponds to a sample volume of 0.247 μL) and (b) representative images of detected particles using the microimaging flow system.

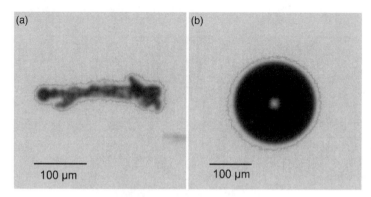

FIGURE 12.8 Morphological particle analysis (a) equivalent circular diameter (ECD) = 102 μm, circularity = 0.35, maximum Feret's diameter = 233 μm, and aspect ratio = 0.21; (b) ECD = 157 μm, circularity = 0.52, maximum Feret's diameter = 162 μm, and aspect ratio = 0.97.

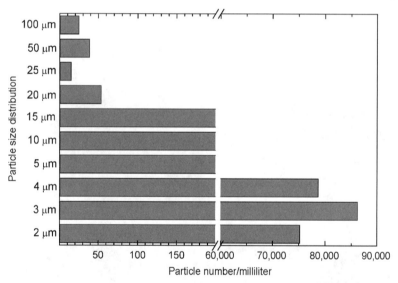

FIGURE 12.9 Particle size distribution of a stressed protein sample. Particle numbers (listed in the figure) obtained using a microflow imaging system (see text).

12.6 INFRARED (IR) MICROSCOPY

Beside the pictured description of particles in biopharmaceuticals (e.g., protein aggregates) by most of the microscopic techniques described so far, it is important to identify particles that may be present in, for example, liquid protein formulations. IR and Raman microscopy are suitable techniques for the identification and characterization of particles as they combine advantages of microscopic methods with fingerprint techniques such as IR and Raman spectroscopy. Raman microscopy is covered in Chapter 11. Below IR microscopy is described.

IR spectroscopy is a vibrational spectroscopic method [54,55] (see Chapter 10). In combination with a microscope, IR spectroscopy can be used as a valuable technique for the identification and characterization of single particles covering a size range from ~20 μm to a few centimeters. In Fig. 12.10, an example for an instrument setup for FTIR microscopy is shown. The FTIR spectrometer is coupled to a microscope, which is equipped with a reflecting Cassegrain objective (×15) (Fig. 12.11) and an attenuated total reflection (ATR) objective (×20) (Figs. 12.12 and 12.13). As the optical path of the visible light is collinear to the IR light, the sample (e.g., single particles) can be viewed via the ocular and can exactly be focused and positioned for IR measurements (Fig. 12.11). With the digital video camera on top of the microscope, pictures of the particles analyzed can be taken for documentation purposes. After passing the sample, the IR spectrum is detected by the mercury–cadmium–telluride (MCT) detector, which

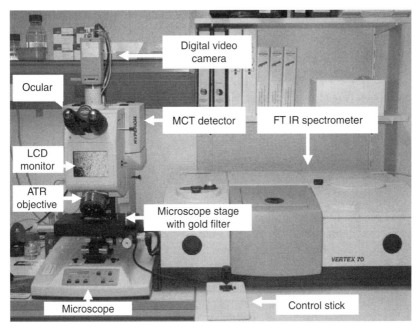

FIGURE 12.10   Instrument setup infrared (IR) microscopy. The FTIR spectrometer (Vertex 70, Bruker) on the right-hand side is coupled to a microscope (Hyperion 2000, Bruker), which is equipped with an IR Cassegrain objective (×15) and an ATR objective (×20, Germanium crystal). The IR beam generated by the spectrometer is directed to the particle on the microscope stage via the IR objective or alternatively via the ATR objective. After passing the sample, the IR spectrum is detected by the MCT detector. Using the microscope (visual mode), particles can be focused for IR measurements. With the digital video camera on the top of the microscope, pictures of the particles analyzed can be taken for documentation purposes.

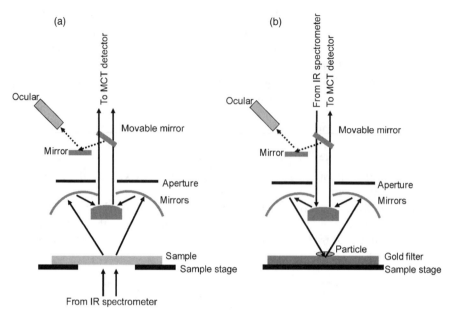

FIGURE 12.11 Schematic presentation of a Cassegrain IR objective and the course of the IR beam in the transmission mode (a) and in the reflection–absorption mode (b). In the reflection–absorption mode (b), the IR beam passes through the particle that lies on the gold filter, is reflected by the gold surface, and passes again through the sample.

is localized at the rear of the microscope and which needs cooling by liquid nitrogen.

Using the Cassegrain objective samples, for example, thin films, can be measured in transmission mode (Fig. 12.11a). A second measurement technique using the Cassegrain objective allows the IR analysis of particles that lie on a metallic surface (e.g., gold filter surface) (Fig. 12.11b). For the comparison of IR spectra, the same reflecting metallic surface should always be used, as different reflecting surfaces influence the IR spectra. A part of the IR light passes through the sample, is reflected by the gold filter surface, and passes again through the sample. This is called *reflection–absorption spectroscopy*. A further part of the IR light is reflected by nature at the upper layer contributing to the spectrum via Fresnel reflection. As reflection at the metal surface is needed, this technique is not suitable for particles that are too thick or for those whose absorbances are too high (this also holds true for the transmission mode). For both measurement techniques, a reference spectrum has to be recorded, which is used for the correction of the sample spectrum.

The ATR, which is also known as *internal reflection spectroscopy*, delivers the IR spectrum from the surface of a sample. Using the ATR objective (Figs. 12.12 and 12.13), particles, including thick and high absorbing particles, can be measured. The principle of ATR is based on the effect that at the interface of two media with different refractive indices, a small part of the reflected radiation in

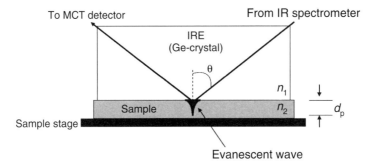

FIGURE 12.12 Scheme of attenuated total reflection (ATR) using the ATR objective. On the top of the ATR objective, a Ge-crystal (IRE, internal reflection element) is mounted, which is brought in direct contact with the sample (e.g., a protein particle). n_1, refractive index of IRE; n_2, refractive index of sample with $n_2 < n_1$; θ, incident angle; and d_p, depth of penetration. On the reflection point, the IR light penetrates into the sample where it is absorbed. *Source:* Adapted from Günzler [57].

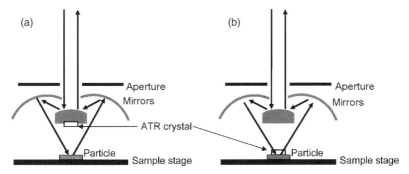

FIGURE 12.13 Schematic presentation of an ATR objective in the visual mode (a) and the measurement mode (b). In the visual mode (a), the ATR crystal is in the upper position and the sample can be focused using the microscope. In the measurement mode (b), the ATR crystal is lowered by means of a crystal holder and is brought into direct contact with the sample enabling the IR measurement by ATR.

the medium with the higher refractive index (n_1), penetrates for a few wavelengths in the medium with the lower refractive index (n_2) [56]. The principle is schematically shown in Fig. 12.12, representing the formation of an evanescent wave due to total internal reflection. The evanescent wave penetrates into the sample and thus interacts with the sample. Therefore, the sample has to be in contact with the internal reflection element (IRE, with refractive index n_1). The depth of penetration (d_p) is dependent on the wavelength: radiation with lower wavelength does not penetrate as much as radiation with higher wavelength, resulting in more intense bands at higher wavelengths compared to lower wavelengths [57]. As the penetration depth is only a few wavelengths, an ATR spectrum normally is independent of the thickness of a sample. Suitable materials as IRE are diamond, ZnSe, Si, or Ge. In the visual mode (Fig. 12.13a), the ATR crystal (Ge) is in the upper position and the sample can be exactly focused. The aperture size has to be adjusted if the measurement spot diameter is smaller than 100 μm. In the measurement mode (Fig. 12.13b), the ATR crystal is lowered and brought into direct contact with the sample. Before the sample is measured, a reference spectrum has to be recorded, which is a single-channel spectrum of the crystal.

In the following, a suitable preparation of samples for IR microscopy is described. If particles can be clearly visually seen, the easiest way for preparation is simply to pick the particles using a pair of tweezers. As this is often not possible, a filtration method is used for liquid protein solutions (e.g., turbid solutions, solutions stored under stressed conditions, and routine samples) using the FiltrAid® device (rap.Id, Germany) (Fig. 12.14a), including a gold filter membrane, available with pore sizes of, for example, 0.8 or 3.0 μm. Preparation is performed in a laminar flow to minimize particle contaminations from the environment. In general, one has to assure that the equipment used is free of contaminating particles, which can be demonstrated by using 0.2-μm filtrated purified water instead of the sample as a negative control. As described above, the surface of the gold filter serves as reflection layer for the reflection–absorption spectroscopy using the Cassegrain objective. On the other hand, IR measurements using the ATR objective are also possible for particles filtrated on the gold filter. In this case, when positioning the Ge-crystal onto the particle, one has to pay attention on not to destroy the gold filter. The liquid sample solution is pipetted onto the middle of the gold filter and filtered by applying a water-jet vacuum pump. Subsequently, the gold filter is washed using 0.2-μm filtered purified water and dried at room temperature. Using this procedure, water-soluble aggregates

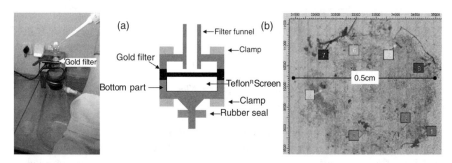

FIGURE 12.14   (a) Sample preparation of liquid protein pharmaceuticals using the FiltrAid® device (rap.Id, Germany). Sample preparation is done in a laminar flow to reduce the risk of secondary contamination of the sample with external particles. The liquid sample is applied by pipetting and filtered through the gold filter by applying a vacuum. Subsequently, the gold filter is washed using 0.2-μm filtered purified water and dried. Particles remaining on the gold filter surface are subjected to FTIR analysis. Using the funnel, the filtration area is defined by 0.5 cm in diameter. (b) Photographic documentation of a liquid sample solution filtered on a gold filter. Numbers indicate particles that were selected for FTIR analysis. (*See insert for color representation of the figure.*)

will not be captured. Depending on the particle load of the solution, the sample volume filtered has to be adapted. Figure 12.14b shows the photographic documentation of a liquid protein solution filtered on a gold filter as described earlier. The picture was recorded using the digital video camera (Fig. 12.10).

Figure 12.15a shows the preparation of a visually turbid protein solution on a gold filter for FTIR analysis. The particles form a "film" and nearly the whole filtration area is covered by particles. On predefined grid positions (Fig. 12.15b), FTIR analysis was performed automatically in reflection–absorption mode using the IR Cassegrain objective. The spectra (Fig. 12.15c) showed typical protein bands (amide I, $1600-1700$ cm^{-1} and amide II, $1480-1575$ cm^{-1}). The obtained spectra were compared with an in-house spectra library and the particles were identified as protein particles.

In Fig. 12.16, the FTIR spectra and the second derivative spectra for the amide I band of a human recombinant IgG4 antibody in solution and an IgG4 aggregate isolated from the IgG4 solution stored for 4 h at 65°C are shown. The FTIR spectra of IgG4 in solution (10 mg/mL, formulated at pH 6) were collected using an AquaSpec cell in the transmission mode. The IgG4 aggregate was isolated from the IgG4 solution stored for 4 h at 65°C by filtration onto a gold filter as described and was measured by the ATR technique. In the second derivative spectrum of the IgG4 antibody in solution, a weak amide I band at 1690 cm^{-1} and a major band at 1639 cm^{-1} is seen, typical for the β-barrel fold in IgG antibodies. In the spectrum of the heat-induced insoluble aggregate, a shift of the major band to 1630 cm^{-1} indicates the loss of the native β-barrel structure and the formation of extended intermolecular β-sheet. Similar results were obtained by Li and Li [58] for an IgG1 antibody. Using IR microscopy Schwegman et al. [59] investigated proteins at the ice/freeze–concentrate interface. For further references, see chapter on IR spectroscopy in this book.

FTIR microscopy is a valuable technique for troubleshooting and characterization rather than for routine analysis. A troubleshooting case is presented in Fig. 12.17. During manufacturing of a protein pharmaceutical, foreign black particles (Fig. 12.17a) were found on a filter used in downstream purification. During the investigations performed, a defective pump seal (Fig. 12.17b) was identified as possible origin of the foreign particles. Using FTIR analysis (ATR technique), it could be shown that indeed the foreign particles originated from the pump seal (Fig. 12.17c).

As the nature and the origin of particles that may be present in protein pharmaceuticals is numerous, it is advisable to construct a spectra library of substances that include proteins (different proteins and different structures, i.e., native, denatured), packaging materials (e.g., glass vials, syringes, and stoppers), and materials used in the manufacturing process (e.g., gaskets, filters, wipes, and storage containers such as tubes).

The size range of particles that can be analyzed and identified by FTIR microscopy is $\sim$25 μm to a few centimeters. Advantages of FTIR microscopy are the fast measurement ($\sim$2 min for the recording of sample and reference spectra) and the possibility to identify particles by comparison with a spectra

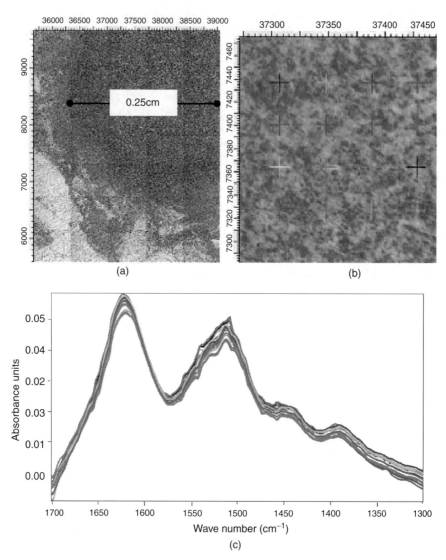

FIGURE 12.15   FTIR microscopy of a turbid protein solution. A turbid protein solution was filtered on a gold filter, resulting in a particle "film" (a). FTIR analysis was performed automatically on predefined "grid" positions (b) in reflection–absorption mode using an IR Cassegrain objective. The FTIR spectra (c) showed typical protein bands (amide I, 1600–$1700\,\mathrm{cm}^{-1}$ and amide II, 1480–$1575\,\mathrm{cm}^{-1}$). The obtained spectra were compared with a spectra library and the particles were identified as protein particles. (*See insert for color representation of the figure.*)

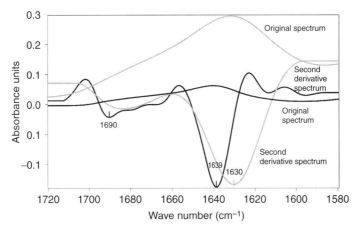

FIGURE 12.16   FTIR spectra and its second derivative spectra of a human IgG4 anti-body in solution (black) and an IgG4 aggregate isolated from the IgG4 solution stored for 4 h at 65°C (gray). FTIR spectra of IgG4 in solution (10 mg/mL, formulated at pH 6) were collected using an AquaSpec cell in transmission mode. The IgG4 aggregate was isolated from the IgG4 solution stored for 4 h at 65°C by filtration onto a gold filter and was measured by the ATR objective.

library (commercial or in-house). Especially for troubleshooting when unwanted particles are present, FTIR microscopy is a valuable technique for the identification of the particles. As shown, FTIR microscopy can be used for the identification and characterization of protein particles (denatured versus native state). On the other hand, FTIR microscopy can be very time consuming when numerous particles are present and the method cannot be validated with respect to the number of particles.

12.7   CONCLUSIONS

In this chapter, selected microscopic techniques for the analysis of protein as well as foreign particles in biopharmaceuticals were described. Microscopic techniques may be used for the specific characterization and/or identification of the origin and nature of particles on a case-by-case basis. Therefore, for routine monitoring of particles, other techniques as described in this book are more appropriate. In most cases, these methods are used as troubleshooting assays. The sample throughput is in most cases very low. Table 12.1 lists an overview of the presented selected microscopic techniques. Among these methods, classical LM with a resolution of about 0.2 μm has the advantages of being a low cost detection technique, which can easily be applied.

For the analysis of particles in the nanometer range, different electron microscopic techniques such as TEM, REM, SEM, and STEM were described. Another high resolution technique is AFM, which also allows the analysis of particles in the nanometer range.

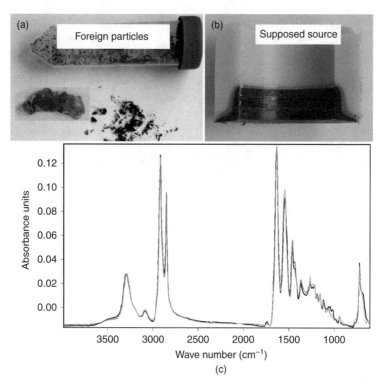

FIGURE 12.17   FTIR spectra of foreign particles. The foreign particles were found on a filter used in downstream purification of a protein pharmaceutical. On the right side the supposed source of the foreign particles (pump seal of a pump used in downstream production). Spectra were collected using the ATR objective. The obtained spectra confirmed that the foreign particles originated from the pump seal (gray: foreign particle; black: pump seal).

A major advantage of microscopic techniques is the single identification of a particle, which depend on the size of the particle and used method.

These high resolution techniques have the disadvantage to be expensive and laborious and are, therefore, used for selected analysis during the development of biopharmaceuticals as well as troubleshooting but not for routine purposes. All these techniques rely on the visualization of the investigated particles, and the identification is based on "experience" or data bases. Most of the presented techniques are nonspecific.

Using FTIR or Raman microscopy (not considered in this chapter), unknown particles may be identified by comparing the particles IR or Raman spectra to spectra libraries.

Two emerging techniques, for example, based on flow imaging microscopy may be useful in the future for the analysis of particles in biopharmaceuticals in the micrometer range, giving information about the particle number, particle size distribution as well as particle morphology, using more or less "high throughput" approaches.

Acknowledgments

We thank Andrea Eiperle, Inge Miller, Maria Trinz, Heidrun Schott, Elisabeth Siegmund, and Susanne Jäger for their helpful technical assistance.

REFERENCES

1. Garidel P, Bassarab S. Impact of formulation design on stability and quality. In: Lycson N, editor.. Quality for biologics: critical quality attributes, process and change control, product variation, characterisation, impurities and regulatory concerns. Hampshire: Biopharm Knowledge Publishing; 2009. pp. 94–113.

2. Garidel P, Kebbel F. Protein therapeutics and protein aggregates characterised by photon correlation spectroscopy: an application for high concentration liquid formulations. Bioprocess Int 2010;8(3):38–46.

3. Gerlach D. Das Lichtmikroskop. 2nd Auflage. Stuttgart: Thieme-Verlag; 1985.

4. Abbe E. Beiträge zur theorie des mikroskops und der mikroskopischen wahrnehmung. Archiv Mikrosk Anat 1873;9:413–487.

5. Bergmann L, Schäfer C, Niedrig H. Lehrbuch der experimental physik, Band 3: Optik, 10, Auflage. Berlin: de Gruyter; 2004.

6. Colliex C. La microscopie électronique. Paris: Presses Universitaires de France; 1998.

7. Van der Ven PFM, Schaart G, Croes HJE, Jap PHK, Ginsel LA, Ramaekers FCS. Titin aggregates associated with intermediate filaments align along stress fiber-like structures during human skeletal muscle cell differentiation. J Cell Sci 1993;106(3):749–759.

8. Liu XQ, Yonekura M, Tsutsumi M, Sano Y. Physicochemical properties of aggregates of globin hydrolysates. J Agric Food Chem 1996;44(10):2957–2961.

9. Kamin-Belsky N, Tomashov R, Shaklai N. Myoglobin induced impairment of structure and function of muscle myofibrils under peroxidative conditions. FASEB J 1997;11(9):A985.

10. Kunkel DD, Lee LK, Stollberg J. Ultrastructure of acetylcholine receptor aggregates parallels mechanisms of aggregation. BMC Neurosci 2001;2 Article No. 19: 12.

11. Hamberg L, Walkenström P, Stading M, Hermansson A-M. Aggregation, viscosity measurements and direct observation of protein coated latex particles under shear. Food Hydrocolloids 2001;15(2):139–151.

12. Krebs MRH, Domike KR, Donald AM. Protein aggregation: more than just fibrils. Biochem Soc Trans 2009;37(4):682–686.

13. Le Brun V, Friess W, Schultz-Fademrecht T, Muehlau S, Garidel P. Insights in lysozyme-lysozyme self-interactions as assessed by the osmotic second virial coefficient: impact for physical protein stabilization. Biotechnol J 2009;4(9):1305–1319.

14. Jones LS, Kaufmann A, Middaugh CR. Silicone oil induced aggregation of proteins. J Pharm Sci 2005;94:918–927.

15. EP (European Pharmacopoeia). 6th ed. 2009. Grundwerk, Band 1, Allgemeiner Teil, Chapter 2.9.19, Deutscher Apotheker Verlag Stuttgart.

16. Demeule B, Gurna R, Arvinte T. Detection and characterisation of protein aggregates by fluorescence microscopy. Int J Pharm 2007;329:37–45.

17. Garidel P. Steady-state intrinsic tryptophan protein fluorescence spectroscopy in pharmaceutical biotechnology. Spectrosc Eur 2008;20(4):7–11.

18. Li B, Flores J, Corvari V. A simple method for the detection of insoluble aggregates in protein formulations. J Pharm Sci 2007;96:1840–1843.

19. Egerton RF. Physical principles of electron microscopy: an introduction to TEM, SEM and AEM. Springer-Verlag, Berlin; 2005.

20. Goldstein J, Newbury D, Joy D, Lyman C, Echlin P, Lifshin E, Sawyer L, Michael J. Scanning electron microscopy and X-ray microanalysis. 3rd ed. New York: Springer-Verlag; 2003.

21. Winter R, Noll F. Methoden der biophysikalischen chemie. Stuttgart: Teubner Studienbücher; 1998.

22. Giepmans BNG. Bridging fluorescence microscopy and electron microscopy. Histochem Cell Biol 2008;130(2):211–217.

23. Meyer HW, Richter W. Freeze-fracture studies on lipids and membranes. Micron 2001;32(6):615–644.

24. Kreplak L, Richter K, Aebi U, Herrmann H. Chapter 15, electron microscopy of intermediate filaments: teaming up with atomic force and confocal laser scanning microscopy. Methods Cell Biol 2008;88:273–297.

25. Mironov AA, Polishchuk RS, Beznoussenko GV. Chapter 5, combined video fluorescence and 3D electron microscopy. Methods Cell Biol 2008;88:83–95.

26. Stahlberg H, Walz T. Molecular electron microscopy: state of the art and current challenges. ACS Chem Biol 2008;3(5):268–281.

27. Farrell HM, Cooke PH, King G, Hoagland PD, Groves ML, Kumosinski TF, Chu B Jr. Particle sizes of casein submicelles and purified κ-casein: comparisons of dynamic light scattering and electron microscopy with predictive three-dimensional molecular models. ACS Symp Ser 1996;650:61–79.

28. Radermacher M. Chapter 1, visualizing functional flexibility by three-dimensional electron microscopy. Reconstructing complex I of the mitochondrial respiratory chain. Methods Enzymol 2009;456(A):3–27.

29. Lindert S, Stewart PL, Meiler J. Hybrid approaches: applying computational methods in cryo-electron microscopy. Curr Opin Struct Biol 2009;19(2):218–225.

30. Studer D, Humbel BM, Chiquet M. Electron microscopy of high pressure frozen samples: bridging the gap between cellular ultrastructure and atomic resolution. Histochem Cell Biol 2008;130(5):877–889.

31. Wall JS, Simon MN, Lin BY, Vinogradov SN. Mass mapping of large globin complexes by scanning transmission electron microscopy. Methods Enzymol 2008;436:487–501.

32. Moores C. Chapter 16, studying microtubules by electron microscopy. Methods Cell Biol 2008;88:299–317.

33. Nagayama K, Danev R. Phase contrast electron microscopy: development of thin-film phase plates and biological applications. Philos Trans R Soc B: Biol Sci 2008;363(1500):2153–2162.

34. Fournier JG. Cellular prion protein electron microscopy: attempts/limits and clues to a synaptic trait. Implications in neurodegeneration process. Cell Tissue Res 2008;332(1):1–11.

35. Müller SA, Engel A. Biological scanning transmission electron microscopy: imaging and single molecule mass determination. Chimia 2006;60(11):749–753.

36. Colton RJ, Engel A, Frommer JE, Gaub HE, Gewirth AA, Guckenberger R, Rabe J, Heckl WM, Oarkinson B. Procedures in scanning probe microscopies. Chichester: John Wiley & Sons; 1998.

37. Müller DJ, Dufrêne YF. Atomic force microscopy as a multifunctional molecular toolbox in nanobiotechnology. Nat Nanotechnol 2008;3(5):261–269.

38. Gadegaard N. Atomic force microscopy in biology: technology and techniques. Biotech Histochem 2006;81(2–3):87–97.

39. Trache A, Meininger GA.. Atomic force microscopy (AFM). Curr Protoc Microbiol 2008;Suppl 8: 2C.2.1–2C.2.17.

40. Giessibl FJ. Advances in atomic force microscopy. Rev Mod Phys 2003;75:949–983.

41. Hauser A, Garidel P, Forster G, Blume A. Atomic force microscopic investigations of the gel phase of phosphatidylcholines containing ω-cyclohexyl fatty acids. Phys Chem Chem Phys 2000;2(20):4554–4558.

42. Silva LP. Imaging proteins with atomic force microscopy: an overview. Curr Protein Pept Sci 2005;6(4):387–395.

43. Yamakoshi Y, Nakazawa K, Tsuchiya T. Protein imaging by atomic force microscopy. Nippon Rinsho Jpn J Clin Med 2007;65(2):270–277.

44. Gaczynska M, Osmulski PA. Chapter 3, atomic force microscopy as a tool to study the proteasome assemblies. Methods Cell Biol 2009;90 (C):39–60.

45. Frederix PLTM, Bosshart PD, Engel A. Atomic force microscopy of biological membranes. Biophys J 2009;96(2):329–338.

46. San Paulo A, García R. High-resolution imaging of antibodies by tapping-mode atomic force microscopy: attractive and repulsive tip-sample interaction regimes. Biophys J 2000;78(3):1599–1605. March.

47. Raab A, Han W, Badt D, Smith-Gill SJ, Lindsay SM, Schindler H, Hinterdorfer P. Antibody recognition imaging by force microscopy. Nat Biotechnol 1999;17: 901–905.

48. Maco B, Fahrenkrog B, Huang NP, Aebi U. Nuclear pore complex structure and plasticity revealed by electron and atomic force microscopy. Methods Mol Biol (Clifton, NJ) 2006;322:273–288.

49. Sysmex FPIA-3000 application note, Flow particle image analysis of size and shape, Malvern. Available at www.malvern.co.uk.

50. Komabayashi T, SpAAngberg LSW. Comparative analysis of the particle size and shape of commercially available mineral trioxide aggregates and Portland cement: a study with a flow particle image analyzer. J Endod 2008;34(1):94–98.

51. Sharma DK, Oma P, King D. Applying intelligent flow microscopy to biotechnology. Bioprocess Int 2009a;7(6):62–67.

52. Sharma DK, Oma P, Krishnan S. Silicone microdroplets in protein formulations. Detection and enumeration. Pharm Technol 2009b;33:74–79.

53. Huang CT, Sharma D, Oma P, Krishnamurthy R. Quantitation of protein particles in parenteral solutions using micro-flow imaging. J Pharm Sci 2009;98:3058–3071.

54. Garidel P, Schott H. Fourier-transform midinfrared spectroscopy for analysis and screening of liquid protein formulations, part 1. Bioprocess Int 2006;4(5):40–46.

55. Garidel P, Schott H. Fourier-transform midinfrared spectroscopy for analysis and screening of liquid protein formulations, part 2. Bioprocess Int 2006;4(6):48–54.

56. Newton I. Opticks. New York: Dover; 1952.

57. Günzler H, Gremlich HU. IR spectroscopy. Weinheim: Wiley-VCH Verlag; 2002.

58. Li CH, Li T. Application of vibrational spectroscopy to the structural characterisation of monoclonal antibody and its aggregate. Curr Pharm Biotechnol 2009;10(4):391–399.

59. Schwegman JJ, Carpenter JF, Nail SL. Evidence of partial unfolding of proteins at the ice/freeze-concentrate interface by infrared microscopy. J Pharm Sci 2009;98(9):3239–3246.

SECTION III
Integrated Approaches to Protein Aggregation and Particles

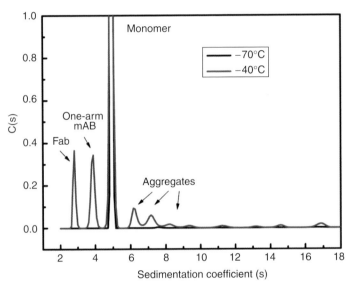

FIGURE 2.3 Sedimentation velocity analysis of an mAb in a liquid formulation after storage at −70 and 40°C for six months. The centrifuge experiments were conducted at 40,000 rpm and 10°C. The data were analyzed by SEDFIT using the continuous c(s) model.

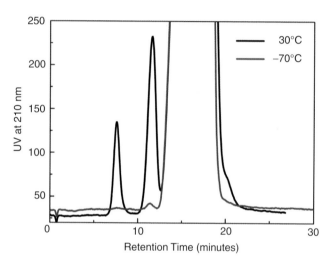

FIGURE 2.7a Flow FFF analysis of an mAb after storage at −70 and 30°C for six month. The eluted peaks were monitored using a UV absorption optical system at a wavelength of 210 or 280 nm. The flow FFF experiments were conducted using a regenerated cellulose membrane with a 10-kDa MW cutoff and a cross flow of PBS at 6 mL/min.

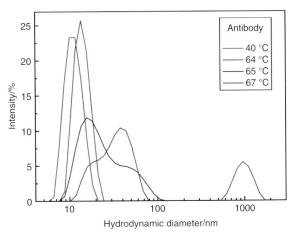

FIGURE 3.12 Size distributions of an antibody (1.2 mg/mL in 20 mM citrate, pH 6.1) at elevating temperatures from 40 to 67°C using the multiple narrow algorithm.

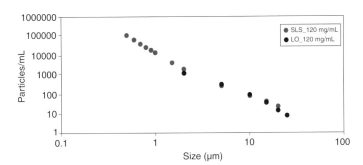

FIGURE 5.4 Particle concentration as a function of size in a protein product, as determined by the SLS method that covers the size range of ≥ 0.5–20 μm and the modified light-obscuration method with the size range of ≥ 2–25 μm. While the absolute particle concentration values as determined by different techniques in the overlapping size range may (as shown in this case) or may not agree (data not shown), the overall distribution profile and pattern—higher concentrations at smaller sizes—are consistent from different techniques.

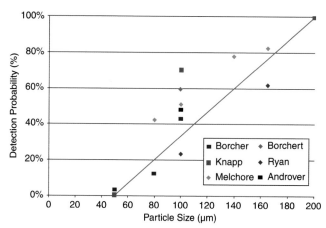

FIGURE 6.1 Detection probability of particles by human inspectors. *Source:* Modified from Ref. 31.

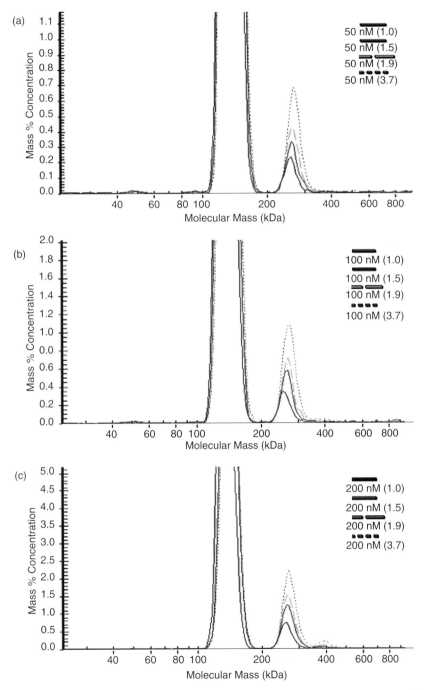

FIGURE 7.3 Macro-IMS spectra of a mAb (IgG1) at (a) 50 nmol/L, (b) 100 nmol/L, and (c) 200 nmol/L using gauge pressures of 1.0, 1.5, 1.9, and 3.7 psi.

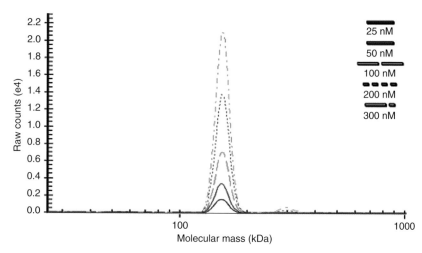

FIGURE 7.4a MacroIMS spectra of a mAb (IgG1) at a concentration of 25-300 nmol/L.

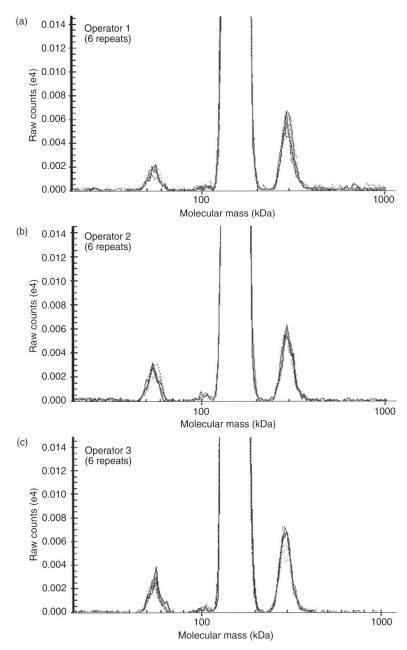

FIGURE 7.5 (a–c) Overlays of six macro-IMS spectrum from three operators run on three separate days.

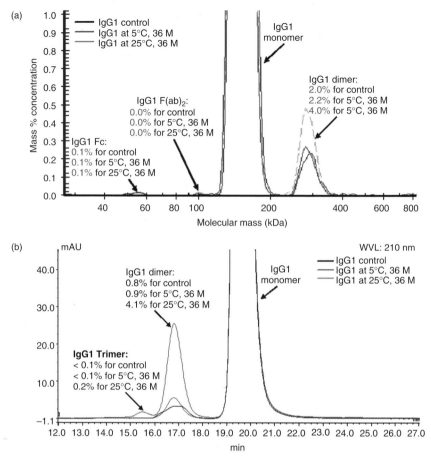

FIGURE 7.6 (a) Macro-IMS analysis of an antibody (IgG1) lyophilisate in vial after storage at 5 and 25°C for 36 months. (b) SEC analysis of an antibody (IgG1) lyophilisate in vial after storage at 5 and 25°C for 36 months.

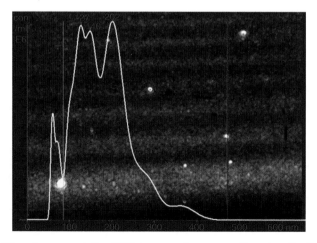

FIGURE 7.18a A representative NTA image and corresponding size distribution of IgG aggregates.

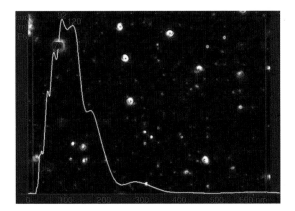

FIGURE 7.19a A representative NTA image and corresponding size distribution of IgM aggregates.

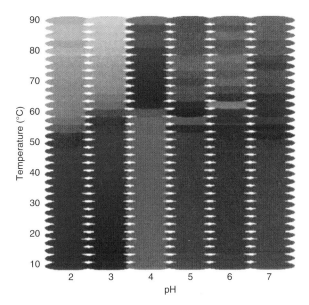

FIGURE 8.4 Temperature–pH phase diagram of bGCSF based on second-derivative absorbance data. Six distinct phases are observed: (1) pH 2–3, T 10–55°C; (2) pH 2–3, T 55–90°C; (3) pH 4, T 10–60°C; (4) pH 4, T 60–90°C; (5) pH 5–7, T 10–50°C; and (6) pH 5–7, T 50–90°C. Blocks of continuous color represent single phases, conditions under which the raw data-derived vectors behave similarly. The colors are arbitrarily chosen. *Source:* Adapted from Kueltzo et al. [44].

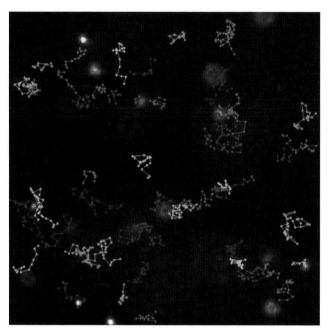

FIGURE 9.9 Fluorescent nanospheres of 200 nm diameter imaged and tracked by SPT. A trajectory starts when the particle moves into the focal plane and ends when it goes out of focus again. The diffusion coefficient (and size) of single particles can be calculated from their trajectories. The field of view is 22.5 μm × 22.5 μm.

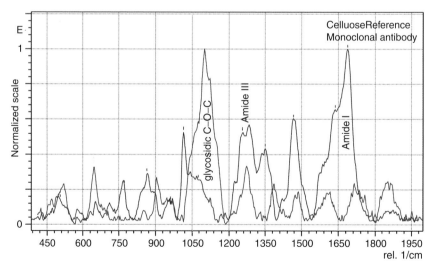

FIGURE 11.7 Overlay of a Raman spectrum of cellulose and a monoclonal antibody. The cellulose spectrum comprises the typical C–O–C–ether band; the monoclonal spectrum exhibits the typical Amide III and Amide I band.

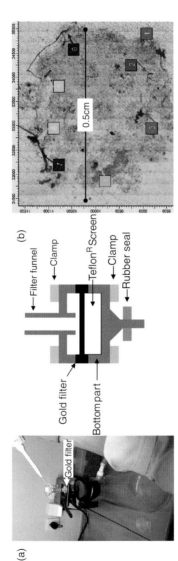

(a)

(b)

Filter funnel
Clamp
Teflon^{R}Screen
Clamp
Rubber seal

Gold filter

Bottom part

Gold filter

0.5cm

FIGURE 12.14 (a) Sample preparation of liquid protein pharmaceuticals using the FiltrAid® device (RapID, Germany). Sample preparation is done in a laminar flow to reduce the risk of secondary contamination of the sample with external particles. The liquid sample is applied by pipetting and filtered through the gold filter by applying a vacuum. Subsequently, the gold filter is washed using 0.2-μm filtered purified water and dried. Particles remaining on the gold filter surface are subjected to FTIR analysis. Using the funnel, the filtration area is defined by 0.5 cm in diameter. (b) Photographic documentation of a liquid sample solution filtered on a gold filter. Numbers indicate particles that were selected for FTIR analysis.

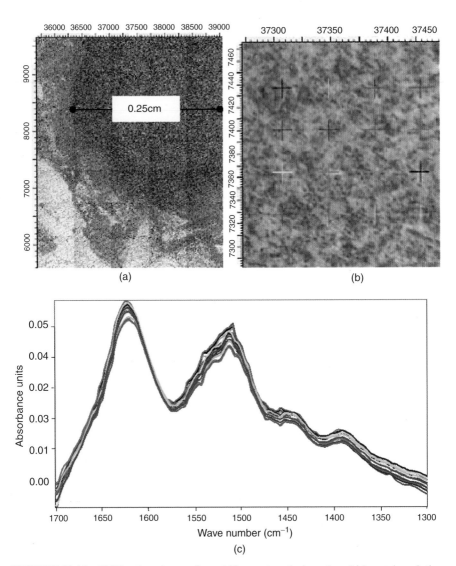

FIGURE 12.15 FTIR microscopy of a turbid protein solution. A turbid protein solution was filtered on a gold filter, resulting in a particle "film" (a). FTIR analysis was performed automatically on predefined "grid" positions (b) in reflection–absorption mode using an IR Cassegrain objective. The FTIR spectra (c) showed typical protein bands (amide I, 1600–1700 cm^{-1} and amide II, 1480–1575 cm^{-1}). The obtained spectra were compared with a spectra library and the particles were identified as protein particles.

13 Comparison of Methods for Soluble Aggregate Detection and Size Characterization

JOHN S. PHILO

Alliance Protein Laboratories, Thousand Oaks, California, USA

13.1 INTRODUCTION

A number of methods for detecting soluble aggregates were described and discussed in Chapter 2. Nonetheless, accurate and practical characterization of soluble aggregates in protein pharmaceuticals remains a formidable challenge for several reasons:

- These aggregates represent an extremely large range of molecular weights, from below 10 kDa for aggregates of peptides and small proteins up to about 1 GDa for an aggregate with a diameter of ~ 0.5 μm (near the lower limit for most "subvisible" particle detectors). No current technique can cover this entire range at a time while providing good separation and quantitation of different species.

- Aggregates exist in a range of types, and multiple types may be present in the same sample. Covalent or fully irreversible noncovalent aggregates have an indefinitely long lifetime and can potentially be fully physically separated from other species and then even subjected to off-line analysis. At the other extreme, rapidly reversible aggregates have only a transient existence and will not be detected by methods that sense only long-lived species. These rapidly reversible aggregates cannot be fully separated from the monomer by separation methods such as size-exclusion chromatography (SEC; SE-HPLC), electrophoresis, or asymmetric flow field-flow fractionation (AF4)—during separation, there is a continuous reequilibration of the oligomer distribution, driven by the law of mass action. "Metastable" aggregates that are reversible but that dissociate only very slowly (hours to days)

Analysis of Aggregates and Particles in Protein Pharmaceuticals, First Edition.
Edited by Hanns-Christian Mahler, Wim Jiskoot.

are also fairly common, and their intermediate lifetime can lead to confusing differences between results from different analytical methods. Further, aggregate characteristics such as hydrophobicity or degree of denaturation can also affect their detectability by some analytical methods.

- Certain product characteristics may degrade the performance of some assays or even preclude their use altogether. Smaller peptides (below ~5 kDa) are difficult for sedimentation velocity (SV) and may present sensitivity issues for light scattering methods, while at the other extreme, it is difficult to find suitable SEC columns for high-mass products such as viruslike particles (VLPs). Very high or very low product concentration presents challenges for many methods. The presence of excipients such as detergents, sugars, polyols, or antimicrobial preservatives can cause significant interference with certain methods. Extremes of pH or even the *absence* of excipients (e.g., very low ionic strength) can also be problematic.

- The various analytical methods for soluble aggregates differ widely in their throughput and cost per sample (total cost including the personnel costs for analyzing and interpreting the data). Thus, for example, some methods are impractical for the large number of samples that are generated during screening of formulation conditions.

- The different analytical methods also differ greatly in their equipment cost, complexity, and robustness. Some methods require extensive training and highly skilled personnel and are simply unsuitable for routine use by QC staff or as lot release assays. Issues of equipment cost and the availability of skilled personnel may also dictate whether particular methods should be outsourced or run in-house.

Thus, regrettably, no single analytical method works well over the entire range of aggregate sizes and types, and some may not be suitable for all stages of product development due to issues of throughput, cost, or regulatory compliance. This chapter discusses the strengths and disadvantages of SEC, electrophoresis, analytical ultracentrifugation (AUC), dynamic light scattering (DLS), multiangle classical light scattering (MALS), and AF4 as an aid to method selection. It also describes how some of the methods that are too expensive, complex, or low throughput for routine use can, nonetheless, be valuable to help qualify and cross validate the assays for routine use and give an example. Finally, a few additional points regarding method selection for formulation and comparability protocols are presented. However, before moving forward to those specifics, it is important to explicitly discuss how and why the measurement itself can change the distribution of aggregates we are trying to measure.

13.2 THE MEASUREMENT CAN CHANGE THE SAMPLE

The ideal aggregation assay would require no pretreatment or modifications to the sample such as dilution, filtration, or modification of solvent conditions. Separation methods, unfortunately, inherently alter the sample because the separation itself will disturb the equilibrium distribution of reversible aggregates. Among the common analytical methods for soluble aggregates, only batch-mode DLS avoids all these issues (at least for those samples where no filtration or centrifugation to remove large particulates is required). Unfortunately, DLS is not suitable as a primary aggregation assay because it has very low resolution and gives poor quantitation of different components; hence, we usually must employ methods that are more perturbing.

13.2.1 Dilution and Separation Effects

All the separation methods produce at least some sample dilution, and in some cases, the dilution is quite large. AF4 produces multiple changes in concentration: an initial dilution as the sample is injected into the channel, followed by reconcentration during the focusing step, and then dilution again during the separation phase. Any change in sample concentration will change the distribution of reversible aggregates (oligomers that exist in mass–action equilibrium with the monomer).[1]

If we dilute a product either before or during the assay, then in general we will not detect all the reversible aggregates that were present in the product vial (and might not detect any of them). When applying a separation method such as SEC, AF4, or SV to a diluted sample, we will, however, detect the irreversible aggregates as well as the relatively stable, long-lived noncovalent aggregates. However, what constitutes "long lived" in this context depends on both the sample history and speed of the separation. If, for example, the reversible aggregates present in the vial dissociate over a timescale of ~1 h, most of them would be detected by an SEC separation that requires only 15 min (assuming we start that separation immediately after any predilution that the SEC protocol requires). However, those same aggregates would not be detected by a slower separation such as SV (typically a 3–5 h run time) and would also not be detected with an SEC protocol that involved predilution followed by a long wait in the autosampler before injection.

What happens if we apply a separation method to a sample undergoing reversible association but where the association–dissociation reactions are very rapid compared to the rate of separation? In this situation, it is *impossible* to separate and quantitate individual oligomers. For a very rapid monomer–dimer equilibrium, for example, if we run SEC or AF4, we would see only a single peak, but that peak actually represents a dynamic mixture of monomer and dimer in the equilibrium proportions corresponding to the local concentration as the peak moves through the column or AF4 channel. A point that causes some confusion is that for some rapidly reversible association schemes we may resolve and detect multiple peaks, but those peaks will, in general, represent

---

[1]Note that, in this chapter, the normal, native nonaggregated state of the protein product is referred to as *monomer*, but for some products that normal state might not actually be a monomer of the expressed sequence.

a dynamic mixture of multiple oligomers rather than a single pure oligomer. As the rates of the reversible association–dissociation reactions get slower and become comparable to the rate of separation of different oligomers, the situation becomes even more complex, and in theory, it is possible to observe more peaks than the total number of different species that are present [1,2]. The influence of the rates of the association and dissociation reactions for monomer–dimer systems has been explored from a theoretical perspective for SEC [3] and recently also for SV [4].

13.2.2 Filtration Effects

Chromatography columns often unintentionally filter out and/or dissociate aggregates. Very large aggregate species may be physically filtered by the frit at the column entrance and/or the column bed itself. It is also quite common for a portion of the injected protein to bind nonspecifically but nearly irreversibly to the column matrix, leading to low sample recovery. Such binding is often enhanced for aggregates, which tend to be "stickier" than the monomer; consequently, it is the aggregates that are preferentially lost to the column surfaces [5–7]. These filtration effects are particularly a concern for SEC columns, and the mechanisms of protein binding and the effects of solvent additives on such binding were recently reviewed [8].

Nonspecific binding to the cross-flow membrane in the channel can also be a problem for AF4, but the surface area for nonspecific binding is orders of magnitude lower than in a column. Some binding to measurement cell surfaces could also potentially occur for SV, but the surface/volume ratio is fairly low relative to the other separation methods. Care may even be needed to be sure all the aggregates ever enter the measurement instrument—this author has seen significant loss of large aggregates in the 50-nm to 1-μm size range to the surfaces of plastic microcentrifuge tubes and pipette tips.

13.2.3 Solvent Effects

Any change of solvent conditions (where "solvent" includes all excipients or other nonprotein components) potentially changes the distribution of all the noncovalent aggregates. For example, SEC mobile phases often have high ionic strength, which can sometimes dissociate aggregates [9] or even induce new aggregates that were not present at lower ionic strength [10]. Solvent conditions such as extremes of pH or addition of organic cosolvents can also dissociate reversible aggregates [9]. Whether aggregates are irreversible or reversible also depends on solvent conditions, so the SEC mobile phase can even cause aggregates that are irreversible in the drug substance (DS) or final formulation buffer to become reversible in the mobile phase and then to completely dissociate [11].

For SEC, the selection of mobile phase during SEC method development typically involves a trade-off between the addition of salts and/or other cosolvents to improve resolution, peak symmetry, and/or enhance sample recovery (to reduce the filtration effects) [8] versus keeping the mobile phase similar to the formulation buffer to minimize changes in the aggregate distribution. That is, changes to the mobile phase that improve the robustness of the chromatography and the precision and reproducibility of the peak areas may actually hurt the *accuracy* of the method (the results are precise but do not reflect the true properties of the sample before injection).

While such solvent effects are particularly a concern with SEC, they are certainly not unique to SEC. Mobile phase optimization to minimize nonspecific binding may also be needed for AF4. Moreover, excipients such as sugars, polyols, and detergents can cause significant interference for SV, and detergent micelles can sometimes cause significant interference for DLS; hence, for these methods, there again may be a trade-off between changing the solvent to optimize the assay versus running a compromised assay without removing the solvent interference.

13.3 STRENGTHS AND LIMITATIONS OF VARIOUS AGGREGATION ASSAYS

13.3.1 Size-Exclusion Chromatography

SEC is by far the most commonly used tool for characterizing the size of soluble aggregates and measuring the fractions of different aggregate species. SEC holds that position because of reasons its many strengths:

1. When used with nondenaturing mobile phases, it can detect and quantitate both covalent and noncovalent aggregates.
2. When used with strongly denaturing mobile phases (e.g., containing SDS, guanidine hydrochloride, or urea), it can specifically detect and quantitate covalent aggregates.
3. It has good sensitivity (peaks representing 0.1% or below by weight can be detected) and good precision.
4. It has fairly high throughput (1–4 samples/h).
5. The equipment and data analysis is highly automated, and the software is often compliant with regulatory requirements for use in GMP environments.
6. It is relatively inexpensive and easy to implement.
7. HPLC equipment and SEC columns are available from a variety of manufacturers.
8. It is suitable for use in a QC environment and can be validated for lot release.

On the other hand, it is clear from Section 13.1 that SEC has some significant limitations and drawbacks. Primary among those is the issue of whether SEC actually detects all the sizes and types of aggregates that were originally present in the sample. That is, are aggregates lost due to filtration, binding to the column, dilution, and/or a change in solvent conditions? As mentioned previously, in some cases, SEC may be inaccurate because the mobile phase has induced the formation of new aggregate species. Changes in aggregate distributions due to dilution and changes in solvent conditions are often aggravated by SEC protocols involving predilution of the sample with the mobile phase, followed by a lengthy incubation period in the autosampler. The nonspecific binding of monomer and aggregates to the column can vary significantly from one column manufacturer to another, even though the resin types are nominally quite similar. Further batch-to-batch variation can be significant even for the same column from the same manufacturer, and changes over time in SEC column properties have forced a number of companies to revalidate their assays used for lot release.

Another limitation of SEC is that only a limited range of aggregate sizes can be analyzed by a particular column (it has limited dynamic range). Column selection always involves a trade-off between resolution and dynamic range. A column type chosen to give good separation of dimer from monomer typically means that all species larger than trimer or tetramer elute as a single unresolved peak at the void (total exclusion) volume. When that is true, the SEC protocol will not distinguish a normal production lot where that peak at the void volume represents tetramer from an abnormal one where it represents a much larger aggregate.

Clearly, another limitation of SEC is that the elution positions are not a reliable guide to the true molecular weight of the eluting species and, therefore, cannot reliably identify the stoichiometry of an aggregate. The elution positions are sensitive to molecular shape (conformation) as well as molecular weight. They will also be affected by any nonspecific interactions of the analyte with the column matrix, and of course, the true molecular weights for glycoproteins and PEGylated proteins cannot be measured based on column calibration with nonconjugated protein standards. Overall though, accuracy of molecular-weight estimates is probably the least important of these drawbacks of SEC, and this shortcoming can usually be readily overcome by the addition of an online classical light scattering detector to directly measure the molecular weights (SEC-MALS).

A final drawback to SEC is that sample recovery, and especially the recovery of the aggregate fractions, is often a strong function of the column history. The recovery is poor for new columns or after extensive washing, but recovery improves with successive injections as those sites become saturated with protein [8]. Thus, good aggregate quantitation often requires a conditioning procedure where multiple sacrificial injections are made of the product (or sometimes a control protein such as bovine serum albumin (BSA)) before injecting unknowns. Unfortunately, the binding to these saturable sites is not completely irreversible, and so the sacrificial protein slowly bleeds off during normal use (potentially contaminating the unknowns) and may be more thoroughly removed by routine column cleaning sequences. Consequently, the conditioning procedure typically needs to be repeated before each group of samples, which makes the method less robust and lowers throughput.

13.3.2 Field-Flow Fractionation

Field-flow fractionation (FFF) encompasses a number of separation paradigms, including separations driven by electrical or sedimentation forces. However, the mode most frequently used for the analysis of protein pharmaceuticals is asymmetrical flow FFF, which commonly goes by the acronyms AfFFF or AF4, and that is the only FFF variant that is discussed here. The capabilities of AF4 and its advantages and disadvantages for aggregation analysis were also recently discussed at length by Cao et al. [12]; an earlier review by Fraunhofer and Winter [13] is also an excellent resource. The specific advantages/disadvantages of coupling AF4 with a MALS detector are discussed in Section 13.3.5.

The "fractograms" produced by AF4 are like chromatograms from HPLC and thus are readily understood, and the peaks are easily integrated to quantitate species fractions. One very important advantage of AF4 over HPLC methods, however, is that in AF4 there is no column matrix with enormous surface area on which aggregates may be lost due to nonspecific binding. This lower potential for surface losses also means that mobile phase choice is generally less restricted than that for SEC. It should be noted, however, that for some proteins nonspecific binding to the semipermeable membrane within the flow channel can be quite problematic. In such cases, the trade-offs between choosing a mobile phase to optimize sample recovery and resolution versus keeping the mobile phase similar to the formulation buffer to minimize changes in the population of noncovalent aggregates are essentially the same as for SEC.

Another strength of AF4 is that it can be applied to species over a very large range of size, from peptides on up to subvisible particles in the 100- to 500-nm range. The range of sizes covered within a given fractogram (the dynamic range) can be very wide [12] and is tunable by varying the rate of cross flow. However, there is an inevitable trade-off between resolution and dynamic range. A final strength of AF4 is that optimized protocols can closely approach the reproducibility and resolution of SEC [12].

Like all separation methods, a drawback of AF4 is that it perturbs the distribution of reversible aggregates due to separation and dilution. A unique aspect of AF4, however, is the fact that the sample concentration may actually rise above the injection concentration during the "focusing" operation, and this may drive formation of new aggregates that were not actually present before injection. Indeed, operating conditions that promote high protein concentrations during focusing, such as the use of higher injection loads or relatively high cross flows, often tend to produce high peak asymmetry, and this effect has been attributed to reversible association [12].

A second drawback of AF4 is that to maintain good resolution and peak symmetry the injection load must usually be kept fairly small (below 10 μg). Consequently, the concentrations of the eluted peaks are low, which can create detector sensitivity issues. Thus, with AF4, it may not be possible to detect very minor species, and lack of sensitivity may more severely limit the use of refractive index (RI) and MALS detectors. For RI detectors, the normal flow switching during the measurement cycle disturbs the detector baseline [14], which further compounds the sensitivity issues.

Perhaps the major drawback of AF4 is that it generally requires a lot of method development and an experienced analyst to obtain good separations and results that are reliable and reproducible [12,14]. There are many experimental parameters to be optimized, including the type of semipermeable membrane, mobile phase composition, channel spacing, channel flow rate, cross-flow rate, injection rate, focusing time, focusing flow rates, and injection load. Furthermore, the required investment in method development does not guarantee a workable method will be obtained or that a successful method will be transferable to other similar molecules. Experienced users at a number of biotechnology companies have told the author that there are certain proteins and peptides for which AF4 simply does not work. There is also some disagreement about the degree of transferability of methods—some AF4 users find methods to be transferable with minor modifications even between different classes of proteins [12], whereas others say that method transfer failed even between closely related proteins.

Another significant drawback of AF4 for aggregate analysis is that inevitably a portion of the injected sample is lost during the focusing phase, and additional sample that was reversibly bound or trapped against the membrane always elutes after the cross flow is stopped at the end of each injection cycle. Opinions differ about whether these "lost" sample fractions may have a composition significantly different from the applied sample, how to measure (or even define) the sample recovery or mass balance, and whether those are even useful concepts for AF4. Overall, it seems difficult to know whether there is uniform recovery of all species.

Other drawbacks of AF4 are that the equipment is considerably more complex than standard LC systems (sometimes requiring rapidly switchable but highly accurate flows from three separate pumps). Consequently, the hardware is less robust than SEC or even AUC, and difficulty in reproducing elution profiles after disassembling the channel to replace the semipermeable membrane appears to be a common complaint. AF4 equipment is also available from very few suppliers. It appears that AF4 is currently being used in QC at several companies, but whether it is used for lot release is unclear.

13.3.3 Electrophoresis

Sodium dodecyl sulfate–polyacrylamide gel electrophoresis (SDS-PAGE) is frequently and routinely used to detect covalent aggregates. It requires little training, is usually easy to implement, has fairly high throughput, and can be validated for lot release. It is inexpensive and the equipment, precast gels, and standards for use as molecular-weight markers are widely available from numerous suppliers. A bonus feature is that the same gel can also often be used to monitor fragments or impurities.

The primary drawback of SDS-PAGE is that it only detects covalently linked aggregates. Another significant weakness is that it is difficult to reproducibly or accurately quantitate the fractions for different bands. In some cases, aggregate bands may be artifacts formed during the assay itself, especially for nonreduced gels of proteins that are highly susceptible to disulfide cross linking. Gel documentation systems and their software may also create regulatory challenges.

Native gel electrophoresis is much less commonly used than SDS-PAGE, but it can also be quite useful for aggregate analysis [15,16]. Because no SDS is used noncovalent as well as covalent aggregates can be detected, but changes in the distribution of noncovalent aggregates due to dilution and/or changes in solvent conditions are possible. Native gels share many of the advantages (and drawbacks) mentioned for SDS-PAGE. One significant difference is that native PAGE often requires significantly more method development—even for proteins of the same size, the protocols will differ substantially depending on the sign and magnitude of the protein's electric charge at the pH of the running buffer. Proteins with an isoelectric point below ~8 can usually be run using a standard Tris-glycine Laemmli gel system. However, the gels typically run for much longer periods than SDS gels (the mobility is lower because the high electric charge from the bound SDS is absent), and the optimum gel type (% cross linking) and run time must be determined experimentally for each different protein. Proteins with a pI above 8 must be run in reverse polarity and require optimization of the buffer and pH as well as the gel type and run length.

Another significant difference between native and SDS gels is that there are no standard molecular-weight markers for native gels, so assigning a stoichiometry to aggregate bands may be difficult. Absolute molecular-weight assignment for the bands requires running gels with different percentage of cross linking and evaluation via a Ferguson plot [42]. The resolution of native gels is usually lower than the corresponding SDS gel because the bands are usually broader.

Finally, it should be mentioned that classic gel electrophoretic methods are now often being replaced by capillary electrophoresis and similar methods employing microfabricated channels rather than capillaries. Such methods are often less labor intensive and more rapid than gels and produce chromatograms that can be easily integrated to give species fractions with a precision much higher than that is possible from gel scanning.

13.3.4   Sedimentation Velocity

There are two primary measurement modes for AUC, SV and sedimentation equilibrium. While sedimentation equilibrium is an excellent tool for characterizing the thermodynamics of reversible association reactions (equilibrium constants and stoichiometries), it is not particularly good at identifying and quantifying small amounts of minor components. SV is far more commonly used in aggregation analysis, and therefore, it is the sole focus of this section, but applications of sedimentation equilibrium to protein therapeutics and its strengths and drawbacks have been reviewed elsewhere [17,18].

The SV data analysis method that is most commonly used for aggregate analysis is the "$c(s)$ method" invented by Peter Schuck at the NIH [19]. This method

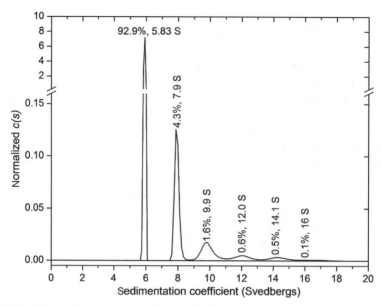

FIGURE 13.1 Sedimentation coefficient distribution for a monoclonal antibody that was subjected to heat stress. The distribution has been normalized, so the area under each peak gives the fraction of that species. *Source:* Data redrawn from Philo [10].

produces a size distribution that is much like a chromatogram. Figure 13.1 shows an example for a stressed monoclonal antibody sample, where five peaks representing aggregates are resolved in addition to the main peak (monomer). The sedimentation coefficients of the aggregate peaks suggest, but do not prove, that these peaks represent dimer, trimer, tetramer, pentamer, and hexamer. One drawback of SV is that it is usually not possible to reliably assign a stoichiometry to the aggregate peaks because sedimentation coefficients depend on molecular conformation (shape) as well as mass and the conformation of the aggregates may be quite different from that of the monomer.

Note that the putative trimer, tetramer, pentamer, and hexamer peaks are fairly well resolved from each other and the dimer, whereas by SEC it is likely that hexamer, pentamer, and tetramer would elute as a single unresolved peak near the void volume. An important strength of SV that a very large range of sizes can be covered (it has a large dynamic range). Monomer and aggregates as large as ~100-mer can be measured in a single analysis (i.e., at a single rotor speed). Unlike chromatography, for SV the effective resolution of different aggregate species varies with their proportion relative to monomer. That is, resolution is related to signal/noise ratio and gets poorer as the fraction of aggregates decreases.

Another strength of SV is that often the experiments can be run without any change in solvent conditions, thus avoiding potential changes in the distribution of noncovalent aggregates. One example where this was important is shown in

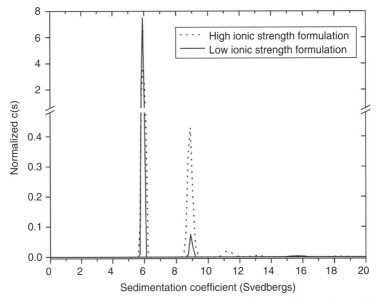

FIGURE 13.2 Sedimentation coefficient distributions for two different formulations of an antibody, one at high ionic strength (dotted line) and the other at low ionic strength (solid line).

Fig. 13.2. The original formulation of this antibody lost bioactivity fairly quickly, and it was thought this was due to aggregation. A new formulation at much lower ionic strength gave much slower loss of bioactivity, but the surprising result was that its aggregation appeared similar to the old formulation when measured by SEC. When SV was run on the two formulations, it was apparent that indeed the new formulation has significantly lower aggregate content. Why did SEC not detect this same difference? The SEC mobile phase was at high ionic strength, which was needed for good recovery of the injected sample. The SEC protocol involved predilution of the samples into the mobile phase, and for the new formulation, this change in solvent conditions induced formation of new noncovalent aggregates while the diluted samples sat for hours in the autosampler.

A final noteworthy strength of SV is that method development is minimal. Other than getting the protein concentration in a workable range, the only major operating variable is the rotor speed, and an experienced analyst can usually select that fairly well simply by knowing the approximate molecular weight of the major species. Thus, it is often possible to obtain high quality SV data the very first time a new protein is run.

One drawback of SV is that its sensitivity and reproducibility for measuring small amounts of aggregates in the dimer–octamer range is inferior to that of SEC. It is difficult to assign a single value for the limit of detection (LOD) or limit of quantitation (LOQ) of SV because these values vary significantly with monomer mass, aggregate stoichiometry, and to some extent with how many other species are present. The LOQ for aggregates in antibody samples appears to be ~1% at best [20,21], and recently, an LOQ of ≥3% was reported for a glycoprotein of ~109 kDa [22]. Even experienced analysts have difficulty achieving reproducible aggregate content for samples containing <2–3% aggregates, and it now appears that much of that variability is related to the quality of centrifuge cell components and difficulties in assuring proper cell alignment in the rotor [23,24]. Consequently when SV is used to cross-check SEC methods, it is best to run aged or stressed samples where the aggregate content is 5% or more.

Another drawback of SV is that certain excipients can cause significant interference. If sugars or polyols are present, their sedimentation will create unwanted gradients in density and viscosity across the measurement cell. These gradients then make the sedimentation rate vary with time and position in the cell. When the concentration of these excipients exceeds a few percentage by weight, these effects can reduce the sensitivity and accuracy of aggregate detection [25] and can also potentially produce false peaks. Micelles of polysorbate 20 or polysorbate 80 usually sediment in the range between 1 and 2 S, rates similar to proteins of about 10–20 kDa. Therefore, for peptides or small proteins, these micelles could be mistaken as aggregates, while for larger proteins, they could be mistaken for product fragments. The strong UV absorbance of some microbial preservatives can also preclude SV measurements using absorbance detection. RI detection is also available, but it generally requires sample dialysis and the use of the dialysate as the reference sample to reduce the interfering signals arising from sedimentation of excipients. Since dialysis will likely change aggregate distributions, absorbance detection is generally used.

Samples for SV can be loaded without filtration and there is little dilution of the sample as the run proceeds (about 30% by the end of the run). There are, however, severe restrictions on applying SV to samples at high concentrations. By using RI detection, it is possible to measure samples up to ~50 mg/mL, but interpreting such data is a major problem. Data analysis and interpretation for SV relies heavily on the underlying theory, but that theory breaks down as solutions become "nonideal" at high concentrations. SV experiments are influenced by both thermodynamic nonideality ("molecular crowding") effects and hydrodynamic nonideality, and these effects become significant at protein concentrations above ~2 mg/mL (and even lower for PEGylated proteins). Qualitative information about sample homogeneity is possible at concentrations approaching 50 mg/mL, but application of sophisticated quantitative approaches such as the $c(s)$ distributions to samples above ~5 mg/mL is inappropriate and likely to lead to spurious results.

An important practical limitation of SV is its low throughput (3 samples/day for absorbance data of the highest quality and 7 samples/day for slightly lower quality). It also requires expensive equipment (available from only a single source) and requires a highly trained analyst. The data analysis and cleaning, assembly, and filling of the measurement cells are fairly labor intensive for that trained analyst. These factors generally mean SV cannot handle the large numbers of samples generated by formulation or process development studies. Both the instrument and the analysis software would be quite difficult to validate for use in a QC environment, and this has apparently never been done.

13.3.5 Multiangle Classical Light Scattering

Classical or "static" light scattering detectors can be operated in either batch mode or flow mode following a separation method. For biotechnology applications, MALS detectors are most commonly used following a separation, and such applications will therefore be the primary focus here, but some aspects of batch-mode measurements are also discussed at the end of this section.

The use of a MALS detector on the output of an SEC column (SEC-MALS) or AF4 channel (AF4-MALS) allows direct measurements of the solution molar mass for each peak. The principal strength of MALS is that these measured masses are based on first principles of physics and are independent of molecular conformation. Furthermore, the masses measured by MALS are also independent of whether the peak elutes at an abnormal position due to unwanted interactions with the column matrix or the membrane in the AF4 channel. Another strength of MALS is that it requires essentially no method development over and above that required to develop a suitable SEC or AF4 protocol.

13.3.6 Does MALS Really Add Value?

While these properties of MALS certainly sound desirable, it is reasonable to ask: for protein pharmaceuticals, is it essential (or even important) to know the true solution mass of the main peak or the minor components? After all, for most applications of SEC or AF4, the goal is simply to quantify the fraction main peak. So is adding a MALS detector really useful, and if so how important is it to use it?

With respect to the main peak, the 2–3% accuracy of MALS (which hereafter in this section will mean either SEC-MALS or AF4-MALS unless one or the other is specified) is usually not sufficient to detect minor differences in primary structure. However, unlike mass spectrometry, MALS measures the mass in solution and can detect relatively unstable noncovalent oligomers. Thus, MALS is useful to clarify whether the normal solution state is monomeric or oligomeric for those cases where the product does not elute normally compared to protein size standards. Many cases are known where highly asymmetric monomers elute at positions that suggest a dimeric state. On the other hand, nonspecific interactions with the column matrix can produce abnormally late elution from an SEC column, and recently, an antibody that elutes like a protein about one-third of its true mass was described [10]. Abnormal elution relative to standards is especially problematic for proteins that are highly glycosylated and for PEGylated products. While it is true that abnormal elution relative to standards does not necessarily invalidate an SEC or AF4 method, in such cases, the qualification and validation of the method may be significantly strengthened by independent confirmation of the mass via MALS.

Another important aspect of MALS characterization of the main peak (but one that is less often exploited) is that it may give important clues about the reversible self-association of the product, even when the association–dissociation rates are so fast that different oligomers cannot be separated. Observing a mass that differs significantly from an integer multiple of the sequence mass, or a mass that varies significantly across the profile of the peak, may be a true indication of reversible association–dissociation behavior and should not simply be dismissed as an artifact or a calibration error. For an antibody example of this behavior, see Fig. 8 in Ref. [10].

With respect to the identification of the stoichiometry for minor aggregate peaks, MALS is not necessarily required or essential since for covalent aggregates this can also be done by collection of peaks for off-line analysis by SDS-PAGE or mass spectrometry. However, the identification of minor peaks via MALS can certainly be useful on its own and as an independent confirmation of off-line methods and may be the only feasible approach for labile aggregate species. As an example, MALS quickly showed that an early eluting "aggregate" peak from SEC was actually not an aggregate at all but a partially unfolded form of the monomer [11].

PEGylated products sometimes contain significant levels of non-PEGylated protein or free PEG, and some products contain monomers with different numbers of PEGs attached. In such cases, potential aggregate species have different ratios of PEG to protein and thus sorting out the chemical nature of each aggregate peak may be challenging. By combining data from MALS, RI, and UV detectors, it is possible to deconvolute the total mass for each peak into its protein and PEG components [26–28] and thus to assign the peaks without collecting them for off-line analysis.

Since SEC peaks eluting near the void volume may contain multiple unresolved species, MALS can be useful to obtain an average mass for those species and to monitor for consistency of that average mass from lot to lot or after process changes. MALS can also sometimes provide information about mechanisms of aggregation, which might be useful during formulation development or in improving the manufacturing process to reduce aggregation. For example, with glycoproteins we sometimes observe via MALS that the aggregates are less glycosylated on average than the monomer, which implies that reducing aggregation may require changes in the cell culture or purification to minimize the amount of underglycosylated material [10].

One unique and emerging MALS application is concentration gradient MALS (CG-MALS). Here, the MALS detector is used in flow mode but is fed by the output of a mixer connected to two or more computer-controlled syringes, an approach pioneered by Allen Minton and coworkers at the NIH. This setup can then create either a series of dilutions of a single-protein stock (to measure reversible aggregation) [29] or various mixtures of two different proteins (to measure binding interactions between them) [30]. Thus, in CG-MALS, one is really making a series of batch-mode measurements using the flow system as a means to easily generate a large number of dilutions or mixtures, and the data being produced is the weight-average molecular weight of each of those dilutions or mixtures. For protein pharmaceuticals, probably the most important aspect of this method is its potential for measuring reversible aggregation in high concentration protein formulations, something that has been a continuing challenge. This possibility arises through recent advances in both theoretical understanding of the strong solution nonideality effects at high concentrations [31] and also of the scattering from highly concentrated solutions [32]. Thus far, the only CG-MALS publications at high concentrations have used only standard proteins; the nonassociating proteins BSA and ovalbumin have been studied up to 125 mg/mL, while reversible monomer–dimer association in chymotrypsin has been studied up to 70 mg/mL [33]. Hopefully, real applications with therapeutic proteins at high concentrations will soon follow. CG-MALS can also be used to characterize functional interactions of protein products, such as the binding of antibodies to their antigens. Another potential application of CG-MALS is to study interactions between the product and excipients.

Thus overall, MALS can be quite a valuable part of the aggregation toolkit, but, on the other hand, currently, it is usually not truly essential and usually does not need to be run on a routine basis. Like SV, it can be a valuable supplementary tool and help to confirm results from other aggregation assays, especially when those results are unexpected. If, however, CG-MALS fulfills its potential to characterize reversible aggregation in high concentration protein formulation, it will probably become a truly essential tool for such products.

13.3.7 Strengths and Weaknesses of MALS

A strength of MALS that has not yet been mentioned is that it requires only a moderate investment in terms of both cost and personnel training. SEC-MALS has been validated for lot release of some products.

The biggest drawback of both SEC-MALS and FFF-MALS is that they inherit the major drawbacks associated with the separation methods: potential changes in the aggregate distribution due to dilution, filtration, and nonspecific binding effects, changes in solvent conditions, and/or the separation itself. The electronics, lasers, and photon detectors within the MALS instruments are generally quite reliable, but the scattering flow cells are subject to fouling and this can sometimes be problematic. The MALS detectors are, unfortunately, also exquisitely sensitive to particles shed from SEC columns, and thus, it is usually necessary to flush the column for at least 12 h to reduce this shedding before data can be collected.

Obviously, the maximum throughput of these methods is limited to that of the separation. However, the data processing is much less automated than in standard HPLC, and it requires a trained and skilled analyst. Thus, often the data processing is the factor that limits how many samples can be run.

MALS detectors can also be used in batch mode, either by employing cuvette adaptors or by direct injection of samples without separation (flow-injection analysis). Obviously, such use avoids all the issues arising from the separation techniques, but without any separation, one can only measure the weight-average molar mass for a sample (and, therefore, cannot measure the fraction or sizes of the aggregates). The major problem with batch-mode analysis is that the data are easily strongly skewed by traces of dust or other large particulates. Thus, reproducible measurements typically require filtration or centrifugation to remove such species, but such pretreatment then again raises the specter of changing the aggregate content one is trying to measure. Another minor problem with batch-mode measurements is that cuvettes that permit measurements over the full angular range usually require a large volume (as much as 4 mL); cuvettes for microliter volumes usually permit measurements at only $90°$ or at best a restricted range of angles.

13.3.8 Dynamic Light Scattering

Like MALS, DLS can be used either as a batch-mode measurement or in flow mode following a separation method. Unlike MALS, batch mode is used most often for DLS. The data analysis for DLS also has two main variations, both of which involve mathematically fitting the autocorrelation function (the raw data from a DLS measurement). A simple cumulant analysis gives an average hydrodynamic size and also sometimes an estimate of the polydispersity (the spread of sizes around the average). While this cumulants approach is mathematically robust and rapid enough for online flow-mode use, average values give no information about the individual size or the proportions of species making up that average.

The alternative data analysis approach instead derives a hydrodynamic size distribution for the sample; this is like a chromatogram, but one that has low resolution and very few data points (usually < 100). This allows resolution of multiple peaks, but it is strictly a mathematical separation, not a physical one, and the resolution is very low. Typically two peaks cannot be resolved unless their hydrodynamic size differs by a factor of two or more, which for spherical particles represents a factor of eight or more in mass. This means that DLS cannot resolve or quantitate small oligomers (dimer to octamer). When multiple peaks are actually resolved, a rough estimate of their weight fractions can usually also be made (based on the assumption that all particles are spherical), but the accuracy and reproducibility of this quantitation is poor. This size distribution analysis is much more complex than the simple cumulant analysis and also less robust and reproducible—it is usual for peaks near the threshold of detection to appear or disappear between sequential measurements of the same sample or with minor changes in software settings. Sometimes the size distribution calculations also fail to give a good fit of the raw data, and if so the results are probably unreliable; hence, it can be helpful for the analyst to inspect the quality of the fitting. Overall, DLS data analysis, like that for AUC, is something of an art and it requires some experience to judge which features of the distributions are significant.

One great strength of batch-mode DLS is its great sensitivity for detecting large aggregates (larger than decamer). Species with sizes of 100 nm and larger can typically be detected at weight fractions in the parts-per-million range. For certain products, we have found that when DLS detects particles in the size range of roughly 20–400 nm these samples will eventually (weeks to months later) form larger subvisible or visible particles (large enough to detect by visual inspection or particle-counting techniques). That is, the smaller particles detected by DLS sometimes are precursors to slowly forming larger ones [6,10]. In such cases, DLS can provide a quick assay useful for tracing back through the manufacturing process to find when these precursor particles are formed or introduced. This approach has, in several cases, led to manufacturing changes that eliminate the formation of the subvisible or visible particles.

A second great strength of DLS is that it can cover an enormous range of sizes in one measurement (∼0.1 nm–1 μm, which corresponds to a range of ∼10^{12} in molecular weight). DLS instruments are much less costly than AUC, the sample size is quite small (usually 2–20 μL), and the measurements usually require only a few seconds to a few minutes per sample. Highly automated instruments that accept samples in 96-, 384-, or 1536-well plates are now available. However, the high throughput of such instruments would likely quickly overwhelm the analyst's ability to interpret size distributions, and thus, probably only the simpler cumulant analysis giving the average size would be feasible for large numbers of samples.

The great sensitivity of DLS to large particles is also one of its greatest weaknesses. When there is large scattering arising from particles larger than a few micrometers, it may be impossible to acquire any interpretable data. Thus, sometimes it becomes necessary to centrifuge or filter the sample to remove such species, but doing so can potentially also remove species that are of interest. High levels of scattering from particles in the ∼20 nm–1 μm range (large but within the normal working range) can also be problematic because the smaller species may get lost in the glare from the large ones and escape detection. This "blinded by the light" phenomenon [6] means that it is common that in samples with strong scattering from particles larger than 20 nm the main component cannot be detected at all. That is, a sample can be more than 99.99% monomer by weight and nonetheless monomer may not be detected. When this happens, it also becomes impossible to estimate weight fractions.

Another aspect of DLS that is both a strength and a weakness is that it does not distinguish the chemical nature of the species creating the scattering. Thus, when traces of large particles are detected, it can be difficult to know whether these represent product aggregates or some external contaminant. One possible test is that if the weight fraction of such species increases with time or stress, then this implies that the normal product is forming (or at least assembling onto) these particles. However, the poor quantitation of weight fractions can make this test difficult to implement. On the other hand, the ability of DLS to detect contaminating particles can be quite valuable. Such particles can potentially serve as nuclei or seeds for the growth of visible or subvisible protein particles (heterogeneous nucleation) [34,35]; therefore, DLS can provide a valuable assay to detect contaminant particles that may be precursors to the larger particles and for tracing the source of the contamination.

It is possible to acquire DLS data for samples at very high protein concentrations, but the interpretation of such data is far from straightforward. Solution nonideality effects at high concentrations can significantly distort the measured hydrodynamic size. Typically, these effects become significant for all protein solutions above 10 mg/mL, but they can be much stronger for samples with high electric charge or low ionic strength. Although interpretation of absolute sizes is problematic at high concentrations, a qualitative change such as an increase in the number of peaks found in the size distribution as the concentration increases would provide strong evidence for reversible association.

A final property of DLS that can sometimes be problematic is that correct calibration of the hydrodynamic sizes depends on the viscosity and RI of the formulation buffer. Thus, for example, screening formulations by DLS measured directly in a 384-well plate will require little analyst time or work to acquire the data, but to correctly compare results across different formulations, the analyst must properly assign these properties for every well in the plate. On the other hand, the correct calibration is not important when comparing aged or stressed samples to a control measurement made in the same buffer.

With respect to validation of DLS methods for lot release, this may have been done in a few cases. If so, it seems likely that cumulant analysis was used rather than size distribution analysis.

13.4 APPROACHES TO ASSAY CROSS VALIDATION OR CROSS QUALIFICATION

Cross validation or cross qualification of aggregate detection and sizing assays is required fairly frequently. One reason for this is that no single method does a good job over the entire range of aggregates sizes and types, and therefore, it is often necessary to confirm whether any given method is adequate to detect the relevant species for that particular product. A second reason for cross validation is that the more complex methods are often not suitable for use in QC. For example, it is now quite common for the regulatory agencies to ask for cross validation of SEC methods used for stability studies, comparability protocols, and/or lot release. Note that the use of the term "cross validation" hereafter is meant to include "cross checking" or "cross qualification" of non-GMP assays.

13.4.1 Method and Sample Selection

Clearly, it is highly desirable for the methods selected for cross validation to be "orthogonal" to the primary method. This usually means choosing a method that works on a fundamentally different principle, but it also may be important to choose one that covers a different range of sizes or aggregate types. Thus,

SEC is orthogonal to SDS-PAGE since it separates via a different mechanism and detects both covalent and noncovalent aggregates. Similarly, SV and/or DLS might be appropriate cross checks for an SEC method since they are based on different principles. A combination of both SV and DLS would be even better because SV can resolve the small oligomers that DLS cannot, while DLS can detect much lower levels of very large aggregates than SV can. Some examples of cross-validation studies involving orthogonal techniques can be found in Refs [11,20,22,23], and [36].

Another important point about method selection for cross validation is that the number of samples required for such studies is usually small (often 10 or less). Such studies also should only need to be done once in the development cycle for each product. This means that it is reasonable to use methods that have low throughput and/or are relatively complex and costly, and it is also practical to employ methods that are not available in-house and, therefore, must be outsourced.

Which samples are appropriate to use in cross-validation studies? One common mistake is to look only at "good" samples with low aggregation, for example, several lots of bulk DS and/or final product. This is not a good choice because an important question to be answered by these studies is whether the method being cross-validated can detect all the relevant aggregate species to which a patient may be exposed. Thus, ideally one would include samples that have reached the end of the product shelf life, ones that represent the extremes of manufacturing variability, and ones that also represent the effects of other stresses that might be encountered such as shipping and handling stress or exposure to light. In practice, however, this full panoply of samples will probably never be available, but hopefully one can at least approximate this by including some appropriately stressed (accelerated stability) samples.

A second reason for including stressed samples may be to push the aggregate levels high enough to be well above the LOQ of all the analytical methods involved in the study. It perhaps should be obvious that one cannot expect to get good quantitative correlation between methods if the aggregate levels are near or below the LOQ of any method, yet nonetheless it is quite common for this point to be overlooked when planning these studies. For example, the normal aggregate levels for unstressed samples of some monoclonal antibodies and cytokines fall well below the LOQ of SV, and therefore, it is essential to select samples with higher aggregate content.

Yet another reason for including stressed samples is to test the method being validated under conditions where it is most likely to perform poorly. If that method works satisfactorily for difficult samples, this will greatly increase our confidence that it will work well for the real product samples. For example, for SEC, usually the aggregates that are most likely to be lost through filtration effects or binding to the column resin are the ones that are larger in size and more denatured. Since stressed samples often contain higher proportions of such species, the stressed samples will provide a much more stringent test for whether SEC can detect all the aggregates that may be present.

13.4.2   When Should Cross Validation Be Done?

It is definitely desirable to cross-validate aggregation assays before Phase 3 clinical trials. However, it is common for companies to wait until they are forced to do this testing by the regulatory agencies. The danger of postponing cross validation is that if the methods turn out to be not suitable for their purpose, then potentially a vast body of work might need to be redone. Depending on the issues that arise and the development stage, this could invalidate the real-time and accelerated stability data or even the formulation development itself, and thus clinical development could be delayed. Therefore, the risk in delaying too long is clearly high.

On the other hand, there is also some risk in doing cross validation too early. Changes in cell line, the purification process, formulation, or packaging could potentially significantly change the types and sizes of aggregates that occur and, therefore, the requirements for the aggregation assay(s). Thus, the danger is that changes at later stages in development might force a repetition of the cross-validation studies. The potential extra time, effort, and/or cost for outsourcing is not trivial, but it does pale in comparison to any risk of clinical delays.

Overall, the optimal time to do the cross validation might be before formulation development. However, the optimum will probably vary slightly depending on the nature of the product, the overall degree of product risk associated with aggregation, the development strategy, and the resources and experience of the company. For example, many companies seem to be adopting strategies aimed at getting the product candidate into humans as quickly and cheaply as possible to weed out products that will fail. Such a strategy may then dictate a minimal formulation effort to get a formulation specifically for early clinical work, and then full formulation studies are done only for promising candidates to create a final product formulation. For such cases, it may be best to postpone the cross-validation study until after creating the final formulation. However, for those products where risks associated with aggregation are high (e.g., a recombinant version of a natural human protein where immunogenicity is a high concern), it may be necessary to do the cross validation before creating the early clinical formulation to satisfy the regulatory agencies.

13.4.3   An Example of Cross Validating an SEC Method

Protein X is a $\sim$20-kDa glycoprotein that is slightly notorious for being "sticky" and easily lost to surfaces. Not surprisingly then, SEC protocols are difficult for this protein, especially with regard to obtaining good recovery. The SEC method that had been in use for some time used a mobile phase that is quite different from the DS and final formulation buffers, and that also contains components that are generally considered to promote protein denaturation. Since this SEC protocol had never been cross validated and because the mobile phase properties suggested a potential for changing the distribution of noncovalent aggregate, it was decided to do some cross validation using SV before trying to develop an improved formulation.

An important aggregation mechanism for protein X is aggregation due to freeze/thaw damage. Therefore, the initial SV study included a sample that had been subjected to four freeze/thaw cycles, and this sample quickly revealed a major discrepancy between SV and SEC. The SV data, taken directly in the DS buffer, gave the size distribution as shown in Fig.13.3a, which indicates 19.9% total aggregates, including some species larger than 50-mer. This result contrasts sharply with the ~4% aggregates measured by SEC. When SV was run on this

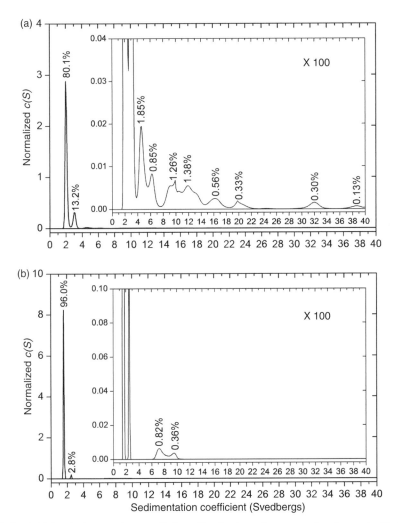

FIGURE 13.3 Sedimentation coefficient distributions for a sample of protein X drug substance after four freeze/thaw cycles. (a) Sample diluted into the drug substance buffer; (b) the same sample diluted into the SEC mobile phase. The insets in each graph show the same data after vertical amplification by ~100-fold, so the minor peaks can be seen. *Source:* Data redrawn from Philo [10].

sample after dilution into the SEC mobile phase, as shown in Fig. 13.3b, the total aggregate content drops to 4%, and all aggregate species larger than ~12-mer disappear. SDS-PAGE on this sample also indicates about 4% aggregates. Thus, the conclusion is that this SEC mobile phase dissociates essentially all the noncovalent aggregates (which constitute roughly 80% of the aggregates) into monomer; thus clearly, the cross validation has disqualified this SEC protocol.

Therefore, a renewed SEC method development effort was launched to find a column and less-denaturing mobile phase that still gave acceptable resolution and aggregate recovery, using the SV results in DS buffer as a guide to the "correct" results. This effort did succeed, as shown by the data in Fig. 13.4. Figure 13.4a shows SEC results for a highly stressed sample using the improved protocol, while Fig. 13.4b shows SV data for this same sample run in the DS buffer. The quantitative agreement for the fraction monomer (63.4% by SEC and 63.2% by SV) is excellent and well within the expected uncertainty for the SV result. The dimer fraction is 12.2% by SEC and 13.8% by SV. Here again, the disagreement for dimer may not be outside the possible uncertainty in the SV result [20,21]. Note that while the recovery of aggregates for this SEC protocol is excellent, the chromatographic separation is not. Thus, it is also possible that quantitation of the "dimer" peak in SEC is inaccurate because of the poor separation from monomer and other species.

This example illustrates one of the inherent difficulties of method cross validation: the resolution of the methods being compared may be substantially different, and therefore, it may not be possible or reasonable to directly compare the quantitation of individual peaks or species. Similarly, since the sensitivity of DLS to larger species far exceeds that of the other methods discussed here, there may actually be no direct way to confirm DLS results by an independent method. This then leads us to another key question: what criterion can we use to decide what level of agreement between the methods is acceptable? Clearly, it is neither necessary nor reasonable to expect total quantitative agreement. Rather, the best we can hope for is high correlation between the methods, and that they give the same rank ordering between "good" and "aggregated" samples. When considering what level of quantitative agreement among methods is needed, it is also very important to keep in mind how well we can quantitate the impact of the aggregates on the safety or efficacy of the product. If one cannot say with certainty that a product containing, for example, 5% aggregates is unsafe, but one containing only 4% aggregates is safe, then there is little point in worrying about the fact that one assay gives 4% while another gives 5%.

A second important criterion is that the method being cross validated should not fail to detect an entire class or size range of aggregates. For example, if SV, AF4, or DLS consistently detect >0.5%[2] of aggregates larger than octamer, but no corresponding peak is present near the void volume in the SEC chromatogram, this could raise significant concerns about the validity of the SEC results. In

---

[2]The 0.5% criterion used here is only for illustrative purposes. It is simply meant to indicate an amount that should be well above the detection threshold for the SEC method and that is also above the usual criterion that all impurities above 0.1 need to be characterized.

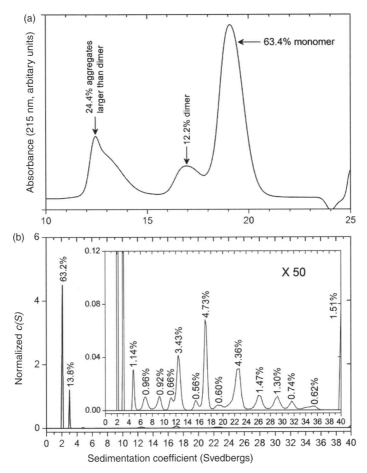

FIGURE 13.4   Cross validation of an improved SEC protocol for protein X against SV. (a) SEC chromatogram for a DS sample highly stressed by freeze/thaw cycles. (b) SV results when this sample is diluted into the drug substance buffer. *Source:* Data redrawn from Philo [11].

such a case, it might be necessary to modify the SEC protocol to improve the recovery of large aggregates. An alternate approach would be to add a second assay specifically to detect those larger species, although for GMP use the choices for such a second assay may be limited.

13.5   AGGREGATION ASSAYS FOR FORMULATION DEVELOPMENT AND COMPARABILITY PROTOCOLS

This section discusses some specific issues related to the selection of aggregation assays for formulation development and for use in comparability protocols.

13.5.1 Formulation Development

Since formulation development inevitably creates a large number of samples to be assayed, the throughput and per-sample costs of the assays are particularly critical. These factors strongly favor the less complex methods such as SEC and electrophoresis.

Two simple but useful types of light scattering tests that were not explicitly discussed previously but are commonly employed in formulation screening are (i) a visual inspection for particles and cloudiness and (ii) some form of batch-mode turbidity assay. The latter can be as simple as measuring the OD at some wavelength where the true protein absorbance is zero or nearly zero (wavelengths of 350–320 nm are commonly used). Such measurements can, of course, be done directly in microtiter plates for high throughput. Such turbidity assays are often used in assessing responses to physical stresses such as shaking, tumbling, or stirring.

Among the more complex methods, AF4 does have the throughput needed for full formulation studies, but whether current instruments are robust enough for such use is an open question [12]. Among the biophysical techniques, SEC-MALS too has the necessary experimental throughput, but its routine use in formulation studies would create a substantial burden of data processing and interpretation. Similarly, the plate-reader format DLS instruments can easily acquire the data for large numbers of samples, but interpretation beyond deriving a simple average radius for each sample would likely be too burdensome. SV, unfortunately, has the lowest throughput among these methods and also requires substantial time from skilled personnel to prepare and load the measurement cells and analyze the data.

Thus, in formulation studies, the biophysical techniques will generally not be used for screening accelerated stability samples from trial formulations. They can, however, play important roles both early and late in formulation development. Before initiating formulation screening, it is highly desirable to fully qualify the primary aggregation screening assay(s) via cross checking against orthogonal methods, as discussed in the previous section. Later after the field has been narrowed to a small number of candidate formulations, it may be appropriate to examine selected accelerated stability samples using a broader array of techniques to confirm the ranking from the screening assay(s). Such data may also help to discriminate between candidate formulations that otherwise seem quite similar.

One of the most difficult aggregation-related issues for formulators is how to compare two formulations which produce aggregates that are qualitatively different. Which is more desirable, a formulation where at the end of the projected shelf life there will be 4% of small oligomers (e.g., dimer, trimer, and tetramer), or one where there will be only 2% of small oligomers but 0.4% of species larger than decamer? Does it matter whether these species larger than decamer include subvisible particles? Does it matter whether the small oligomers are covalent in one formulation and noncovalent in another? These are difficult questions indeed, but the difficulty arises primarily because the formulation scientist usually has no quantitative information about how aggregates of particular sizes or types affect safety and efficacy.

13.5.2   Comparability Protocols

There is often a need to compare product or bulk DS lots from a new manufacturing process, manufacturing site, formulation, or dosage form ("A") to a previous one ("B"). Similarly, there is always a need to compare a new biosimilar product to a reference-listed drug. For simplicity here, all such comparisons will be called "comparability protocols," although that does not conform to formal regulatory definitions. Aggregation assay selection for comparability protocols is much easier because the number of samples involved is usually small—such protocols often involve only three lots each from the two processes being compared. This means that it is reasonable to use the full array of techniques, even if that means outsourcing them. The one exception may be AF4 if this has not been used previously for this product, since it would likely involve considerable effort to develop a new AF4 protocol.

When designing comparability protocols, it is important to keep in mind that aggregation levels and the details of the aggregate distribution usually vary significantly from batch to batch even within a single process. ("Significantly" in this context means significantly compared to the reproducibility of the assays.) These normal variations can make setting acceptance criterion (what passes as "comparable") rather difficult, but basically the situation is similar to that for glycoproteins, where current methods of glycan analysis invariably detect batch-to-batch variations. Consequently, "comparable" for aggregates usually means (i) a comparable range of aggregate content and (ii) a comparable distribution of aggregate sizes and types. In particular, one hopes not to see a qualitative change in the aggregate distribution (the new A batches contain a whole class of aggregates that was not present in the old B batches). Thus, some of the issues around how to compare aggregate distributions that are qualitatively different (discussed above for formulations) should also be considered when setting acceptance criteria for comparability.

Clearly, if one needs to establish that the *range* of aggregate content and distribution is similar, then statistical considerations dictate that it will be helpful to have more batches to compare. Even with three batches each from A and B, it can sometimes be quite difficult to distinguish real differences from those merely due to sampling error, especially when the batch-to-batch variability is relatively high and for assays such as SV where the intrinsic assay variability may also be relatively high. This also means that it is important to understand the assay variability to help distinguish which differences are real. Nonetheless, it is surprisingly common to see protocol designs where only a single batch of A and B are to be measured and with no replicates of any sample to establish assay variability. Unless the samples contain no detectable aggregates, the almost inevitable conclusion of such studies is that A and B are different, and nearly always follow-up studies of additional batches are then required.

Some special considerations arise when trying to show comparability of a biosimilar or "follow-on" product to an existing marketed product. The manufacturer of the biosimilar will not have access to the bulk DS of the innovator product. However, comparisons of aggregation for final product samples may be difficult or impossible due to interference from excipients such as human serum albumin (HSA), detergents [37,38], or antimicrobial preservatives. It has been reported in conference presentations that the comparability assessment for some biosimilars currently marketed in the EU involved repurifying DS from the final product. However, the validity of that approach is questionable, since for erythropoietin it has been shown that such attempts to regenerate the bulk DS produce additional aggregate species, and that putting two products with the same nominal composition through the same repurification protocol did not produce equivalent changes in the repurified product [39].

13.6 CONCLUDING REMARKS

Hopefully, this chapter has helped to clarify the capabilities, strengths, and weaknesses of the most widely used analytical methods for soluble aggregates. Clearly, there is still a need for improved methods and especially ones that can be used routinely and validated for lot release.

One continuing challenge is characterizing the reversible association for the many high concentration products currently under development (and controlling it to limit the product viscosity). It is not always appreciated that often the principal difficulty is not in acquiring the necessary experimental data, but rather in having the proper theoretical framework to correctly interpret the complex behavior of "crowded" solutions. The fact that the same theoretical difficulties apply to all the physical methods, not just AUC or light scattering, is also not yet widely understood. Another major unresolved issue for the industry is whether reversible oligomers that form at high concentrations are ever really relevant to safety or efficacy.

A second challenge is how to "connect the dots" between soluble aggregates and visible and subvisible particles, since sometimes conditions that cause greater accumulation of one have little effect on the other. The fact that the methods for particles usually give outputs in particles per milliliter while those for smaller aggregates generally give weight concentration contributes to this disconnect. In many cases, no accumulation of intermediates between these two size classes is observed, which is consistent with nucleation-controlled growth mechanisms, but the behavior of at least some products does not really fit such mechanisms. Mechanistic understanding of the particle growth usually requires monitoring mass flows, but that is seldom possible with current analytical methods. Typically, there is a considerable time delay between the stress or event that triggers the formation of large particles and their first detectable appearance, which also makes it difficult to understand mechanisms and differentiate cause from effect.

A final point to consider is whether as an industry is the time and effort spent on analyzing soluble aggregates really focused on the most important species?

Usually, the analytical methods are optimized for separating monomer from dimer and other small oligomers. Typically, these small oligomers do represent the majority of the total aggregates and, hence, will probably have the most potential impact on product efficacy. However, it is not clear that the small oligomers are really the aggregates that pose the greatest risk to patient safety, especially with respect to immunogenicity, since the larger aggregates (roughly octamer or decamer and larger) are thought to be more immunogenic [40,41]. Thus, it may be worthwhile to develop and validate a lot release assay that is specifically focused on detecting low levels of these larger aggregates. AF4 is certainly one possible candidate for such an assay. However, it seems surprising that currently companies never seem to consider developing a second SEC protocol for this specific purpose, using a resin of larger pore size (and hence sacrificing good quantitation of small oligomers), and choosing a resin type and column size for optimal detection of large aggregates rather than good resolution or good throughput. Ideally, the mobile phase for such an assay should be the formulation buffer, and the wider selection of resin types made possible by the lower resolution requirement should greatly increase the likelihood that this is possible. The use of a different resin type and/or mobile phase for such an assay would also make it at least partly orthogonal to the other (high resolution) SEC assay, which may also help to mitigate regulatory concerns about relying solely on a single SEC assay for lot release.

REFERENCES

1. Belford GG, Belford R. Sedimentation in chemically reacting systems. II. Numerical calculations for dimerization. J Chem Phys 1962;37:1926–1932.
2. Oberhauser DF, Bethune JL, Kegeles G. Countercurrent distribution of chemical reacting systems. IV. Kinetically controlled dimerization in a boundary. Biochemistry 1965;4:1878–1884.
3. Yu CM, Mun S, Wang NH. Theoretical analysis of the effects of reversible dimerization in size exclusion chromatography. J Chromatogr A 2006;1132:99–108.
4. Correia JJ, Stafford WF. Extracting equilibrium constants from kinetically limited reacting systems. Methods Enzymol 2009;455:419–446.
5. Ejima D, Yumioka R, Arakawa T, Tsumoto K. Arginine as an effective additive in gel permeation chromatography. J Chromatogr A 2005;1094:49–55.
6. Arakawa T, Philo JS, Ejima D, Tsumoto K, Arisaka F. Aggregation analysis of therapeutic proteins, part 2: analytical ultracentrifugation and dynamic light scattering. Bioprocess Int 2007;5:36–47.
7. Watson E, Kenney WC. High-performance size-exclusion chromatography of recombinant derived proteins and aggregated species. J Chromatogr 1988;436:289–298.
8. Arakawa T, Ejima D, Li TS, Philo JS. The critical role of mobile phase composition in size exclusion chromatography of protein pharmaceuticals. J Pharm Sci 2009;99:1674–1692.
9. Kamberi M, Chung P, DeVas R, Li L, Li Z, Ma XS, Fields S, Riley CM. Analysis of non-covalent aggregation of synthetic hPTH (1–34) by size-exclusion chromatography and the importance of suppression of non-specific interactions for a precise quantitation. J Chromatogr B Analyt Technol Biomed Life Sci 2004;810:151–155.

10. Philo JS. A critical review of methods for size characterization of non-particulate protein aggregates. Curr Pharm Biotechnol 2009;10:359–372.

11. Philo JS. Is any measurement method optimal for all aggregate sizes and types?. AAPS J 2006;8: E564–E571.

12. Cao S, Pollastrini J, Jiang Y. Separation and characterization of protein aggregates and particles by field flow fractionation. Curr Pharm Biotechnol 2009;10:382–390.

13. Fraunhofer W, Winter G. The use of asymmetrical flow field-flow fractionation in pharmaceutics and biopharmaceutics. Eur J Pharm Biopharm 2004;58:369–383.

14. Arakawa T, Philo JS, Ejima D, Sato N, Tsumoto K. Aggregation analysis of therapeutic proteins, part 3: principles and optimization of field-flow fractionation (FFF). Bioprocess Int 2007;5:52–70.

15. Arakawa T, Philo JS, Ejima D, Tsumoto K, Arisaka F. Aggregation analysis of therapeutic proteins, part 1: general aspects and techniques for assessment. Bioprocess Int 2006;4:42–49.

16. Betts S, Speed M, King J. Detection of early aggregation intermediates by native gel electrophoresis and native western blotting. Methods Enzymol 1999;309:333–350.

17. Philo JS. Analytical ultracentrifugation. In: Jiskoot W, Crommelin DJA, editors. Methods for structural analysis of protein pharmaceuticals. Arlington (VA): AAPS Press; 2005. pp. 379–412.

18. Liu J, Shire SJ. Analytical ultracentrifugation in the pharmaceutical industry. J Pharm Sci 1999;88:1237–1241.

19. Schuck P. Size-distribution analysis of macromolecules by sedimentation velocity ultracentrifugation and Lamm equation modeling. Biophys J 2000;78:1606–1619.

20. Liu J, Andya JD, Shire SJ. A critical review of analytical ultracentrifugation and field flow fractionation methods for measuring protein aggregation. AAPS J 2006;8: E580–E589.

21. Gabrielson JP, Randolph TW, Kendrick BS, Stoner MR. Sedimentation velocity analytical ultracentrifugation and SEDFIT/c(s): limits of quantitation for a monoclonal antibody system. Anal Biochem 2007;361:24–30.

22. Hughes H, Morgan C, Brunyak E, Barranco K, Cohen E, Edmunds T. Lee K. A multitiered analytical approach for the analysis and quantitation of high-molecular-weight aggregates in a recombinant therapeutic glycoprotein. AAPS J 2009;11:335–341.

23. Pekar AH, Sukumar M. Quantitation of aggregates in therapeutic proteins using sedimentation velocity analytical ultracentrifugation: practical considerations that affect precision and accuracy. Anal Biochem 2007;367:225–237.

24. Arthur KK, Gabrielson JP, Kendrick BS, Stoner MR. Detection of protein aggregates by sedimentation velocity analytical ultracentrifugation (SV-AUC): sources of variability and their relative importance. J Pharm Sci 2009;98:3522–3539.

25. Gabrielson JP, Arthur KK, Kendrick BS, Randolph TW, Stoner MR. Common excipients impair detection of protein aggregates during sedimentation velocity analytical ultracentrifugation. J Pharm Sci 2008;98:50–62.

26. Wen J, Arakawa T, Philo JS. Size-exclusion chromatography with on-line light-scattering, absorbance, and refractive index detectors for studying proteins and their interactions. Anal Biochem 1996;240:155–166.

27. Kendrick BS, Kerwin BA, Chang BS, Philo JS. Online size-exclusion high-performance liquid chromatography light scattering and differential refractometry methods to determine degree of polymer conjugation to proteins and protein-protein or protein-ligand association states. Anal Biochem 2001;299:136–146.

28. Arakawa T, Wen J. Determination of carbohydrate contents from excess light scattering. Anal Biochem 2001;299:158–161.

29. Attri AK, Minton AP. New methods for measuring macromolecular interactions in solution via static light scattering: basic methodology, and application to nonassociating and self-associating proteins. Anal Biochem 2005;337:103–110.

30. Fernandez C, Minton AP. Automated measurement of the static light scattering of macromolecular solutions over a broad range of concentrations. Anal Biochem 2008;381:254–257.

31. Minton AP. The effective hard particle model provides a simple, robust, and broadly applicable description of nonideal behavior in concentrated solutions of bovine serum albumin and other nonassociating proteins. J Pharm Sci 2007;96:3466–3469.

32. Minton AP. Static light scattering from concentrated protein solutions, I: general theory for protein mixtures and application to self-associating proteins. Biophys J 2007;93:1321–1328.

33. Fernandez C, Minton AP. Static light scattering from concentrated protein solutions II: experimental test of theory for protein mixtures and weakly self-associating proteins. Biophys J 2009;96:1992–1998.

34. Philo JS, Arakawa T. Mechanisms of protein aggregation. Curr Pharm Biotechnol 2009;10:348–351.

35. Chi EY, Krishnan S, Randolph TW, Carpenter JF. Physical stability of proteins in aqueous solution: mechanism and driving forces in nonnative protein aggregation. Pharm Res 2003;20:1325–1336.

36. Gabrielson JP, Brader ML, Pekar AH, Mathis KB, Winter G, Carpenter JF, Randolph TW. Quantitation of aggregate levels in a recombinant humanized monoclonal antibody formulation by size-exclusion chromatography, asymmetrical flow field flow fractionation, and sedimentation velocity. J Pharm Sci 2007;96:268–279.

37. Heavner GA. Reaction to the paper: interaction of polysorbate 80 with erythropoietin: a case study in protein-surfactant interactions - rebuttal letter. Pharm Res 2006;23:643–644.

38. Hermeling S, Schellekens H, Crommelin DJA, Jiskoot W. Micelle-associated protein in epoetin formulations: a risk factor for immunogenicity?. Pharm Res 2003;20:1903–1907.

39. Heavner GA, Arakawa T, Philo JS, Calmann MA, Labrenz S. Protein isolated from biopharmaceutical formulations cannot be used for comparative studies: follow-up to "a case study using Epoetin Alfa from Epogen and EPREX". J Pharm Sci 2007;96:3214–3225.

40. Rosenberg AS. Effects of protein aggregates: an immunologic perspective. AAPS J 2006;8:E501–E507.

41. Fradkin AH, Carpenter JF, Randolph TW. Immunogenicity of aggregates of recombinant human growth hormone in mouse models. J Pharm Sci 2009;98:3247–3264.

42. Rodbard, D, Chrambach, A. Estimation of molecular radius, free mobility, and valence using polyacrylamide gel electrophoresis. Anal Biochem 1971;40:95–134.

14 Protein Purification and Its Relation to Protein Aggregation and Particles

ROBERTO FALKENSTEIN, STEFAN HEPBILDIKLER,
WOLFGANG KUHNE, THORSTEN LEMM,
HANS ROGL, and EVA ROSENBERG

Bioprocess Development, Purification, Pharma Technical Development
Biologics Europe, Roche Diagnostics GmbH, Penzberg, Germany

GERHARD WINTER

Department of Pharmacy, Pharmaceutical Technology and
Biopharmaceutics, Ludwig-Maximilians-University Munich, Munich,
Germany

FRANK ZETTL

Bioprocess Development, Purification, Pharma Technical Development
Biologics Europe, Roche Diagnostics GmbH, Penzberg, Germany

RALF ZIPPELIUS

Pharma Biotech Production, Roche Diagnostics GmbH, Penzberg,
Germany

14.1 INTRODUCTION

Protein drugs are prone to chemical and physical instability during manufacturing, shipping, and storage. Chemical instability means any process that involves modification of the protein regarding covalent bond formation or cleavage, thereby generating a new chemical entity. Physical instability is related to conformational changes, adsorption to surfaces, aggregation, and precipitation [1,2]. Finding a balance between protein stability, protein purity, and process reproducibility possess a challenge especially for the purification or the so-called downstream

Analysis of Aggregates and Particles in Protein Pharmaceuticals, First Edition.
Edited by Hanns-Christian Mahler, Wim Jiskoot.
© 2012 John Wiley & Sons, Inc., Published 2012 by John Wiley & Sons, Inc.

processing (DSP) of the therapeutically applied proteins. Several parameters including protein concentration, pH, ionic strength, temperature, redox potential, and cosolvents have to be properly evaluated to separate the active pharmaceutical ingredient (API) from process-related impurities such as cell debris, lipoproteins, cell culture media components, host cell proteins (HCPs), host cell DNA and RNA, or viruslike particles. Moreover, product-related impurities encompassing, for example, isoforms, fragmented molecules, or protein aggregates have to be removed, which mostly exhibit only marginal differences in physical and chemical properties [3,4]. Thus, usually environmental conditions are applied during the purification process, which are far from physiological. Therefore, proper process development is needed to find a combination of parameters that ensures both stability and maximum purity at the same time. Furthermore, during bioprocessing, the protein is exposed to air–liquid interfaces, to surfaces of different hydrophobic and hydrophilic materials, to freeze-thaw stress, to temperature variations, and to UV irradiation or mechanical stress known to potentially provoke aggregation and particle formation [5–9].

Protein aggregates are considered as having the potential to cause severe immunological responses. In particular, patients may form antibodies against the drug that reduce therapeutic efficacy and, in rare cases, induce autoimmunity by cross reacting with the endogenous counterpart of the drug [6,10,11]. Studies have revealed potential driving forces and mechanisms underlying the behavior of protein aggregation, including conformational, colloidal, and also nucleation aspects [12–14]. Owing to the fact that the mechanisms of aggregation are not yet fully elucidated and factors improving or adversely affecting the stability of a certain protein are neither predictable nor transferable, protein stability has to be ensured at all stages in the manufacturing process to achieve the required quality of the drug substance.

Protein molecules that have been slightly altered in physical and/or chemical properties during early stage purification can be removed in subsequent purification steps. However, especially at the interface of final polishing and formulation, it is rarely possible to remove these product-related impurities. This chapter addresses the importance of purification process steps focusing especially on both the removal of aggregates as well as the process control as a powerful tool to minimize protein aggregation and particle formation.

14.2 DOWNSTREAM CONCEPTS FOR THE PURIFICATION OF THERAPEUTIC PROTEINS

The development of techniques and methods for protein purification has been an essential prerequisite for many of the advances made in biotechnology during the last decades.

Within protein research, the availability of highly purified protein material is vital for physicochemical characterization and the elucidation of structure–function relationships of the molecule of interest. With regard to the manufacturing of therapeutic proteins, the requirements for purity of the molecule are even higher to ensure maximum safety and efficacy of the resulting drug for the patient.

Depending on the intended use of the molecule, protein purification processes may include only rather crude techniques such as precipitation steps or, if high purity of the molecule is to be achieved, a sequence of highly efficient column chromatography steps with different selectivity. For instance, a typical purification process for a therapeutic antibody usually requires three consecutive chromatography steps. In most cases, these consist of an affinity (capture) column and two subsequent ion-exchange columns with oppositely charged functional groups. In addition, a number of different filtration steps are generally implemented in such a process for the purpose of intermediate concentration, rebuffering, and clarification of the protein solution.

Besides affinity and ion-exchange chromatography (IEC), hydrophobic interaction chromatography (HIC), hydroxyapatite chromatography (HAC), size-exclusion chromatography (SEC), and immobilized metal-affinity chelate (IMAC) chromatography are considered as the most prominent chromatography types used in protein purification.

The key to successful and efficient protein purification during process development is always to select the most appropriate techniques, optimize their performance, and combine them in a logical way to maximize yield and purity. Knowledge of the molecular properties of the protein of interest, for example, molecular mass and isoelectric point (IP), certainly facilitates the development of a new purification process.

Today, well-characterized and productive recombinant expression cell lines are used in general as the source for the manufacture of therapeutic proteins. At the end of the fermentation process, the cell-free supernatant, which contains the expressed protein of interest, is used as the starting material for the purification process. The established purification process should provide high yields and must be suitable for removing quantitatively process- and product-related impurities.

As outlined above, the protein of interest might be subjected to stress factors at several stages purification. Therefore, suitable analytical methods have to be in place during process development and manufacturing to monitor the quality of the protein of interest (product) during the purification process. For the release of the API of a protein pharmaceutical, specifications are set that address all types of process- and product-related impurities. Only API batches that meet the respective specifications can be applied for drug product manufacturing [4].

14.3 CONTROLLING AND MONITORING THE AGGREGATE LEVEL OF THERAPEUTIC PROTEINS DURING PURIFICATION PROCESSING

14.3.1 Preparative Chromatography

Chromatography is the most widely used method to remove protein aggregates from process fluids. Aggregated proteins differ in size and various biophysical parameters from the native protein. These differences can be used to separate the native protein from the aggregated ones by preparative chromatography. The most common techniques are SEC and IEC. If these techniques are not efficient enough in aggregate removal, alternative separation principles such as HIC and HAC are available [15].

Owing to its simple size-based separation mechanism, SEC is a very robust technique. While it is often used for analytical purposes, its use in preparative chromatography is limited. The major drawback of this method is its limited capacity. Since only 5–10% of the column volume can be applied per run, this step may turn out to be a true process bottleneck, especially if large amounts of a therapeutic protein per dose are needed, as it is the case for monoclonal antibodies (mAbs). Consequently, SEC plays no role in the industrial purification of products such as mAbs. However, it might be considered for final polishing of therapeutic products where relatively low amounts of API are needed such as hormones or viral vectors for gene therapy.

IEC uses different surface charges of aggregated and native proteins. Cation-exchange (CEX) chromatography is widely used for this purpose in the purification of mAbs [16,17]. Since vendors have significantly improved the capacity of these matrices, this method offers a relatively high mass throughput. Nevertheless, the screening of different matrices might be necessary to identify a gel that offers the required selectivity combined with high capacity. In many cases, the CEX step for the removal of aggregates is very sensitive with regard to pH and conductivity changes. Thus, it might be helpful to evaluate suitable process parameters by a design of experiment (DoE) approach. The benefit of this approach is that the single influence of pH and conductivity is not addressed separately; however, the interaction of the two parameters is investigated. Performing such DoE studies results in a design space for the relevant process parameters. Figure 14.1 gives an example of such a design space, illustrating the high sensitivity of yield and aggregate removal to pH and conductivity changes in CEX chromatography. A quite narrow pH and conductivity range needs to be maintained to ensure a certain level of soluble aggregates determined by SEC in the pool. If the set points for pH and conductivity are outside the design space (white area), this will result in an insufficient aggregate removal as well as a low recovery. Narrow design spaces are a significant challenge with regard to the process monitoring and control technology, especially in large-scale manufacturing.

In the last years, chromatography media vendors have developed new resins that carry both hydrophobic and ion-exchange moieties. The variants that are available include the combination of hydrophobic and anion-exchange functionality, as well as CEX functionality. These so-called mixed mode resins may also be suitable for the removal of aggregates, either in flow through or in binding mode [18]. Owing to the multifactorial dependency of binding and elution, it is difficult to develop a robust chromatography step for such resins. DoE studies are highly recommended to identify and characterize the necessary buffer conditions and process parameters. In summary, mixed mode resins offer a high selectivity,

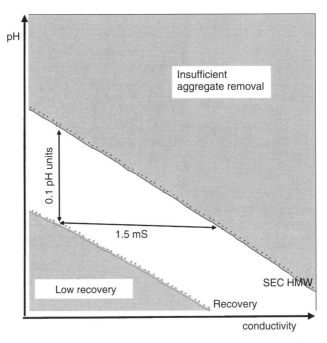

FIGURE 14.1 Design space (white) of a CEX chromatography step with regard to pH and conductivity.

but have to be often evaluated case by case and are not suitable for platform approaches, which are often aspired in mAb processes due to economical reasons. Thus, these resins are mostly used, when other techniques did not lead to a satisfactory reduction of the aggregate levels.

HIC or reversed-phase chromatography (RPC) uses the different hydrophobicity of the monomeric and aggregated forms of the protein. In general, these methods are very effective in the removal of aggregates [19,20]. A variety of the relevant functional groups of different hydrophobic strength, such as propylene–glycol, phenyl, or butyl phases, needs to be screened to end up with a robust chromatography step suitable for large-scale industrial applications as well as robust aggregate removal. Moreover, the process parameters have to be carefully evaluated considering protein stability, since either higher salt conditions or the use of organic solvents are required.

HA, a special form of calcium phosphate, has been widely used for protein purification since the early 1950s [21]. Protein binding to HA is mediated by electrostatic interactions of carboxyl and amino functions with Ca^{2+} and PO_4^{3-} groups of the crystal lattice [22–24]. Since the availability of a ceramic form of HA (CHT® Ceramic Hydroxyapatite), the resin has evolved as an alternative to conventional CEX chromatography and HIC for preparative polishing purification of mAbs [25]. Especially the CHT Type I material easily allows fast method development with respect to efficient aggregate removal from monoclonal IgG

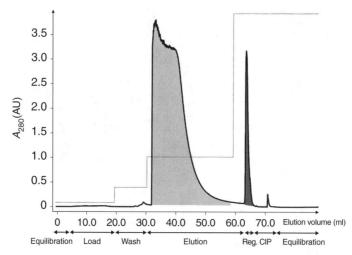

FIGURE 14.2 Aggregate removal on ceramic hydroxyapatite (CHT) Type I, 40 μm, 20 × 1 cm. Process conditions: flow rate 300 cm/h, load 50 mg IgG/mL CHT Type I (∼90% DBC), equilibration 2 mM $Na_2HPO_4 \times 2H_2O$, pH 6.8, 5 CV, load Protein A eluate (pH adjusted to pH 6.8), wash 35 mM $Na_2HPO_4 \times 2 H_2O$, pH 6.8, 2 CV, elution 120 mM $Na_2HPO_4 \times 2 H_2O$, pH 6.8 (∼6 CV), regeneration 0.5 M $Na_2HPO_4 \times 2 H_2O$, pH 6.8, 3 CV, cleaning in place 1 M NaOH, 2 CV. Dotted line, conductivity; ▨, IgG monomer; and ■, IgG aggregates.

preparations by applying phosphate gradient elution. Figure 14.2 shows a typical elution profile for the intermediate purification (post protein A) of an IgG1. After method development using phosphate gradient elution, the chromatography on CHT was optimized to isocratic elution conditions, resulting in effective monomer and aggregate separation. The initial content of approximately 1% antibody aggregates could be reduced to <0.2%.

14.3.2 Filtration

In general, there are two ways to operate filtration equipment: normal flow filtration (NFF) or dead-end mode filtration and tangential flow filtration (TFF) or often called *cross-flow filtration*. TFF works more effectively than NFF, especially when the solid or colloidal feed fraction increases. The shear flow over the membrane surface causes an inertial lift of, for example, deposited protein, particles, and solutes off the processed membrane, leading to lateral migration of the deposit, which is then transported back to the bulk solution by the axial drag of the tangentially flowing stream [26–30] (Fig. 14.3 adapted according to [30]).

Thus, the volumetric rate of fluid flowing through the membrane (permeate flux) is increased in comparison to filtrations performed in dead-end mode.

14.3.2.1 Normal Flow Filtration (NFF)   Minimizing transmission of infectious pathogens is an overall strategy during processing of biological products. By applying membrane pore sizes of 0.1–0.2 μm, NFF is commonly used to

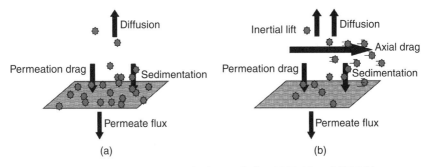

FIGURE 14.3 Hydrodynamic forces during NFF (a) and TFF (b).

reduce the bioburden of process intermediates and support the absence of germs in the finally formulated drug product. In addition, nanofiltration is performed during processing of recombinant products such as mAbs from mammalian cell lines, which may contain endogenous retroviruses, or adventitious viruses, which can enter the process stream. Typically membrane pore sizes of 20(−50) nm are applied (Section 14.3.3). Depth filtration can remove nonproteinaceous particles or larger protein aggregates of product- or process-related impurities such as host cell DNA or HCPs.

NFF is characterized by the feed flow going perpendicular to the filter surface [31]. The fluid is processed either under constant flow or constant pressure conditions. Depth filtration is preferably performed at constant pressure since the applied filter potentially releases particles and fibers under high pressure peaks, which can then enter the bulk material. During constant pressure depth filtration, a decrease in the filtrate flow rate over time indicates deposition of retained solute components, forming a cake on the membrane and causing fouling at the inner surface. Hence, increasing the feed flow rate is required to maintain permeate flux. This, in turn, may affect the integrity of the filtration device. To circumvent a breakthrough of protein aggregates, particles, or other impurities that are adversely affecting bulk quality, the maximum filtrate volume needs to be determined, which ensures the retention of the impurities. Therefore, during filtration experiments, samples are drawn from the filtrate and the rise of differently sized aggregates, particles, and other impurities can be monitored by applying suitable analytical methods. Figure 14.4 shows that at a defined processed filtrate volume, the turbidity increases and nearly reaches the value of 30 NTU of the unfiltered bulk. Concomitantly to the turbidity break through observed at a filtration volume beyond $100 L/m^2$, a second species with a mean hydrodynamic diameter of about 190 nm was detected by dynamic light scattering (DLS). Therefore, a maximum volume of $100 L/m^2$ membrane area should be filtered in this case to ensure the retention of differently sized aggregates by the filter module used.

14.3.2.2 Tangential Flow Filtration (TFF) In TFF, the feed is going tangentially to the membrane surface [31]. Two streams leave the filtration device, the so-called retentate and permeate.

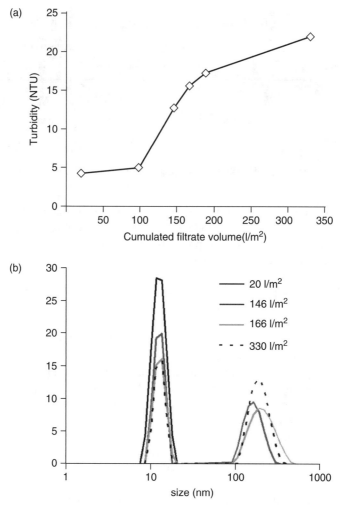

FIGURE 14.4   Accumulated filtrate volume versus turbidity (a) and DLS relative intensity of mAb monomer (about 10 nm hydrodynamic diameter) and an aggregated species >100 nm hydrodynamic diameter (b) of collected fractions during depth and 0.2 µm filtration of a capture pool.

In manufacturing of biopharmaceuticals, a TFF step may be used to separate cells from the culture fluid [32] or during refolding of solubilized inclusion bodies (IBs), when denaturant and reducing agent have to be removed (Section 14.3.4). During the multistep purification of mAbs polymeric ultrafiltration (UF), membranes with a nominal molecular-weight cutoff (NMWC) of 10–50 kDa are frequently applied, retaining the mAb reliably in the retentate and letting the buffer and small solutes passing through the membrane pores into the permeate.

UF in TFF mode is usually conducted between orthogonal chromatographic steps to concentrate the protein, exchange buffer, remove low molecular-weight impurities, or reduce the salt concentration [33]. Moreover, a second UF step is usually required after the final polishing step to diafiltrate the molecule of interest into a suitable formulation buffer ensuring sufficient stability during shipping and storage. Especially in mAb processes, a further concentration step is usually implemented to reduce the volume of the bulk. This results in reduced storage and shipping cost as well as in a reduced administration volume of the formulated solution, since high dosing of these molecules is required [34]. The capability to remove any kind of impurity from the bulk after the dedicated chromatographic steps is limited to larger insoluble aggregates and particles, which can be usually addressed by microfiltration. Therefore, this second UF step at the interface of DSP and final formulation needs to be carefully evaluated considering the induction of differently sized aggregates. This evaluation encompasses both environmental conditions and several operational parameters during UF processing to prevent the protein from aggregation.

Since protein aggregation is known to depend on total protein concentration [34,35], ambient temperature, storage period, pH, and the type and concentration of solutes used [2,36–39], these environmental conditions are of special interest during UF optimization. Ionic strength, pH, and buffer composition of the processed solutions during UF can significantly influence their aggregate pattern. It is reported that IgG aggregates, monitored by SE-HPLC and DLS, were formed due to lowering the ionic strength during UF diafiltration. An increase in conductivity by adding salt to the diafiltration buffer was suitable to reduce the formation of aggregates during buffer exchange [40].

It is known from current literature that during dialysis of different therapeutic proteins, the concentration of the diffusible buffer forming solutes changes on the retentate side compared to the permeate side [41]. This thermodynamic nonideality is based on electrostatic interactions of the protein at nonisolectric pH and the charged solutes in its vicinity, leading to unequal partitioning of these solutes across the semipermeable membrane [42]. This effect is called the *Donnan effect*, which was first pointed out by Frederic G. Donnan in 1911 [43].

The Donnan effect is potentially relevant during UF operation of IgGs, especially at very high protein concentrations. Postdiafiltration as well as postconcentration assays of an IgG solution at 200 mg/mL showed a molar histidine concentration (determined by analytical CEX chromatography) up to 50% lower than those of the diafiltration buffer. Deviations were also observed when the IgG was dialyzed and concentrated in an acetate buffered environment. Here, a molar acetate concentration (determined by analytical RP chromatography) up to 50% higher was found after UF concentration (Fig. 14.5a).

Concomitantly, pH and conductivity were not stable during the UF concentration process (Fig. 14.5b). In the case of histidine, an increase in pH and conductivity was obvious. Since pH and buffer composition are known to influence protein stability, the formation of aggregates was monitored by employing several analytical methods, such as SE-HPLC, turbidity measurements, and light

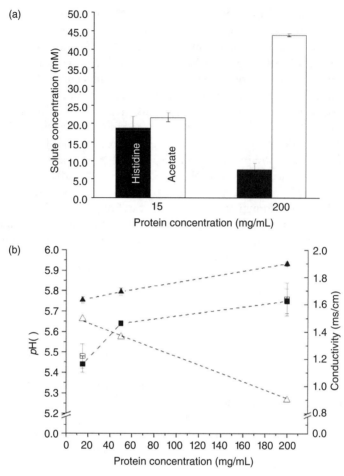

FIGURE 14.5 Loss of histidine and accumulation of acetate during UF of an IgG solution at pH 5.5: molar concentration of histidine (black bars) and acetate (white bars) before UF processing at 15 mg/mL protein concentration and after UF processing at 200 mg/mL protein concentration (a); pH (squares) and conductivity (triangles) during UF concentration of solutions containing 20 mM histidine (black symbols) or 20 mM acetate (plain symbols) before the UF starts (b); experimental data is presented as mean values of three measurements ± SD.

obscuration, to investigate the formation of differently sized aggregates. IgG solutions before UF (15 mg/mL, 20 mM histidine pH 5.5) and after UF (200 mg/mL) were investigated during quiescent storage at 40°C for eight weeks. Concentrated solutions containing only 10 mM of histidine and concentrated solutions containing 20 mM histidine after UF processing were investigated. The solutions before UF were known to exhibit a good physical stability in a buffer containing 20 mM histidine at pH 5.5 (Fig. 14.6).

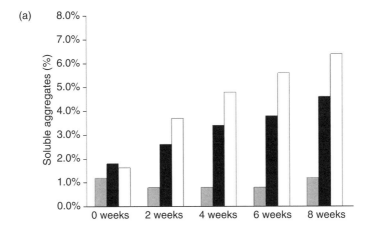

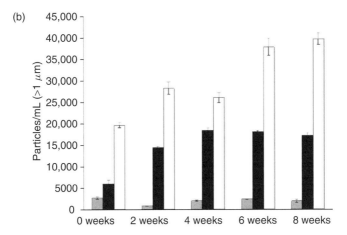

FIGURE 14.6 Percent soluble aggregates monitored by SE-HPLC (a) and number of particles larger 1 μm determined by light obscuration of IgG solutions (b) before starting the UF concentration process (15 mg/mL, 20 mM histidine pH 5.5: gray bars) and after UF (200 mg/mL, 20 mM histidine pH 5.5: black bars and 200 mg/mL, 10 mM histidine pH 5.8: white bars) at 40°C over eight weeks.

An increase in soluble aggregates as well as in the number of particles larger 1 μm was recognized for both concentrates at 200 mg/mL protein concentration. However, the concentrates having a higher level of histidine after UF showed a better aggregate profile compared to the concentrates containing only 10 mM histidine. The histidine concentration of 20 mM was achieved by applying a higher histidine concentration before starting the UF concentration and thus balancing the loss of this solute during processing. Concomitantly, the pH during UF was observed to be stable at pH 5.5 when a higher molar concentration of histidine was present, which is considered to support the stability of the protein during and after UF.

Instead of balancing the solute concentration during UF processing to achieve the evaluated buffer conditions ensuring product stability, the UF step may be conducted at a pH closely to the IP of the protein to suppress the Donnan effect or the buffer conditions may be adjusted after the UF process step by using a suitable conditioning buffer. However, this is not recommended since the colloidal stability at a pH near the IP of the protein is, in general, more compromised than under electrostatic repulsive conditions [12], and a therefore more compact packing of the molecules on the UF membrane leads to a strong decrease in permeate flow through and thus increasing UF processing time unfavorably [44]. The conditioning considering pH or solute concentrations needs to be carefully evaluated as well, since the corrective solution itself can compromise the stability of the protein due to temporarily high local pH or solute concentrations.

During the concentration process, the protein accumulates in the retentate, reaching very high concentrations potentially exceeding 100 mg/mL when material is needed for the supply of highly concentrated mAb preparations for subcutaneous administration. Figure 14.7 shows turbidity values at 350 nm and the level of particles larger 1 µm determined in the retentate during UF by employing light obscuration measurements. The samples were taken every time the

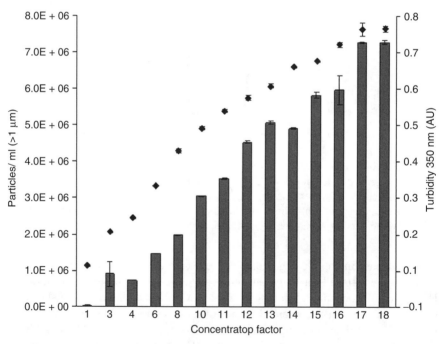

FIGURE 14.7   Turbidity measurement (triangles, referring to the right scale) and number of particles larger than 1 µm (bars, referring to the left scale) during the UF concentration process of an IgG solution starting with a protein concentration of 5 mg/mL in 20 mM histidine buffer pH 6.0 (concentration factor = 1); experimental data is presented as mean values of three measurements ± SD.

retentate concentration doubled and aliquots with a particle content higher than 120,000 mL^{-1} were diluted using 0.2-μm filtered histidine buffer to match the specific capacity of the applied sensor (particle counter SVSS-C, PAMAS Partikelmess- und Analysesysteme, Rutesheim, Germany). The particles formed during UF concentration were shown to be of proteinaceous nature by using a filtration/staining method as described by Li et al. [45]. Figure 14.8 shows these insoluble protein aggregates separated from the ultrafiltrated concentrates at 90 mg/mL by 0.1 μm filtration and subsequent washing and staining by using the metal chelate stain pyrogallol red-molybdate, which is known to be able to stain proteins immobilized on solid-phase supports [46] and not unspecific particulate matter. During the UF processing, not only proteinaceous particles can be generated but also particles of nonproteinaceous nature can be potentially leached or abraded from the bioprocessing equipment, encompassing tubings, fittings, or pump heads [47].

Beside the high concentration reached in the retentate, a very high protein concentration is reached near the UF membrane, forming the so-called polarization layer where aggregation is considered to be facilitated as well. Owing to this accumulation of the processed protein and potentially its aggregates, being largely rejected by the membrane, the buffer flow through the membrane, called *permeate flux*, is significantly reduced leading to an undesirable increase in process times [31,48]. Moreover, because of the tangential operation mode, the formed aggregates may be removed and transported back to the retentate affecting product quality adversely.

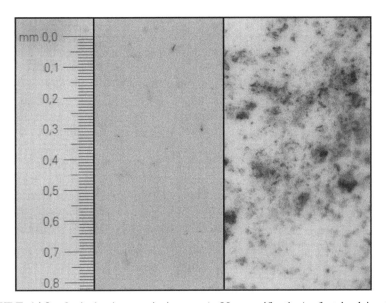

FIGURE 14.8 Optical microscopic images (×80 magnification) of stained insoluble aggregates after 0.1 μm filtration of an IgG solution before UF processing at 5 mg/mL and after UF concentration at 90 mg/mL.

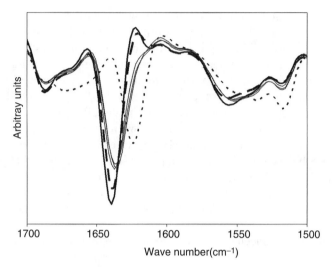

FIGURE 14.9 Comparison of the second derivative FTIR spectra of a native mAb solution at 5 and 90 mg/mL (black line), the protein attached to the cellulose-based UF membrane (bold dashed black line), the separated insoluble aggregates (gray lines), and the heat treated solution of 90 mg/mL (dotted line).

Insoluble IgG particles separated from a highly concentrated bulk after UF by centrifugation exhibit conformational changes investigated by FTIR spectroscopy (Fig. 14.9). The diminished bands at 1639 and 1690 cm^{-1} as well as the shift of the band at 1639 cm^{-1} to a lower wave number revealed perturbation in secondary structure, that is, a loss in the proportion of β-sheet motifs. This was shown to be much more pronounced by heating, which is in accordance with current literature [49,50]. The protein that was directly adsorbed to the membrane after processing remained nearly in its native secondary conformation. This was also reported by Maruyama and coworkers who found that the simple adsorption of a model protein to hydrophilic UF membranes induced only a negligible perturbation in its secondary structure [51]. However, the aggregated protein that was accumulated in the gel layer near the membrane after concentrating the solution in a stirring cell exhibits significantly denatured protein as detected by FTIR [52].

Regarding operational parameters during UF processing that potentially influence the aggregate level of the concentrated bulk, it was found that the applied pressure drop between inlet and outlet (Δp) during the UF has to be considered as an impact factor. Aggregation was monitored by using SE-HPLC, turbidity measurements, DLS (Fig. 14.10), and light obscuration (Fig. 14.11). All analytical techniques revealed that a higher Δp during UF concentration experiments with an IgG in 20 mM histidine pH 6.0 results in an increased level of differently sized aggregates in the concentrated solutions. In general, a higher level of soluble aggregates was observed with increasing protein concentration from 15 to 90 mg/mL, as determined by SE-HPLC. Moreover, a higher turbidity, as well as an increase in DLS relative intensity, was recognized. However, a slight increase in the level of soluble aggregates, accompanied by an increase in turbidity and DLS

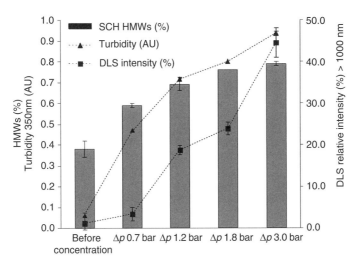

FIGURE 14.10   Aggregates analyzed by SE-HPLC (gray bars, referring to the left scale), turbidity at 350 nm (black triangles, referring to the left scale), and relative intensity of the peak >1000 nm hydrodynamic diameter determined by DLS (black squares, referring to the right scale); an IgG solution at 5 mg/mL (before concentration) and at 90 mg/mL protein concentration obtained after UF applying a Δp of 0.7, 1.2, 1.8, and 3.0 bar; experimental data is presented as mean values of three measurements $\pm$ SD.

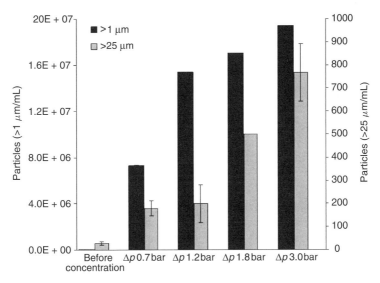

FIGURE 14.11   Particles per milliliter larger 1 μm (black bars, referring to the left scale) and 25 μm (gray bars, referring to the right scale); determined by light obscuration at 5 mg/mL (before concentration) and 90 mg/mL protein concentration obtained from UF applying a Δp of 0.7, 1.2, 1.8, and 3.0 bar; experimental data is presented as mean values of three measurements $\pm$ SD.

TABLE 14.1 Selection of Dedicated Viral Clearance Steps in mAb Downstream Processes

Dedicated Viral Clearance Steps	Primary Principle	Applicable to
Solvent/detergent treatment —Low pH treatment —Detergent treatment —Combination of low pH and detergent treatment	Inactivation	Lipid-enveloped viruses
—Nanofiltration	Removal by size exclusion	Nonenveloped and enveloped viruses (depending on size)
—UV-C irradiation	inactivation	Nonenveloped viruses

relative intensity, was obvious when the Δp increased from 0.7 to 3.0 bar. At the same time, with increasing Δp values, a steady rise of particles monitored by light obscuration can be observed, underlining the need to restrict the Δp in UF processes (Fig. 14.11). Other operational parameters that can potentially impact the level of aggregates in the retentate, encompassing transmembrane pressure (TMP) and flow velocity, were kept constant at comparable levels during processing [53].

Other parameters known to potentially impact the quality of the processed bulk regarding the level of aggregates are temperature, types of pumps used, processing time, and type of processed surfaces and their leachates as well as particles abraded from the applied bioprocessing equipment [5,47,54,55].

In summary, environmental conditions as well as operational parameters need to be evaluated to diminish the risk of provoking aggregation during processing. Suitable analytical methods are needed to address differently sized aggregates that may occur during TFF to establish a well-evaluated manufacturing process, thus ensuring the stability of the processed bulk material.

14.3.3 Dedicated Virus Inactivation/Removal

Retrovirus-like particles are endogenous particles observed in the cell culture supernatant, which enter the purification process. Although not infective when CHO cells are used, it has to be shown that these potential impurities can be removed and/or inactivated during processing to avoid a theoretical infection of patients treated with the purified protein therapeutic. Therefore, in accordance to the guidelines of the health authorities, patient safety has to be considered in the design of purification processes for therapeutic proteins. Overall, removal/inactivation capacity is recommended to reduce retrovirus-like particles below one particle in a million doses. In addition, adventitious viruses which potentially enter the manufacturing process, e.g. as raw material contaminants have to be removed by the purification process. Therefore, purification processes contain steps that are dedicated to viral clearance in accordance with regulatory guidance documents. Four of these process steps are described in Table 14.1).

Potential virus contaminants can be inactivated by detergent treatment and low pH treatment bundled under the term solvent/detergent treatment.

Detergents are efficient inactivating agents for lipid-enveloped viruses. Detergent treatment is well characterized and widely used in manufacturing of plasma-derived biologics. Since detergents are introduced into the process, their removal by DSP has to be ensured as long as they are not part of the formulated product solution. The same is true for organic solvents such as ethanol or isopropanol. Again, lipid-enveloped viruses are more sensitive to these inactivating agents than non-enveloped viruses.

Low pH treatment is a fast, efficient, and widely used method to inactivate lipid-enveloped viruses, for example, retrovirus-like particles. Within well-characterized ranges for pH, temperature, and time, this process step is effective and robust in inactivation of lipid-enveloped viral particles. For efficient inactivation of enveloped viruses, a combination of pH ≤ 3.6, incubation time ≥ 30 min, and room temperature is recommended, for example, as described in the article by Brorson et al. [56].

Low pH treatment is easily implemented into the purification process of mAbs following Protein A affinity chromatography as a capture step that uses low pH buffer for product elution. Depending on the sensitivity of the molecule, an increase in aggregate level may be observed during incubation at the pH required for efficient inactivation of retroviruslike particles.

As a precaution, the process intermediate stability at different pH conditions is investigated during purification process development, and the tolerable pH range needs to be determined, as shown in Fig. 14.12.

In general, analytical SE-HPLC is applied to monitor the potential induction of soluble aggregates, since the removal capacity for these species is limited during the following preparative chromatographic steps. A robust removal of these soluble aggregates by cation exchange chromatography, encompassing soluble dimers and oligomers, can be challenging if their level exceeds a few percentage in product mass [57]. In addition, the type of aggregates formed may influence the setting of process conditions (Table 14.2): for example, aggregation that is reversible on pH increase is considered less critical at this stage of the process. At the same time, oligomers such as tri- or tetramers may be easier to remove in DSP than dimers.

Any aggregates potentially formed during low pH treatment need to be removed during subsequent purification steps of the DSP to meet the product quality specification of the therapeutic product.

Virus-retentive filtration is a widely used method for removal of viral contaminants. Due to the mechanism of virus reduction this process step is orthogonal to the inactivation of potential viral contaminants by solvent/detergent treatment. This step removes all potential viral contaminants larger in diameter than the nominal pore size of the separation media used. The separation mechanism is simple and size based: the smaller the pore size, the wider the range of viral particles that can be removed. Therefore, it is considered a strong and robust contribution to viral safety of therapeutic proteins.

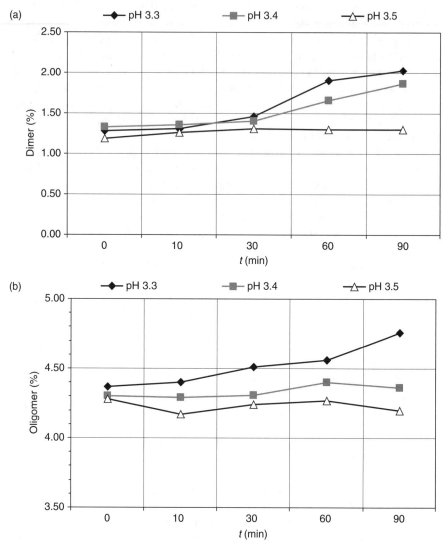

FIGURE 14.12 Effect of mAb incubation at pH 3.3, 3.4, and 3.5 on the level of (a) dimer and (b) oligomer according to SE-HPLC (area percentage).

TABLE 14.2 Removal of Aggregate Species by Two Different Cation Exchange Resins according to SE-HPLC (Area-%)

Cation Exchange Resin	Aggregates in Load Material (Area-%)		Aggregates in Product Pool (Area-%)	
	Oligomer	Dimer	Oligomer	Dimer
CEX 1	6.8	2.9	2.7	2.5
CEX 2			1.0	1.0

Considering the diameter of solubilized mAbs of ~10 nm, there is an obvious challenge to construct membranes that allow unhindered passage of the therapeutic protein while reliably retaining viral particles of down to 20 nm in diameter. Currently, nanofiltration modules with a nominal pore size of 20 nm are available on the market. Many of these devices show performance limitations either with regard to flow rate, capacity, and/or robustness. Moreover, it is observed that impurities can significantly reduce flow rate and capacity. Impurities, of course, include protein aggregates. Hence, a low level of aggregates and impurities is in general beneficial for performance and capacity of nanofilter media.

In any case, nanofiltration is a bottleneck for the purified product solution. It is recommended to reduce product aggregates to a minimum, for example, <1 area-% in SE-HPLC, before applying the product solution to a nanofilter to improve the capacity of the filtration device.

Therefore, while this process step does not directly remove product aggregates, reduction of aggregates and impurities upstream of this process step is required to efficiently use the extremely expensive single use virus-retentive. The purification process is optimized accordingly to reduce all impurities in the protein solution applied to the virus-retentive.

UV-C irradiation is an interesting complementary approach to other more widely used virus removal/inactivation technologies. UV-C light is able to modify the nucleic acid of viral particles [58]. Therefore, this technology preferably inactivates viruses carrying no lipid envelope such as murine minute virus (MMV). The non-enveloped viruses are physicochemically resistant and usually smaller than enveloped viruses. Thus, they represent a higher challenge for removal/inactivation in purification processes.

Infectivity of lipid-enveloped viruses is reduced as well. However, a significant higher irradiation dose is required than that for non-enveloped viruses. A systematic design of a UV-C irradiation process for pharmaceutical proteins in large-scale batches is described by Li et al. [59].

The exposure of proteins to light and the subsequent chemical and physical degradation have been studied for many years. The review of Kerwin and Remmele describes major pathways of photodegradation for proteins revealing potential changes in primary, secondary, and tertiary structure [7]. UV-C irradiation can also lead to protein aggregation as shown in Fig. 14.13.

If aggregation is an issue, the type of aggregate and modification of amino acid side chains need to be determined. The protein residues that potentially undergo primary photooxidation include tryptophan, tyrosine, phenylalanine, methionine, histidine, and cysteine/cystine [7]. The capacity of the purification steps to remove the aggregates and other undesired species that have been potentially generated needs to be tested. Thus, a low irradiation dose is desirable.

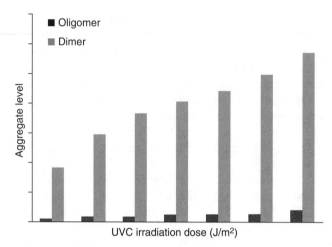

FIGURE 14.13   Effect of increasing UV-C irradiation dose on aggregate level of an mAb process intermediate.

Owing to the risk of aggregation at high irradiation doses combined with the protective effect of a lipid envelope, the use of this technology to inactivate endogenous retrovirus-like particles from cell culture is limited.

Only a small number of purification processes for therapeutic proteins contain the technique of UV-C irradiation, although it provides a complementary approach for inactivation of nonenveloped viruses. Implementation in a purification process may be considered, especially if the risk of patient infection with human pathogenic viruses is evident.

In any case, virus inactivation steps using solvent/detergent treatment or UV irradiation have the potential to provoke protein aggregation and have to be evaluated case by case during the development of purification processes.

14.3.4   Refolding

Different host systems are available today and the gram-negative bacterium *Escherichia coli* and other prokaryotes are still the first choice if posttranslational modifications are not a prerequisite for protein function. The recombinant gene product can be expressed within short cultivation times and at high concentration levels; however, it usually accumulates in the cell in a nonnative form building dense particles called *IBs* [60]. Different methods are discussed in the literature to optimize the in vivo production of the soluble and active form of the protein [61]; however, in vitro solubilization, purification, and refolding of the target protein from the IBs are mostly applied to receive the soluble and active protein with adequate high yield. The optimum conditions of the in vitro refolding process are usually evaluated case by case considering solubility, yield, aggregation, and bioactivity of the target protein. The specific amino acid sequence of a protein determines simultaneously folding, function, and degradation [62]. Thermodynamic considerations of stability and folding of protein domains have been extensively discussed [63]. After the isolation of the IBs from the disrupted cells, the protein is exposed to a chemical denaturant. Often strong denaturants such as urea or guanidine hydrochloride are employed [64], but some IBs can be dissolved under controlled alkaline conditions without affecting the backbone integrity of the target protein.

The refolding of the target protein is usually initiated by dissolution of the chemical denaturant. This can be achieved by simple dilution of the bulk or by dialysis. Unfortunately, during this dilution process, the protein may form aggregates, which further complicates the isolation and purification process. Therefore, it is essential to optimize the conditions during refolding to minimize the formation of aggregates. Aggregation continues potentially due to the exposure of the hydrophobic amino acid residues to the surfaces of the protein, and this may be the major reason for the failures in protein refolding [65].

When developing a refolding process, it is important to consider the amount of disulfide bridges included in the native structure of the protein, since the number of possible combinations increases with the number of cysteine residues present in the sequence. To promote correct disulfide bond formation, the addition of a redox system, for example, reduced and oxidized glutathione (GSH-GSSG) may be important. No generic methods for the refolding of the protein delivered from IBs exist, due to the unique entity of each target protein. Thus, finding the most suitable conditions for the refolding procedure may follow a random strategy [66,67].

Molecular chaperones have been employed in only a few cases using GroEL, the most applied chaperone system. Artificial chaperone systems such as cyclodextrins have also been developed [69,70].

To improve the refolding yield, different types of additives are used in the refolding buffer. Some examples are ammonium sulfate, polyols, sugars, and certain amino acids such as glycine, proline, and arginine [60,66,68,71–74]. There is an optimum concentration of the different additives, at which the maximum refolding yield is reached. Moreover, pH, conductivity, and protein concentration can have major effects on refolding efficiency.

Arginine is one of the most widely used refolding additives. This amino acid has a very basic side chain that possesses a similarity to guanidine. Arginine has been found to increase the refolding yields of humantype tissue plasminogen activator [75,76].

Experiments with an interferon mutant have shown that the arginine concentration applied in the buffer plays an important role in the refolding yield as well. By increasing the concentration of arginine up to 0.8 M, the yield of correctly folded protein was nearly doubled during renaturation over 72 h (Fig. 14.14).

In addition, experiments using increasing concentrations of Brij[®] (between 0.01% and 0.1%) were performed over 72 h. Higher yields of the correctly folded protein were obtained with 0.05% and 0.1% detergent added to the renaturation buffer containing arginine. The combination of 0.8 M arginine and 0.05% Brij in the renaturation buffer offered the best results concerning yield during 72 h renaturation time.

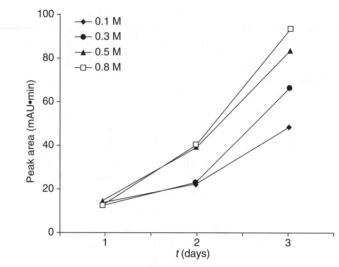

FIGURE 14.14   Effect of increasing concentration of arginine during renaturation on the yield of an interferon mutant. Correctly folded protein was determined by reversed-phase (RP) HPLC in comparison to a standard sample.

In summary, higher yields of the correctly refolded interferon mutant were obtained by using a combination of Brij and arginine in the renaturation buffer. These additives suppress the formation of aggregates, which could significantly reduce the protein yields.

14.3.5   Freeze-Thaw Steps at the Interface of DSP and Final Formulation

After finalization of the DSP, the API obtained in solution has to be stored until the final formulation and bulk filling steps are conducted. Process intermediate solutions during the purification process and the intermediate API bulk are usually stored refrigerated at $2-8°C$. This restricts the growth of certain microorganisms such as bacteria or fungi and contributes to the stability of the protein [77]. In most cases, concomitant storage of the liquid solution at reduced temperatures can only be applied over a short time as many proteins are prone to chemical and physical instability, which is frequently attributed to nonenzymatic reactions in purified solution [2]. Obviously, the applied purification process needs to ensure the absence of enzymes that may degrade the protein in solution during storage. Adequate stability especially after the purification process is an obligate prerequisite since product-related impurities such as aggregates cannot be removed any further. Moreover, the specification tolerance for the product material is narrow. Storage of the final formulated drug substance is usually conducted frozen or in cases of $2-8°C$ non-frozen. Owing to the absence of water, freeze-dried bulk may also be favored; however, drying techniques are currently not routinely applied for protein bulk in large scale. Freezing of the bulk solution requires far less energy and technological expenses than drying, for example, lyophilization or drying of large volumes up to several hundred liters. Therefore, large-scale freezing is commonly used for long-term storage of bulks in the pharmaceutical industry. By freezing the bulk to temperatures below the glass-transition temperature, a tremendous advantage for the manufacturer in terms of flexibility and availability of supplies over an enhanced product life cycle is gained.

Concomitantly, freezing and thawing of protein solutions are additional stress factors leading to stability issues including aggregation or precipitation. A major stress factor is the exposure of the protein to the ice surface [78,79] and the container surface [80] potentially leading to a perturbation of their native structure. Moreover, the phenomenon of protein cold denaturation and physicochemical changes of the solution during freezing and thawing steps is discussed to induce changes in protein structure. Cold denaturation may lead to aggregation as a consequence of unfolding due to weakened noncovalent electrostatic and hydrophobic interactions within the molecule at lower temperatures and has been described for some specific globular proteins and enzymes [81,82].

More frequently, protein aggregation or precipitation is caused by the physicochemical changes and phase transition. During the freezing process of a protein solution, the material usually supercools to a temperature up to $15°C$ below the freezing point before ice nucleates and crystallizes for the first time. After crystallization has begun, the temperature rises close to the freezing point and decreases slowly until the water has completely crystallized. During the freezing and crystallization process, solute molecules, for example, additives such as sucrose, salts, or macromolecules (as the protein), are preferably excluded from the ice crystals as they would cause defects in the ice crystals. This leads to an enriched concentration of solute molecules in the remaining unfrozen solution, a phenomenon which is called *cryoconcentration*.

In the presence of sodium chloride, eutectic formations can be observed, which may delay a complete freezing of the solution to temperatures of $-20°C$ and below. Solutes that crystallize easily from aqueous solution may crystallize simultaneously with water; however, most carbohydrates and proteins remain amorphous. At the end of the freezing process, these compounds are present in a matrix containing relatively large amounts of unfrozen water [83]. When freezing is completed, all components are embedded in a highly viscous glassy matrix and the prevailing temperature is below the characteristic temperature called *glass-transition temperature* (T'_g), above which the matrix is regarded as "rubbery." Below T'_g that may be passed at temperatures of -30 to $-40°C$, the product is transformed into a stable state phase where diffusive processes within the matrix are prevented due to restricted molecular mobility [84].

Additionally, physicochemical changes of the buffer can lead to significant pH changes. In particular, buffers containing sodium phosphate are affected by this phenomenon (Fig. 14.15). This pH shift during freezing can reduce protein stability and can lead to aggregation. By changing the buffer system to a buffer without significant pH shift, the protein stability can be increased and aggregation reduced (Fig. 14.16).

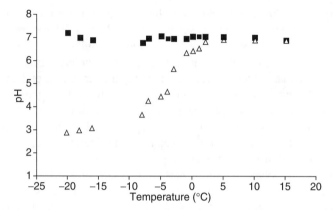

FIGURE 14.15 pH shift of sodium phosphate (△) and potassium phosphate (■) buffer solutions.

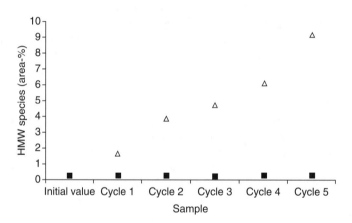

FIGURE 14.16 Increase of HMW species content (SE-HPLC) after several freeze-thaw cycles ($-20°C/+20°C$) of a monoclonal antibody (IgG) in sodium phosphate (△) and potassium phosphate (■) buffer solutions (pH 7.0 at $+20°C$).

To summarize, during the freezing process, the protein is potentially exposed to significant changes in pH, concentration, and ionic strength, and a stable state is not reached until passing the specific glass-transition temperature T_g'.

The period of time, during which proteins are subjected to adverse conditions, depends primarily on the volume-to-surface area ratio of the used containers. For the last few years, production scales and yields have increased considerably, resulting in large volumes of protein solutions, which have to be stored. For economic reasons, the protein solutions are preferably frozen in large vessels, offering only a small surface area in relation to their volume, and therefore leading to very long processing times for freezing and thawing. This bears an increased risk for aggregation or precipitation, as the protein is exposed to stress factors for a long time.

Two major starting points to avoid protein aggregation and precipitation during freezing and thawing have been described: first, the use of formulation buffers that do not show a pronounced pH or conductivity shift. Furthermore, the addition of stabilizing excipients, the so-called cryoprotectants, is recommended. If stability problems are detected in the course of freezing process scale-up, changes of the formulation cannot be considered any more since they are mostly associated with additional development activities leading to additional costs and, in the worst case, causing a delay in time to market. Freeze and thaw equipment needs to be applied, which is representative for large-scale systems considering among other things heat and mass transfer, time–temperature profiles, and the final ice-interfacial area [85].

14.3.6 Purification Process Scale-Up and Transfer to GMP Manufacturing

The risk of aggregate formation on purification process scale-up or process transfer to a GMP facility can be attributed to differences in the mode of operation, on the one hand, and differences between small- and large-scale equipment, on the other hand.

During process development and characterization, critical process parameters such as pH, conductivity, protein concentration, and temperature are identified with respect to the biochemical nature of the molecule. Therefore, while scaling up to manufacturing scale, it is unlikely that an unexpected quantity of differently sized aggregates will occur.

The appearance of large insoluble aggregates can be observed by flocculates, precipitate, or blockage of sterile filters. These effects may appear more pronounced at manufacturing scale since large volumes and long optical flow paths increase the detectability by sight. In contrast, the use of nontransparent material (stainless steel, opalescent bags, and tubing) may obscure the detection of this type of aggregates.

The impact of the mode of operation at large scale is pronounced if shear stress is generated. This may be the case for piping or tubing with a diameter that is not sufficient for the flux applied. A wide range of different tubing diameters along the flow path may also contribute to shear stress. This risk should be particularly considered in plants where manual connections are allowed.

Another source of stress which is related to operational conditions is the air–liquid interface. The protein can accumulate at a large hydrophobic air–water interface and expose hydrophobic amino acid residues to air; hence, the formation of aggregates can be initiated sometimes accompanied by denaturation [86,87]. Only a small expansion of the native state surface rather than a complete unfolding seems to be necessary to precede aggregation [88,89].

In general, the air–liquid interface is increased by turbulence in fluid transport. Common risk factors are excessive shaking and mixing. Additionally, vessel inlets may be placed far away from the bottom of the vessel or too close to a stirrer. If the flow rate is not adapted to the inner diameter of the inlet the protein solution will abruptly expand and mix with air on release from the inlet in addition to the shear stress in the tubing itself.

Mixing at an optimized speed or avoiding solutions dripping down several meters toward the bottom of a large container is an appropriate measure to address this issue.

Proper mixing is very important, particularly when adjusting the pH of a protein solution with acid or base or adding other solutions that are a priori known to induce aggregates or protein denaturation because of high local concentrations of the critical agent.

During refolding, for example, by pulse dilution, it was shown that either the soluble protein is achieved or the formation of insoluble aggregate is favored [90]. For this reason, careful control and evaluation of the mixing speed and the used container geometry is mandatory, as well as the velocity of the addition of solutions and the duration of the whole process.

Technical failure in a process plant can also contribute to an aggregation issue. A potential reason is the malfunction of a particular device besides the possibility of error in programming by the operator. Common examples are valves that are not properly opening or closing. This, in turn, may lead to enhanced shear stress or to inadequate contact and mixing of solutions, most importantly high salt additives or acids and bases. As there are numerous valves and connections in a process plant built for flexible use, it is essential to have skilled and experienced personnel to identify the source in such a case.

However, the mode of operation may even be specially designed to deal with precipitate and aggregates. One of the most prominent examples is the drain out of a container if the solution contains aggregates. As aggregates settle to the bottom, a subsequent filter is immediately clogged if the solution is taken straight from the bottom valve. Alternatively, there can be one or several side valves or even a flexible suction tube coming in from the top. It is particularly important when transferring a process from one plant to another to include the required mode of operation in the manufacturing instruction.

As indicated at the beginning of this section, differences in the equipment itself used at small and large scale can also affect aggregate formation. The main potential risk factors are described in the following.

Usually, a purification process is developed at laboratory scale and is then scaled up linearly to manufacturing scale. This means, for example, the linear flow rate and bed height are maintained in a chromatography step, whereas the column diameter is increased [91]. Thus, identical chromatography performance can be expected at both scales. The GMP facility may require process adaptations if equipment is lacking or if it differs significantly from the equipment used in process development. These process adaptations may increase the risk of aggregate formation.

Pumping procedures are critical with regard to aggregation at all scales. For biological molecules, it is recommended to employ those types of pumps and pump heads that cause the least stress for the protein, for example, membrane pumps. However, at manufacturing scale, mostly different types of pumps have to be used as in the small scale due to the required working range. For example, rotary lobe pumps are often applied at manufacturing scale, since membrane pumps are more difficult to clean and sanitize and suitable dimensions of the pump that would fit into the plant are sometimes not available. In contrast, membrane pumps are preferred at smaller scales since protein aggregation is often increased when rotary lobe pumps are applied.

Pumps are also critical in terms of the heat they introduce into the process solution. Especially the local heating of the solution that is inside the pump head may induce aggregates. Temperatures of up to 50°C have been measured with certain pumps, which is high for biological molecules. With regard to heat, the temperature control system itself should, of course, also be designed appropriately: the temperature of the surface that is actually exchanging the heat should be in a range that is compatible with the biological molecule.

Exposure to different surface types is another point to be considered when working at process scale: in DSP, stainless steel is usually exposed to chloride-containing solutions. This can lead to corrosion if steel surfaces are not maintained regularly or if steel quality is not adequate. Depending on the nature of the protein molecule, iron that is leached from a corroded steel surface may serve as a catalyst for protein oxidation and potentially may lead to subsequent aggregation. Moreover, abraded steel particles may serve as nuclei initiating aggregation, which has been reported for steel particles shed from a piston pump [47]. When discussing surfaces, the large surfaces in a process created by filtration membranes and chromatography gels should be taken into account. The effects are in general very well evaluated during process development. In addition, suppliers of these materials provide carefully selected hydrophilic surfaces of membranes and gel beads that show little interaction with biomolecules [51].

In spite of the factors described that may induce aggregation, experience shows that the observation of aggregates is, in most cases, not linked to a loss of protein yield. This means that only a small fraction of the total protein has contributed to those aggregates. Still, filter blocking may be a consequence of aggregation. In a production process under GMP, this as well as the mere observation of turbidity requires adequate attention. Immediately on observation, the filter area may be increased. Preferably the filter area should be chosen based on V_{max}/P_{max} experiments at small scale during process development. These experiments should consider manufacturing process conditions, if applicable even in previous process steps.

In summary, there are a few issues that need to be considered when scaling up a purification process or transferring it to a GMP facility. Generally, at large scale, the surface-to-volume ratio is more favorable, that is, lower, than that at small scale. Therefore, usually lower levels of aggregates are observed at large compared to small scale.

To minimize the risk of aggregate formation at manufacturing scale, a proper process development and characterization will employ scale-down models of the individual process steps that adequately reflect the manufacturing conditions. When developing the scale-down models, it is recommended to consider both equipment and the mode of operation applied at manufacturing scale. Scaling up exercises during process development and, in accordance with the QbD/PAT approach, the implementation of in-line or at-line analytics monitoring differently sized aggregates are suitable means to reduce the risk of increased aggregate levels in a GMP manufacturing campaign.

14.4   SUMMARY: STRATEGIES TO REDUCE AGGREGATES DURING DSP

One of the main focuses in the development of purification processes is the removal of product aggregates. Aggregates can be one of the most abundant impurity in the course of the purification process of mAbs after capturing the target molecule. Besides the routinely monitoring of soluble product aggregates by SE-HPLC, the analysis of higher oligomers and even subvisible and visible particles may be also considered in DSP development laboratories as well as in GMP manufacturing, since it is typically done with final formulated product. A considerable part of the development activities and decisions are driven by aggregate removal capacity. Whatever the root cause of aggregate formation and the source of aggregates may be, in DSP, many versatile and well-characterized tools are available for aggregate removal.

However, process steps dedicated to product quality polishing or viral clearance such as low pH treatment, buffer exchange, and concentration of the protein solution between process steps or final formulation, exposure to different surfaces and interfaces, as well as simple storage of process intermediates bear a risk of aggregate formation. The harsh conditions applied may affect product molecule integrity. This, in turn, may lead to product aggregation.

Finally, a well-developed purification process is designed to remove aggregates, while the risk of aggregate formation during the process is reduced to a minimum. Especially at the interface of DSP and final formulation this is essential, because product- and process-related impurities will not further be removed from the final product.

REFERENCES

1. Brange J. Physical stability of proteins. In: Frokjaer S, Hovgaard L, editors. Pharmaceutical formulation development of peptides and proteins. New York (NY): Academic Press; 2000. 89–112.

2. Manning MC, Patel K, Borchardt RT. Stability of protein pharmaceuticals. Pharm Res 1989;6:903–918.

3. Hejnaes K, Matthiesen F, Skriver L. Protein stability in downstream processing. In: Subramanian G, editor. Volume 2, Bioseparation and bioprocessing: a handbook. Weinheim: Wiley-VCH; 1998. pp. 31–65.

4. International Conference on Harmonization of Technical Requirements for Registration of Pharmaceuticals for Human Use, ICH specifications: Test procedures and acceptance criteria for biotechnological/biological product (Q6B), www.ich.org, 1999

5. Cromwell M, Hilario E, Jacobson F. Protein aggregation and bioprocessing. AAPS J 2006;8:572–579.

6. Rosenberg AS. Effects of protein aggregates: an immunologic perspective. AAPS J 2006;8:501–507.

7. Kerwin BA, Remmele RLJ. Protect from light: photodegradation and protein biologics. J Pharm Sci 2007;96:1468–1479.

8. Roy S, Mason BD, Schöneich CS, Carpenter JF, Boone TC, Kerwin BA. Light-induced aggregation of type I soluble tumor necrosis factor receptor. J Pharm Sci 2009;98:3182–3199.

9. Paborji M, Pochopin NL, Coppola WP, Bogardus JB. Chemical and physical stability of chimeric L6, a mouse-human monoclonal antibody. Pharm Res 1994;11:764–771.

10. Schellekens H, Casadevall N. Immunogenicity of recombinant human proteins: causes and consequences. J Neurol 2004;251:4–9.

11. Schellekens H. Immunogenicity of therapeutic proteins: clinical implications and future prospects. Clin Ther 2002;24:1720–1740.

12. Chi EY, Krishnan S, Kendrick BS, Chang BS, Carpenter JF, Randolph TW. Roles of conformational stability and colloidal stability in the aggregation of recombinant human granulocyte colony-stimulating factor. Protein Sci 2003;12:903–913.

13. Chi EY, Weickmann J, Carpenter JF, Manning MC, Randolph TW. Heterogeneous nucleation-controlled particulate formation of recombinant human platelet-activating factor acetylhydrolase in pharmaceutical formulation. J Pharm Sci 2005;94:256–274.

14. Dong A, Prestrelski SJ, Allison SD, Carpenter JF. Infrared spectroscopic studies of lyophilization- and temperature-induced protein aggregation. J Pharm Sci 1995;84:415–424.

15. Shukla AA, Hubbard B, Tressel T, Guhan S, Low D. Downstream processing of monoclonal antibodies-application of platform approaches. J Chromatogr B 2007;848:28–39.

16. Ansaldi D, Lester P. Separation of protein monomers from aggregates by use of ion-exchange chromatography. EP1500661 A1. 2005.

17. Falkenstein R, Kolb B, Sebald M. Method for the purification of antibodies. WO2006125599. 2006.

18. Gagnon P. IgG aggregate removal by charged-hydrophobic mixed mode chromatography. Curr Pharm Biotechnol 2009;10:434–439.

19. Guse AH, Milton AD, Schulze-Koops H, Müller B, Roth E, Simmer B, Wächter H, Weiss E, Emmrich F. Purification and analytical characterization of an anti-CD4 monoclonal antibody for human therapy. J Chromatogr A 1994;661:13–23.

20. Lu Y, Williamson B, Gillespie R. Recent advancement in application of hydrophobic interaction chromatography for aggregate removal in industrial purification process. Curr Pharm Biotechnol 2009;10:427–433.

21. Tiselius A, Hjertén S, Levin Ö. Protein chromatography on calcium phosphate columns. Arch Biochem Biophys 1956;65:132–155.

22. Gorbunoff MJ. The interaction of proteins with hydroxyapatite: I. Role of protein charge and structure. Anal Biochem 1984;136:425–432.

23. Gorbunoff MJ. The interaction of proteins with hydroxyapatite: II. Role of acidic and basic groups. Anal Biochem 1984;136:433–439.

24. Gorbunoff MJ, Timasheff SN. The interaction of proteins with hydroxyapatite: III. Mechanism. Anal Biochem 1984;136:440–445.

25. Gagnon P. Monoclonal antibody purification with hydroxyapatite. New Biotechnol 2009;25:287–293.

26. Davis RH, Leighton DT. Shear-induced transport of a particle layer along a porous wall. Chem Eng Sci 1987;42:275–281.

27. Romero CA, Davis RH. Global model of crossflow microfiltration based on hydrodynamic particle diffusion. J Membr Sci 1988;39:157–185.

28. Altena FW, Belfort G. Lateral migration of spherical particles in porous flow channels: application to membrane filtration. Chem Eng Sci 1984;39:343–355.

29. Belfort G, Davis RH, Zydney AL. The behavior of suspensions and macromolecular solutions in crossflow microfiltration. J Membr Sci 1994;96:1–58.

30. Chan R. Fouling mechanisms in the membrane filtration of single and binary protein solutions. Sydney: School of Chemical Engineering and Industrial Chemistry, The University of New South Wales; 2002. p. 290.

31. Cheryan M. Ultrafiltration and microfiltration handbook. Boca Raton (FL): CRC Press; 1998. p. 539.

32. Wang A, Lewus R, Rathore AS. Comparison of different options for harvest of a therapeutic protein product from high cell density yeast fermentation broth. Biotechnol Bioeng 2006;94:91–104.

33. Herb L, Raghunath B. Ultrafiltration process design and implementation. In: Shukla AA, Etzel MR, Gadam S. editors. Process scale bioseparation for the biopharmaceutical industry. Boca Raton (FL): CRC Press; 2007. pp. 297–332.

34. Dani B, Platz R, Tzannis ST. High concentration formulation feasibility of human immunoglubulin G for subcutaneous administration. J Pharm Sci 2007;96:1504–1517.

35. Rivas G, Fernandez JA, Minton AP. Direct observation of the self-association of dilute proteins in the presence of inert macromolecules at high concentration via tracer sedimentation equilibrium: theory, experiment, and biological significance. Biochemistry 1999;38:9379–9388.

36. Manning MC, Matsuura JE, Kendrick BS, Meyer JD, Dormish JJ, Vrkljan M, Ruth JR, Carpenter JF, Sheftert E. Approaches for increasing the solution stability of proteins. Biotechnol Bioeng 1995;48:506–512.

37. Wang W. Protein aggregation and its inhibition in biopharmaceutics. Int J Pharm 2005;289:1–30.

38. Carpenter JF, Kendrick BS, Chang BS, Manning MC, Randolph TW. Inhibition of stress-induced aggregation of protein therapeutics. Methods Enzymol 1999;309:236–255.

39. Chi EY, Krishnan S, Randolph TW, Carpenter JF. Physical stability of proteins in aqueous solution: mechanism and driving forces in non-native protein aggregation. Pharm Res 2003;20:1325–1336.

40. Ahrer K, Buchacher A, Iberer G, Jungbauer A. Effects of ultra-/diafiltration conditions on present aggregates in human immunoglobulin G preparations. J Membr Sci 2006;274:108–115.

41. Stoner MR, Fischer N, Nixon L, Buckel S, Benke M, Austin F, Randolph TW, Kendrick BS. Protein-solute interactions affect the outcome of ultrafiltration/diafiltration operations. J Pharm Sci 2004;93:2332–2342.

42. Tanford C. Physical chemistry of macromolecules. New York, London, Sydney: John Wiley & Sons; 1967. p. 710.

43. Donna FG. Theorie der membrangleichgewichte und membranpotentiale bei vorhandensein von nicht dialysierenden elektrolyten. Ztg Elektrochem 1911;17:572–581.

44. Nakatsuka S, Michaels AS. Transport and separation of proteins by ultrafiltration through sorptive and non-sorptive membranes. J Membr Sci 1992;69:189–211.

45. Li B, Flores J, Corvari V. A simple method for the detection of insoluble aggregates in protein formulations. J Pharm Sci 2007;96:1840–1843.

46. Shojaee N, Patton WF, Lim MJ, Shepro D. Pyrogallol red-molybdate: a reversible, metal chelate stain for detection of proteins immobilized on membrane supports. Electrophoresis 1996;17:687–693.

47. Tyagi AK, Randolph T, Dong A, Maloney KM, Hitscherich CJ, Carpenter JF. IgG particle formation during filling pump operation: a case study of heterogeneous nucleation on stainless steel nanoparticles. J Pharm Sci 2008;98:94–104.

48. Porter MC. Concentration polarization with membrane ultrafiltration. Ind Eng Chem Prod Res Dev 1972;11:234–248.

49. Pelton JT, McLean LR. Spectroscopic methods for analysis of protein secondary structure. Anal Biochem 2000;277:167–176.

50. Matheus S, Friess W, Mahler H-C. FTIR and nDSC as analytical tools for high-concentration protein formulations. Pharm Res 2006;23:1350–1363.

51. Maruyama T, Katoh S, Nakajima M, Nabetani H, Abbott TP, Shono A, Satoh K. FT-IR analysis of BSA fouled on ultrafiltration and microfiltration membranes. J Membr Sci 2001;192:201–207.

52. Maruyama T, Katoh S, Nakajima M, Nabetani H. Mechanism of bovine serum albumin aggregation during ultrafiltration. Biotechnol Bioeng 2001;75:233–238.

53. Rosenberg E, Hepbildikler S, Kuhne W, Winter G. Ultrafiltration concentration of monoclonal antibody intermediate solutions: development of an optimized method minimizing aggregation. J Membr Sci 2009;342:50–59.

54. Winter CM. Process for concentration of antibodies and antibody derivatives. 2006051347. 2006.

55. Bee JS, Chiu D, Sawicki S, Stevenson JL, Chatterjee K, Freund E, Carpenter JF, Randolph TW. Monoclonal antibody interactions with micro- and nanoparticles: adsorption, aggregation, and accelerated stress studies. J Pharm Sci 2009;98:3218–3238.

56. Brorson K, Krejci S, Lee K, Hamilton E, Stein K, Xu Y. Bracketed generic inactivation of rodent retroviruses by low pH treatment for monoclonal antibodies and recombinant proteins. Biotechnol Bioeng 2003;82:321–329.

57. Karlsson E, Ryden L, Brewer J. Ion-exchange chromatography. In: Janson J-C, Ryden L, editors. Protein purification: principles, high resolution methods, and applications. New York (NY): Wiley; 1998. pp. 145–205.

58. Hollaender A, Daniels F, Loofborrow JR, Pollister AW, Stadler LJ. Radiation biology. New York (NY): McGraw-Hill; 1955. p. 593.

59. Li Q, MacDonald S, Bienek C, Foster PR, MacLeod AJ. Design of a UV-C irradiation process for the inactivation of viruses in protein solutions. Biologicals 2005;33:101–110.

60. Fahnert B, Lilie H, Neubauer P. Inclusion bodies: formation and utilisation. Adv Biochem Eng/Biotechnol 2004;89:93–142.

61. Baneyx F. Recombinant protein expression in *Escherichia coli*. Curr Opin Biotechnol 1999;10:411–421.

62. Wetlaufer DB. Folding of protein fragments. Adv Protein Chem 1981;34:61–92.

63. Jaenicke R. Stability and folding of domain proteins. Prog Biophys Mol Biol 1999;71:155–241.

64. Summers CA, Flowers RA II. Protein renaturation by the liquid organic salt ethylammonium nitrate. Protein Sci 2000;9:2001–2008.

65. De Bernardez Clark E. Refolding of recombinant proteins. Curr Opin Biotechnol 1998;9:157–163.

66. Chow MKM, Amin AA, Fulton KF, Whisstock JC, Buckle AM, Bottomley SP. An analytical database of protein refolding methods. Protein Expr Purif 2006;46:166–171.

67. Hamada H, Shiraki K. L-Argininamide improves the refolding more effectively than l-arginine. J Biotechnol 2007;130:153–160.

68. Cabrita LD. Protein expression and refolding - a practical guide to getting the most out of inclusion bodies. Biotechnol Annu Rev 2004;10:31–50.

69. Liu Y, Zhao D, Ma R, Xiong Da, An Y, Shi L. Chaperone-like cyclodextrins assisted self-assembly of double hydrophilic block copolymers in aqueous medium. Polymer 2009;50:855–859.

70. Rozema D, Gellman SH. Artificial chaperones: protein refolding via sequential use of detergent and cyclodextrin. J Am Chem Soc 1995;117:2373–2374.

71. Kumar TK, Samuel D, Jayaraman G, Srimathi T, Yu C. The role of proline in the prevention of aggregation during protein folding in vitro. Biochem Mol Biol Int 1998;46:509–517.

72. Maeda Y, Yamada H, Ueda T, Imoto T. Effect of additives on the renaturation of reduced lysozyme in the presence of 4M urea. Protein Eng 1996;9:461–465.

73. Mishra R, Seckler R, Bhat R. Efficient refolding of aggregation prone citrate synthase by polyol osmolytes: How well are protein folding and stability aspects coupled? J Biol Chem 2005;280:15553–15560.

74. Ou W-B, Park Y-D, Zhou H-M. Effect of osmolytes as folding aids on creatine kinase refolding pathway. Int J Biochem Cell Biol 2002;34:136–147.

75. Rudolph R, Opitz U, Kohnert U, Fischer S. Preparation of a plasminogen activator expressed in procaryotic cells. EP361475 A1. 1990.

76. Rudolph R, Fischer S. Verfahren zur renaturierung von protein. DE3611817 A1. 1987.

77. Wang W. Instability, stabilization, and formulation of liquid protein pharmaceuticals. Int J Pharm 1999;185:129–188.

78. Chang BS, Kendrick BS, Carpenter JF. Surface-induced denaturation of proteins during freezing and its inhibition by surfactants. J Pharm Sci 1996;85:1325–1330.

79. Strambini GB, Gabellieri E. Proteins in frozen solutions: evidence of ice-induced partial unfolding. Biophys J 1996;70:971–976.

80. Kueltzo LA, Wang W, Randolph TW, Carpenter JF. Effects of solution conditions, processing parameters, and container materials on aggregation of a monoclonal antibody during freeze-thawing. J Pharm Sci 2008;97:1801–1812.

81. Privalov PL. Cold denaturation of proteins. Crit Rev Biochem Mol Biol 1990;25:281–305.

82. Jaenicke R, Heber U, Franks F, Chapman D, Griffin MCA, Hvidt A, Cowan DA. Protein structure and function at low temperatures. Philos Trans R Soc Lond 1990;326:535–553.

83. Pikal MJ. Mechanisms of protein stabilization during freeze-drying and storage: the relative importance of thermodynamic stabilization and glassy state relaxation dynamics. In: Rey L, May JC, editors. Freeze-drying/lyophilization of pharmaceutical and biological products. New York (NY): Marcel Dekker; 1999.

84. Duddu SP, Zhang G, Dal Monte PR. The relationship between protein aggregation and molecular mobility below the glass transition temperature of lyophilized formulations containing a monoclonal antibody. Pharm Res 1997;14:596–600.

85. Singh SK, Kolhe P, Wang W, Nema S. Large-scale freezing of biologics. Bioprocess Int 2009;7:34–42.

86. Sluzky V, Tamada J, Klibanov A, Langer R. Kinetics of insulin aggregation in aqueous solutions upon agitation in the presence of hydrophobic surfaces. Proc Natl Acad Sci U S A 1991;88:9377–9381.

87. Cleland JL, Powell MF, Shire SJ. The development of stable protein formulations: a close look at protein aggregation, deamidation, and oxidation. Crit Rev Ther Drug Carrier Syst 1993;10:307–377.

88. Fink AL. Compact intermediate states in protein folding. Annu Rev Biophys Biomol Struct 1995;24:495–522.

89. Kendrick BS, Carpenter JF, Cleland JL, Randolph TW. A transient expansion of the native state precedes aggregation of recombinant human interferon-gamma. PNAS 1998;95:14142–14146.

90. Jaenicke R. Folding and association versus misfolding and aggregation of proteins. Philos Trans R Soc Lond B 1995;348:97–105.

91. Aldington S, Bonnerjea J. Scale-up of monoclonal antibody purification processes. J Chromatogr B 2007;848:64–78.

15 Formulation Development and Its Relation to Protein Aggregation and Particles

MIRIAM PRINTZ and WOLFGANG FRIESS

Department of Pharmacy, Pharmaceutical Technology and
Biopharmaceutics, Ludwig-Maximilians-University Munich,
Munich, Germany

15.1 INTRODUCTION

Parenteral protein formulations not only have to be physiologically acceptable but must also maintain the stability of the protein molecules. A limited spectrum of formulation variables, including pH, ionic strength, the addition of surfactants, or a restricted number of other stabilizers are used to meet the demands of protein pharmaceuticals. One major concern in protein formulation is the formation of protein aggregates that may be inactive or potentially cause adverse effects and, therefore, have to be minimized. Aggregates may be formed during manufacturing, storage, or transportation.

Typically, an integrated approach to the analysis of protein aggregates and particles has to be accomplished during formulation development, considering various types of protein aggregates. Triggers and causes for aggregation and particle formation may be a variation in temperature, agitation stress such as stirring, pumping, and shaking as well as the exposure to different surfaces.

During protein formulation development, a bunch of analytical methods is required to analyze the entire size range and types of protein aggregates. Hence, the current European Medicines Agency (EMA) draft guideline suggests the use of orthogonal methods, which means the use of a combination or a variety of different analytical methods, each having its own characteristic measuring principle, for example, by size, quantification, structure, etc. [1] For quantification and/or size estimation, typically methods such as high performance liquid chromatography (HPLC); asymmetrical flow field-flow

Analysis of Aggregates and Particles in Protein Pharmaceuticals, First Edition.
Edited by Hanns-Christian Mahler, Wim Jiskoot.
© 2012 John Wiley & Sons, Inc., Published 2012 by John Wiley & Sons, Inc.

fractionation (AF4) applying various detectors, e.g., UV, fluorescence, and multiangle laser light scattering (MALLS)detector; analytical ultracentrifugation (AUC); and sodium dodecyl sulfate–polyacrylamide gel electrophoresis (SDS-PAGE) are used. In addition, static and dynamic light scattering (DLS), light obscuration, UV spectroscopy, and turbidity are commonly used analytical tools in formulation development. For characterization of protein aggregates and structural analysis of proteins, spectroscopic methods such as circular dichroism (CD), Fourier-transform infrared (FTIR) spectroscopy, second-derivative UV absorption spectroscopy, and fluorescence spectroscopy are applied.

An additional challenge during formulation development can arise from the availability of only small amounts of protein and limited time, so that not all analytical tools can be fully applied. Thus, accelerated stability studies of protein pharmaceuticals are implemented and extrapolation, as far as practicable, of the gained data is performed to identify the most suitable formulation. However, as aggregation kinetics do not typically follow Arrhenius' behavior, the extrapolation to predict aggregation and stability behavior at lower storage temperature over longer storage time remains challenging [2]. In the context of limited availability of material as well as for high throughput formulation screening approaches, it appears necessary to select analytical methods enabling miniaturization. Consequently, methods for aggregate analysis that can be adapted to well plate systems are of interest, which includes UV–vis and fluorescence spectroscopy, nephelometry, turbidity, DLS, SE-HPLC, and laboratory on a chip gel electrophoresis [3]. These setups allow the use of robotic systems, and the application of different stress methods can be combined with factorial design of experiment or also enable the evaluation of lyophilized formulations in microplates [4,5].

Other questions have to be raised in the context of freeze-thaw stability testing. Freeze-thaw stability testing is advised to be performed at genuine scale, but might have to be conducted with much smaller volumes as the availability of protein material is limited in early stages. Therefore, the obtained data might contingently not correlate to the freeze-thaw behavior and stability data at manufacturing scale [1]. Furthermore, agitation stress has to be simulated. By using mechanical stress testing devices such as horizontal or vertical shakers [6], stirred reactors [7], and pumps [8], accelerated mechanical stress situations are imitated. However, it remains difficult to predict the extent of mechanical stress that a protein is confronted with during manufacturing and transport [1]. All of this also has to be considered against the background of the differences in type and quality of surfaces of containers, stoppers, or tubings used in the various stages of product development and manufacturing. Another aspect in this context are environmental factors, which could change during development and manufacturing and, thereby, influence the quality of the product, such as temperature fluctuations, influence of light exposure, and a possible dilution effect in infusion liquids.

15.2   STABILITY OF LIQUID PROTEIN PHARMACEUTICALS DURING STATIC STORAGE

During formulation development of liquid protein pharmaceuticals, a main focus is the stability of the protein in solution (for dried products, see Section 15.6), especially under static conditions. The intended storage temperature is typically set between 2 and 8°C for liquid protein pharmaceuticals and dried proteins, whereas drug substance (bulk) is frequently stored frozen. In the case of accelerated temperature studies during formulation development, typically temperatures such as 25, 30, and 40°C are used for protein pharmaceuticals, in accordance to the conditions of the International Conference on Harmonization of Technical Requirements for Registration of Pharmaceuticals for Human Use (ICH) guidelines.

One can undisputably state that there is no single protein aggregation pathway but a variety of pathways resulting in different aggregation end states (see Chapter 1). As a consequence, the type of aggregates formed a protein molecule on quiescent storage can be different depending on the solution conditions. The stabilizing effects of cosolutes as described by Timasheff are attributed to the protein–solvent interaction and not directly to the protein–excipient interplay [9]. The molecules are preferentially excluded from the surface of the native protein [10] and lead to a thermodynamically unfavorable situation and an entropically unfavorable state. As denaturation would lead to an enhanced contact surface between protein and additive, which is thermodynamically even more disadvantageous, the native monomer structure is preferred, which is one major aspect of protein stability.

Owing to this complexity, a broad aggregate analysis approach is essential, covering a wide range of aggregate sizes and structures [1,6,11–13] and a limited application of, for example, only size-exclusion (SE) chromatography or visible inspection leaves many open questions. Although SE-HPLC is considered the working horse in protein formulation development, various challenges have been described using SE-HLPC. The single use of an SE-HPLC method could lead to artifacts due to dilution [14], adsorption of protein to the column [10], and the influence of high salt concentration in the mobile phase [15]. Every technique not only offers a bunch of benefits but also goes along with its restrictions. For instance, using SDS-PAGE, the detection of noncovalently linked aggregates is not possible, as they are split during sample preparation [16]. AF4 is currently orthogonally used to SE-HPLC, but here artifacts due to the measuring principle have also been described [15]. AUC might be disturbed by stabilizers such as sugars [18]. DLS is not capable to quantify aggregates and exogenous particles interfere [1]. At least a combination of small soluble aggregate analysis, for example, by SE-HPLC supplemented by orthogonal methods covering the several nanometers to micrometer range, for example, by turbidity testing or subvisible and visible particle analysis is necessary [19,20].

Recently, it was shown that freeze thaw, thermal, shaking, and stirring stresses in liquid formulations lead to different aggregates in quality, quantity, and morphology [6,12,21]. Although shaking and freeze-thaw stress led to pronounced formation of subvisible particles observed by light obscuration, the increase in soluble aggregates detectable by SE-HPLC was only slight [21]. However, aggregation on static storage at elevated temperature could not be substantiated by visual inspection, turbidity measurements, or light obscuration. Only SE-HPLC detected changes. Significant differences in physicochemical characteristics of aggregates induced after thermal and freeze-thaw stress were also reported by Hawe et al. Thermal stress led to an increased formation of dimers and soluble oligomers traceable by SE-HPLC and AF4. Evolved aggregates smaller than 30 nm after thermal stress were measured by DLS, as well as slightly elevated particle levels in the micrometer range by light obscuration. Aggregates created by heating were in part covalently linked as seen in SDS-PAGE and made up of conformationally perturbed monomers as observed in CD, ATR-FTIR, and extrinsic dye fluorescence. Thus, a clear picture of the aggregation characteristics could be derived. In contrast, freeze-thawing stress primarily induced particles in the micrometer range. These aggregates were noncovalently linked (SDS-PAGE) and composed of nativelike monomers (CD, ATR-FTIR, and extrinsic dye fluorescence spectroscopy) [12].

Regarding formulation properties, pH and ionic strength are considered to be the most important parameters for aggregation. However, for example, for the stability of FK506-binding protein, it could be shown that in the pH range of 5–9, the pH dependence of the unfolding free energy from residual charge–charge interactions in the unfolded state was negligible. The negligible contribution was attributed to the lack of sequentially neighboring charged residues around groups that are titrated in this pH range. Salt lowered both conformational and colloidal protein stability at low salt concentrations, but raised stability at high concentrations, which could be explained by two opposing types of protein–salt interactions: the Debye–Hückel type, modeling the response of the ions to protein charges, favors the unfolded state, while the Kirkwood type, accounting for the disadvantage of the ions moving toward the low dielectric protein cavity from the bulk solvent, disfavors the unfolded state [22]. The initial decrease in folding stability with increasing salt concentration could be attributed to a stronger effect of the Debye–Hückel type interaction over the Kirkwood type. As the concentration increases further, the relative strengths of the two types of interactions reversed and a net stabilization was obtained. In contrast, for hydrophobic cytokines, charge shielding with increasing salt concentrations leads to substantial aggregate formation [19]. Electrostatic repulsion has been shown to be responsible for the absence of aggregation of RNAse using low pH [23]. The influence of pH is consequently complex. At low and high pH, charges increase leading to repulsion and reduced conformational stability. Consequently, most proteins have maximal thermodynamic stability around the isoelectric point. However, if a protein is already unfolded, the aggregation of the denatured molecules could be enhanced if the electrostatic repulsion is reduced at a pH close to the isoelectric point.

15.3 MECHANICAL STRESS STABILITY DURING FORMULATION AND SHIPMENT

During processing and handling of proteins as well as during transport of protein solutions, the protein may be exposed to various kinds of mechanical or interfacial stresses. Such mechanical stress conditions are known to potentially induce protein aggregation. Aggregates formed by mechanical and interfacial stresses can appear in a variety of morphologies, requiring the analysis of the full spectrum of potential aggregates [6,7]. So far there are only few general guidelines regarding extent and accomplishment of mechanical stress to mimic the protein exposure to interfacial and agitational stress during processing, fill and finish, and shipment. The American Society for Testing and Materials (ASTM) addresses issues related to process control, design, and performance, as well as quality acceptance/assurance tests for the pharmaceutical manufacturing industry and published guidance regarding standard test methods for, say, vibration testing for shipping containers (D 999-01) or standard practice for performance testing of shipping containers and systems (D 4169-08). Beyond, the International Safe Transit Association (ISTA) provides test procedures (ISTA 1A 2001 packaged products 150 Ib (68 kg) or less) [24–26]. Typically, horizontal and vertical shakers, stirred reactors, rotation, vortexing, and pumps are used as mechanical stress methods during formulation or process development [6]. Mechanical stress studies on various proteins revealed that agitation methods such as shaking- and stirring-induced diverse species, sizes, and quantities of noncovalent aggregates. Shaking involves an enhanced interplay of protein with air–and glass–liquid interfaces, which leads to aggregation and an enhanced transportation of aggregated proteins into the solution [27]. In contrast, stirring may provoke shearing, interfacial effects between the protein and stirrer bar/glass bottom, cavitation, local thermal effects, and rapid transportation of either aggregated or adsorbed protein into solution [6]. Shear stress alone is not supposed to cause unfolding [27].

Surfactants such as polysorbates are commonly employed to stabilize the protein against aggregation through agitation, but their mechanism of protection is still under discussion. By adding surfactants, an adsorption competition between surfactant and protein to these interfaces is described. Protein is displaced from the interfaces and thereby protected from the surface-induced denaturation and aggregation [11]. Another theory describes the interaction between surfactant and exposed hydrophobic areas of the protein. The hydrophobic surfaces of the proteins are supposed to be covered by surfactants and aggregation of protein is therewith inhibited [11]. However, typically these interactions are very weak and the effect may actually favor unfolding due to preferential interaction of structures exposing more hydrophobic sites [28]. Another theory is in the potential ability of surfactants to act as chaperones and facilitate the refolding of partially unfolded proteins [29,30]. Surfactants are typically applied at concentrations slightly close to or above the critical micelle concentration to ensure surface coverage [31]. Most frequently used nonionic surfactants in protein pharmaceuticals are polysorbate 20 and 80 [6,30,32–34]. They appear to be less effective in stabilization of protein exposed to stirring stress [6].

In addition, negative effects of polysorbates on protein stability are mentioned in the literature. After long-term storage at elevated temperatures increased protein aggregation was observed [34]. Peroxide contamination of polysorbates might be a reason for oxidation of proteins [35–37]. The surfactant–protein ratio seemed to be essential for stabilizing effects, as at low polysorbate 80 concentration destabilization can occur [6,38–40].

Different stabilizing effects were mentioned by Matheus et al. working on the selection of the optimal buffer system at pH 6.0 for a 100 mg/mL IgG formulation (Figs. 15.1 and 15.2) [38]. Although protein in acetate buffer was characterized by a low level of larger aggregates and precipitates during horizontal shaking, the increase in degradation products in SE-HPLC and SDS-PAGE after exposure to accelerated temperature conditions was rather high. In citrate

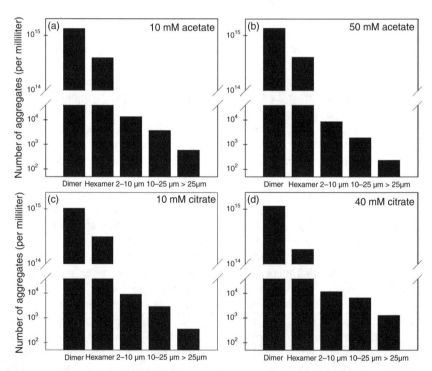

FIGURE 15.1 The number of soluble aggregates, as measured by SE-HPLC, and of subvisible particles (2–10, 10–25, and ≥25 µm), as measured by light obscuration of different 100 mg/mL IgG1 formulations in (a and b) 10/50 mM acetate, (c and d) 10/40 mM citrate, (e and f) 10/50 mM histidine, or (g and h) 10/50 mM phosphate buffer, at pH 6.0 after 168 h shaking [38].

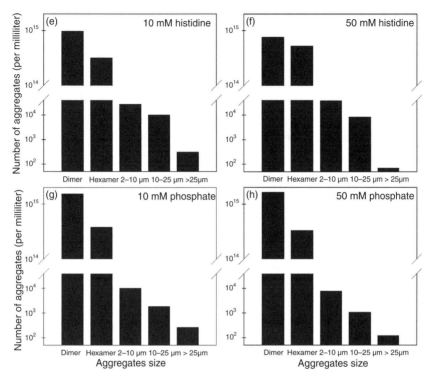

FIGURE 15.1 (*Continued*)

buffer, the monomer fraction could be kept at the highest level during exposure to accelerated temperatures, particularly at 40 mM citrate. However, the increased susceptibility of this formulation to the formation of large-sized aggregates on mechanical agitation as well as to deamidation was a major obstacle for citrate buffer. The histidine-buffered protein solutions behaved in a similar manner as that of the citrate-buffered ones, since protein aggregation during storage at 40°C/75% RH could be reduced, but in contrast, the unfavorable formation of medium to large size aggregates was extremely pronounced during shaking and even more at accelerated thermal storage conditions. Thus, the 10 mM phosphate buffer system was chosen as a "golden mean" to maintain protein stability in a liquid 100 mg/mL formulation, keeping both aggregate formation and protein degradation under stress conditions at a moderate rate. The effect appeared to be less related to ionic strength, but a stabilizing increased positive charge density in the presence of histidine was discussed. Furthermore, the reduced buffer strength was found sufficient to maintain the pH.

Slight differences in protein structure affect the aggregate formation behavior on mechanical stress as shown for IgG1 antibodies [40]. The amount of insoluble, visible particles of an IgG1 was increased after mechanical stress, but there was no increase in soluble aggregates observed by SE-HPLC or turbidity [40], whereas an increase in soluble aggregates was reported for a different

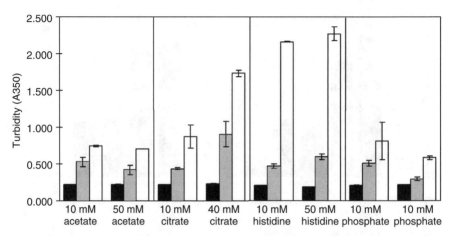

FIGURE 15.2   Turbidity of 100 mg/mL IgG1 pH 6.0 in different buffer formulations before (black columns) and after applying shaking stress for 24 h (gray columns) or 168 h (blank columns) [38].

IgG1 [6,33]. Another impact factor on protein aggregation characteristics in its final container is the fill volume and with that the headspace. It was shown that surfactant-free formulations without headspace in vial—similar to a prefilled syringe—remained essentially free of aggregates on shaking similar to a formulation with 0.005% polysorbate 20 with headspace [13]. The same formulation in vial with headspace with less polysorbate showed substantial formation of nativelike aggregates detectable by SE-HPLC, turbidity, light obscuration, and visual inspection. During stirring, less polysorbate 20 was necessary to inhibit the formation of large particles, whereas higher amounts of surfactant were required to suppress the creation of smaller particles [13].

15.4   STABILITY DURING FREEZE THAW

Protein solutions, both as bulk substance and as final product, may undergo freezing or freeze-thawing processes either during manufacturing or later shipment and/or storage either intended (as part of the process) or accidentally. During freezing, several changes occur to the protein microenvironment. As ice crystals evolve, the concentration of both protein and excipients increases, which can come along with a drastic decrease in pH at the eutectic point, depending on chosen buffer, bulk volume, and freezing rates [41–43]. If the excipients, which are concentrated to high concentrations while freezing, show a preferential binding to the protein surface, the protein may be destabilized and denatured during freezing. Moreover, the cooling and warming rates show an impact on the loss of protein activity during freezing and thawing as well. An inverse correlation between cooling rate and loss of protein activity is mentioned in several articles

[42,44,45]. Various studies have shown that freeze-thaw stress induces the formation of small quantities of nativelike insoluble aggregates [12,46–49]. Hawe et al. showed that visible aggregates formed on freeze thaw in an antibody solution but only about 0.15% of the total protein content became aggregated. CD and extrinsic fluorescent dye analysis of the whole samples and FTIR of the precipitates confirmed that the native structure of the IgG was retained to a high degree [12]. It has been found that excipients have similar positive or negative effects on protein stability both in solution and during freeze thawing due to the postulated same mechanism of preferential exclusion [50]. Bhatnagar studied the individual contribution of ice formation and freeze concentration on the stability of a sucrose- and citrate-containing LDH solution during freezing and could identify ice formation itself as the critical destabilizing factor [51]. In addition to optimized pH, ionic strength, and cosolute supplementation, cryoprotectants can be employed to protect proteins against denaturation on freeze thaw such as sugars, polyols, amino acids, polymers, and diverse other substances (Section 15.6).

15.5 SPECIAL CHALLENGES IN HIGH CONCENTRATION PROTEIN FORMULATIONS

The use of protein formulations for subcutaneous delivery has attracted substantial attention as it is more convenient and facilitates home administration. As a consequence, for example, for some antibodies, high protein concentration in subcutaneous formulations containing 100 mg/mL and more might be desired because of limitation of the volume for subcutaneous administration. Challenging aspects of highly concentrated protein formulations are, on the one hand, higher viscosity, which can make the formulation difficult to manufacture or administer. On the other hand, concentration-dependent reversible self-association, also considered as "nativelike aggregation," resulting in opalescent solution or precipitation occurs [16,52,53]. Reversible self-association can be described as intermolecular interaction of native protein molecules and precipitated protein associates can be redissolved and yield native protein molecules again. Solubility of a protein as the thermodynamic activity at the equilibrium of a saturated solution is difficult to measure and indirect analysis methods may be required [54]. Tangential flow filtration (TFF) is the industry standard for buffer exchange and concentrating proteins. The viscosity of high concentration products should be controlled, since viscous protein solutions can significantly increase the process time and might lead to higher back pressure during TFF. Some of these viscosity-related problems may be manageable by improving equipment, design, operation, and formulation parameters [16,53]. Depending on the protein's propensity to aggregate or precipitate, this could lead to decreased flux and eventually membrane clogging [54,55–57]. Rosenberg et al. presented an optimized method for ultrafiltration, with adapted transmembrane pressure and cross-flow conditions, resulting in minimized aggregate formation for three monoclonal antibodies [55]. The formation of aggregates was monitored by turbidity, SE-HPLC, light obscuration, DLS and a microscopic method, and the aggregate structure analyzed by FTIR. The analytics revealed that mostly large insoluble and structurally perturbed aggregates form during the ultrafiltration/concentration process. The optimized method did not significantly reduce the high molecular-weight species, as detected by SE-HPLC, but substantially reduced large aggregate formation as studied by turbidity and DLS.

Measuring the second virial coefficient (B22) could be relevant for the prediction of protein aggregation as well as viscosity. Until now, there is only rare information on the correlation between B22 and protein aggregation [58–60]. A study on lysozyme could show a correlation of B22 and physical protein stability as analyzed by turbidity [60]. Comparing B22 of an IgG1 with stability over 12 weeks at 40°C demonstrated that histidine 5 mM was the most promising buffer candidate according to B22 and showed a slightly better physical stability as assessed by turbidity and SE-HPLC compared to the other tested formulations. The effect of buffer species on the stability of interferon-tau (IFN-tau) was compared to B22 determined by self-interaction chromatography [58]. At pH 7 and 20 mM buffer systems, IFN-tau formulated at 1 mg/mL and thermally stressed formed aggregates in the 20–40 nm range in phosphate and Tris buffer, but not in histidine buffer. In SE-HPLC, the aggregate formation rate was the highest in phosphate buffer, whereas both Tris and histidine resulted in less aggregate formation. Only slight differences in B22 were measured, suggesting that modulation of protein–protein interactions is probably a minor component of the stabilization mechanism for IFN-tau, at least with respect to thermally induced aggregation [58].

Protein self-association is an important factor to consider in high concentration protein formulations [54]. Most aggregation reactions are reported to be of second or higher order and would be enormously accelerated in high concentration protein formulations [1,2,6,8,61]. On the basis of the mechanism of excluded volume, an increased volume fraction is occupied by the protein molecules themselves at higher protein concentrations. The related decrease in the effective volume available and, in turn, the higher apparent protein concentration push the reaction equilibrium of protein self-association toward the associated state [54]. In contrast, the reaction rate of macromolecular association can be limited either by the conversion of the activated complex to a fully formed dimer or by the diffusion-controlled formation of the activated complex. Owing to the larger and/or more asymmetric form of the denatured state, the equilibrium of the protein unfolding reaction is driven toward the compact native conformation by the volume exclusion as a consequence of increasing protein concentrations [62]. Consequently, crowding would increase the reaction rate of self-association, whereas, if the system is diffusion limited, a diminished reaction rate results, owing to the fact that crowding considerably lowers the diffusional mobility of macromolecules (Fig. 15.3) [62,63]. Therefore, an increase in protein concentration could actually stabilize the protein against the formation of insoluble aggregates [64,65] or with respect to agitation-induced aggregation [34,66]. Thus, the relationship between protein concentration and aggregation tendency has to be evaluated on

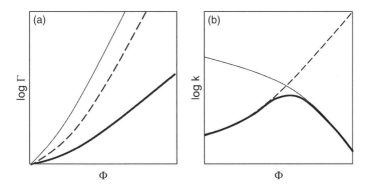

FIGURE 15.3   Effect of the fractional volume occupancy Φ on the nonideality factor Γ (a) for various degrees of association ($n = 2$ solid line; $n = 3$ dashed line; and $n = 4$ lighter line) and on the reaction rate constant k (solid line) (b), k being transition state limited at low volume occupancy (dashed line) and diffusion limited at high volume occupancy (lighter line) [38].

a case-to-case basis and formulation development at the concentration of interest is essential.

Another challenge in formulation development of high concentration protein pharmaceuticals is that dilution for analysis may influence the concentration-dependent aggregation and might induce artifacts [68]. Therefore, protein pharmaceuticals should be analyzed at their original concentration wherever possible, and one should look for alternative analytical tools that enable to measure at high concentration [16,54,68].

Matheus et al. studied the influence of protein concentration (2, 10, 50, and 100 mg/mL) and formulation buffer (PBS pH 7.2, citrate pH 5.5) on antibody aggregation on shaking [69]. Although an almost unchanged monomer fraction of more than 99% was observed in SE-HPLC, opalescence was altered depending on protein concentration and formulation buffer. Subvisible protein aggregates quantified by light obscuration analysis did not depend on protein concentration at $t = 0$, whereas after shaking stress, the number of particles >10 and >25 µm were influenced by protein concentration and formulation buffer. For citrate buffer formulations, the highest number of subvisible particles was measured in the highest concentration (100 mg), whereas for PBS buffer formulations, the number of subvisible particles >25 µm decreased with increasing protein concentration possibly attributed to an increase in large precipitates at the expense of smaller sized subvisible and light scattering particles. An inverse concentration and aggregation relationship seen at lower concentrations might be explained by a reduced ratio of the air/water interface to protein with increasing concentration [34].

The formation of native protein aggregates could also be important with respect to nonnative protein aggregation. The aggregates may serve as nuclei, undergo conformational changes, and subsequently grow rapidly to form insoluble precipitates [59,61,70]. Irreversible noncovalent aggregates can be detected, qualified, and quantified by SE-HPLC. However, the nativelike aggregates are often overlooked and poorly analyzed [16]. Indeed, the analytical tools for reversible aggregates are not satisfying. Static light scattering and DLS as well as AUC appear to be more beneficial to monitor the phenomenon of self-association, as the concentration and the primary microenvironment can be maintained during measurement. A new method to rapidly detect protein self-association simultaneously with the determination of the second viral coefficient, a measure of solution nonideality, using SE-HPLC was described by Bajaj et al. [71] for β-lactoglobulin. The simultaneous measurement of concentration and scattered light intensity by using a novel flow cell could be a useful tool for high throughput characterization of protein association during early stages of protein formulation.

15.6 SPECIAL CHALLENGES IN DRIED PROTEIN PHARMACEUTICALS

Freeze drying is considered the method of choice to stabilize proteins that show substantial stability problems in liquid. About 50% of currently marketed protein drugs are provided in lyophilized form [72]. However, lyophilization may induce protein damage due to freezing and drying stress. The effect of freezing and the use of cryoprotectants have been described earlier. In addition, as water is removed, alternative partners for hydrogen-bond formation are considered to be necessary, which is termed *water replacement* [73]. This is provided by lyoprotectants, mostly sugars, polyols, and amino acids. For lyoprotection, the sugar stabilizers need to be in a proper ratio to the protein to satisfy water binding sites, which in practice means that a mass ratio of about 1:1 is usually needed [72,74,75].

Protein aggregation cannot be assessed directly in the lyophilized formulation, but can be measured after reconstitution with the methods used for the analysis of protein solutions. Analytics performed on the lyophilized materials typically focus on material properties such as glass-transition temperature, modification, or residual moisture. By FTIR, the interactions of dried proteins and carbohydrates were observed. It could be shown that hydrogen binding occurs between proteins and carbohydrates, and this water replacement is necessary to keep the proteins in the native state during drying [76]. Additionally, these lyoprotectants stabilize the protein by immobilizing them in a glassy matrix, which strongly reduces their mobility. Glass formation alone is insufficient as seen, for example, for protein samples freeze dried with dextran, which are completely amorphous and form glasses with high glass-transition temperature but show loss of native protein structure [77]. Furthermore, there is evidence by FTIR measurements that only proteins that kept their native state in the dried form were able to regain most of their biological activity after reconstitution. A loss of native structure during drying seems to be, in several cases, irreversible and leads, therefore, to denaturation and aggregation after reconstitution [78,79] or to poor storage stability.

Protein aggregation involves collisions between protein molecules and is considered to be closely related to molecular mobility [80]. Analysis of the difference between storage temperature and glass-transition temperature, as a rough measure for the global mobility, indicated a good correlation between mobility and monomer loss analyzed by SE-HPLC [81,82]. The solid-state chemistry and protein stability was thoroughly elaborated by Pikal in a set of papers studying the structural relaxation of lyophilisates and both the chemical and physical stability of human growth hormone (hGH) [83–86]. The unfolding of hGH in the dried state could be well modeled by a three-state kinetic model, which is a two-state unfolding model followed by aggregation. Using data for denaturation temperature, heat of denaturation, and heat capacity of denaturation, free energy versus temperature curves were calculated. Even formulations with saccharides added are thermodynamically unstable near ambient temperature, but significant denaturation in the solid state is prevented by low mobility. Directly comparing aggregation (SE-HPLC and DLS) of a hydrophobic cytokine in liquid solution in a prefilled syringe versus lyophilized in a vial in a mannitol–sucrose combination during static storage indicated that for this aggregation-prone protein the overall aggregation profile was similar in both dosage forms [19]. Another general point to consider is that the protein also affects its environment, for example, by concentration-dependent change in excipients crystallinity and polymorphism [87]. A detailed study on the effect of lyophilisate collapse on antibody stability indicated that protein stability on storage is still warranted, if not even improved compared to noncollapsed samples. SE-HPLC and AF4 indicated no difference immediately after freeze drying, but more subvisible and visible particles had formed in partially collapsed lyophilisates. A trend to enhanced stability in the collapsed systems could be shown with a less pronounced storage-related increase in soluble aggregates as well as in particle numbers, turbidity values, DLS Z-average diameter, and polydispersity index [88].

15.7 SUMMARY

Typically, available protein and time are limited during formulation development. However, to thoroughly characterize and understand protein aggregation as a main route of protein instability, different stress tests using a combination of analytical methods are mandatory. Numerous formulation factors such as the selection of pH or the addition of surfactants have to be balanced and an optimum has to be found. An additional challenge derives from the fact that aggregation typically does not follow Arrhenius behavior and extrapolation of static storage stability data to predict aggregation is associated with uncertainties. This applies even more so to mechanical stress study data. Various types of aggregates may be induced by different stress conditions and setups. Frequently, SE-HPLC as the analytical workhorse in small aggregate analysis does not allow adequate conclusions when used as a single method. Especially freeze thaw and mechanical stress frequently induce no changes in SE-HPLC monomer content but larger aggregates form that can only be detected applying another set of analytical methods. Supplemented by characterization of the aggregate structure, such a comprehensive picture allows a better understanding of the underlying mechanism of aggregate formation and a rational formulation approach.

REFERENCES

1. Mahler HC, Friess W, Grauschopf U, Kiese S. Protein aggregation: pathways, induction factors and analysis. J Pharm Sci 2009;98(9):2909–2934.

2. Cleland JL, Powell MF, Shire SJ. The development of stable protein formulations: a close look at protein aggregation, deamidation, and oxidation. Crit Rev Ther Drug Carrier Syst 1993;10(4):307–377.

3. Capelle MAH, Gurny R, Arvinte T. High throughput screening of protein formulation stability: practical considerations. Eur J Pharm Biopharm 2007;65(2):131–148.

4. Hui Z, Graf O, Milovic N, Luan X, Bluemel M, Smolny M, Forrer K. Formulation development of antibodies using robotic system and high-throughput laboratory (HTL). WO 2008/157278 A1. 2008.

5. Grant Y, Matejtschuk P, Dalby PA. Rapid optimization of protein freeze-drying formulations using ultra scale-down and factorial design of experiment in microplates. Biotechnol Bioeng 2009;104(5):957–964.

6. Kiese S, Papppenberger A, Friess W, Mahler HC. Shaken, not stirred: mechanical stress testing of an IgG1 antibody. J Pharm Sci 2008;97(10):4347–4366.

7. Colombie S, Gaunand A, Lindet B. Lysozyme inactivation under mechanical stirring: effect of physical and molecular interfaces. Enzyme Microb Technol 2001;28(9–10):820–826.

8. Cromwell ME, Hilario E, Jacobson F. Protein aggregation and bioprocessing. AAPS J 2006;8(3):E572–E579.

9. Timasheff SN. The control of protein stability and association by weak interactions with water: how do solvents affect these processes. Annu Rev Biophys Biomol Struct 1993;22:67–97.

10. Arakawa T, Prestrelski SJ, Kenney WC, Carpenter JF. Factors affecting short-term and long-term stabilities of proteins. Adv Drug Deliv Rev 2001;46(1–3):307–326.

11. Mahler HC, Muller R, Friess W, DeLille A, Matheus S. Induction and analysis of aggregates in a liquid IgG1-antibody formulation. Eur J Pharm Biopharm 2005;59(3):407–417.

12. Hawe A, Kasper JC, Friess W, Jiskoot W. Structural properties of monoclonal antibody aggregates induced by freeze-thawing and thermal stress. Eur J Pharm Sci 2009;38(2):79–87.

13. Friess W, Kiese S, Mahler HC, Pappenberger A. Method for stabilizing a protein. US patent Application 2008275220. 2008. (Germany).

14. Moore JMR, Patapoff T, Cromwell MEM. Kinetics and thermodynamics of dimer formation and dissociation for a recombinant humanized monoclonal antibody to vascular endothelial growth factor. Biochemistry 1999;38(42):13960–13967.

15. Liu J, Andya J, Shire S. A critical review of analytical ultracentrifugation and field flow fractionation methods for measuring protein aggregation. AAPS J 2006;08(03):E580–E589.

16. Shire SJ, Shahrokh Z, Liu J. Challenges in the development of high protein concentration formulations. J Pharm Sci 2004;93(6):1390–1402.

17. Wang W, Singh S, Zeng DL, King K, Nema S. Antibody structure, instability, and formulation. J Pharm Sci 2006;96(1):1–26.

18. Gabrielson JP, Arthur KK, Kendrick BS, Randolph TW, Stoner MR. Common excipients impair detection of protein aggregates during sedimentation velocity analytical ultracentrifugation. J Pharm Sci 2009;98(1):50–62.

19. Hawe A, Friess W. Development of HSA-free formulations for a hydrophobic cytokine with improved stability. Eur J Pharm Biopharm 2008;68(2):169–182.

20. Sek D, Warne NW, Ho K, Luisi DL, Kantor A. Use of sucrose to suppress mannitol-induced protein aggregation. PCT/US2008/052115. 2008.

21. Printz M, Friess W. Simultaneous detection of changes in protein tertiary structure and aggregation by SEC with post column addition of Bis-ANS. Poster AAPS National Biotechnology Conference Seattle, USA. 2009.

22. Spencer DS, Ke X, Logan TM, Zhou HX. Effects of pH, salt, and macromolecular crowding on the stability of FK506-binding protein: an integrated experimental and theoretical study. J Mol Biol 2005;351(1):219–232.

23. Tsai AM, van Zanten JA, Betenbaugh MJ. II Electrostatic effect in the aggregation of heat denatured RNase A and implications for protein additive design. Biotechnol Bioeng 2000;59(3):281–285.

24. American Society for Testing and Materials (ASTM) Designation: D 999—01. Standard Test Methods for Vibration Testing of Shipping Containers. 2001

25. American Society for Testing and Materials (ASTM) Designation: D 4169—08. Standard Practice for Performance Testing of Shipping Containers and Systems. 2008.

26. International Safe Transit Association(ISTA); ISTA 1 Series: Non-Simulation Integrity Performance Test; Procedure 1A: Packaged-Products weighing 150lb (68kg) or Less, 2001.

27. Maa YF, Hsu CC. Protein denaturation by combined effect of shear and air-liquid interface. Biotechnol Bioeng 1997;54(6):503–512.

28. Garidel P, Hoffmann C, Blume A. A thermodynamic analysis of the binding interaction between polysorbate 20 and 80 with human serum albumins and immunoglobulins: a contribution to understand colloidal protein stabilisation. Biophys Chem 2009;143(1–2):70–78.

29. Bam NB, Cleland JL, Yang J, Manning MC, Carpenter JF, Kelley RF, Randolph TW. Tween protects recombinant human growth hormone against agitation-induced damage via hydrophobic interactions. J Pharm Sci 1998;87(12):1554–1559.

30. Bam NB, Randolph TW, Cleland JL. Stability of protein formulations: investigation of surfactant effects by a novel EPR spectroscopic technique. Pharm Res 1995;12(1):2–11.

31. Katakam M, Bell LN. Effect of surfactants on the physical stability of recombinant human growth hormone. J Pharm Sci 1995;84(6):713–716.

32. Charman SA, Mason KL, Charman WN. Techniques for assessing the effects of pharmaceutical excipients on the aggregation of porcine growth hormone. Pharm Res 1993;10(7):954–962.

33. Kreilgaard L, Frokjaer S, Flink JM, Randolph TW, Carpenter JF. Effects of additives on the stability of recombinant human factor XIII during freeze-drying and storage in the dried solid. Arch Biochem Biophys 1998;360(1):121–134.

34. Treuheit MJ, Kosky AA, Brems DN. Inverse relationship of protein concentration and aggregation. Pharm Res 2002;19(4):511–516.

35. Ha E, Wang W, Wang YJ. Peroxide formation in polysorbate 80 and protein stability. J Pharm Sci 2002;91(10):2252–2264.

36. Donbrow M, Azaz E, Pillersdorf A. Autoxidation of polysorbates. J Pharm Sci 1978;67(12):1676–1681.

37. Kerwin BA. Polysorbates 20 and 80 used in the formulation of protein biotherapeutics: structure and degradation pathways. J Pharm Sci 2008;97(8):2924–2935.

38. Matheus S. Preparation of high concentration cetuximab formulations using ultrafiltration and precipitation techniques [PhD thesis]. Germany: University of Munich; 2006. 140–179.

39. Ziegler K, Schwartz D, Frieß W. Agitation-induced aggregation behavior of an IgG antibody: effect of protein and surfactant concentration. Abstract 6th World Meeting on Pharmaceutics, Biopharmaceutics and Pharmaceutical Technology Barcelona, Spain;2008.

40. Mahler H-C, Senner F, Maeder K, Mueller R. Surface activity of a monoclonal antibody. J Pharm Sci 2009;98(12):4525–4533.

41. Chilson OP, Costello LA, Kaplan NO. Effects of freezing on enzymes. Fed Proc 1965;24:55–65.

42. van den Berg L, Rose D. Effect of freezing on the pH and composition of sodium and potassium phosphate solutions; the reciprocal system KH2PO4-Na2-HPO4-H2O. Arch Biochem Biophys 1959;81(2):319–329.

43. Gómez G, Pikal MJ, Rodríguez-Hornedo N. Effect if initial buffer composition on pH changes during far-from equilibrium freezing of sodium phosphate buffer solutions. Pharm Res 2001;18:90–97.

44. Whittam JH, Rosano HL. Effects of the freeze-thaw process on alpha amylase. Cryobiology 1973;10(3):240–243.

45. Fishbein WN, Winkert JW. Parameters of biological freezing damage in simple solutions: catalase. I. The characteristic pattern of intracellular freezing damage exhibited in a membraneless system. Cryobiology 1977;14(4):389–398.

46. Printz M, Friess W. SEC with UV and fluorescence detection by BisANS and the influence of PS 20. Poster Protein Stability Conference, Breckenridge, USA; 2009.

47. Kiese S. Protein aggregation - Induction, analytical methods and inhibition in biopharmaceutical formulations. [PhD thesis]. University of Munich, Germany; 2009. 227–250.

48. Chang BS, Kendrick BS, Carpenter JF. Surface-induced denaturation of proteins during freezing and its inhibition by surfactants. J Pharm Sci 1996;85:1325–1361.

49. Natalello A, Santarella R, Doglia SM, de Marco A. Physical and chemical perturbations induce the formation of protein aggregates with different structural features. Protein Expr Purif 2008;58:356–361.

50. Carpenter JF, Crowe JH. The mechanism of cryoprotection of proteins by solutes. Cryobiology 1988;25(3):244–255.

51. Bhatnagar BS, Pikal MJ, Bogner RH. Study of the individual contributions of ice formation and freeze concentration on isothermal stability of lactate dehydrogenase during freezing. J Pharm Sci 2008;97:798–814.

52. Minton AP. Influence of macromolecular crowding upon the stability and state of association of proteins: predictions and observations. J Pharm Sci 2005;94(8):1668–1675.

53. Wilf J, Minton AP. Evidence for protein self-association induced by excluded volume. Myoglobin in the presence of globular proteins. Biochim Biophys Acta 1981;670(3):316–322.

54. Friess W, Mahler H-C, Jörg S. Highly concentrated protein formulations. In: Mahler HC, Luessen H, Borchard G, editors. Protein pharmaceuticals - formulation, analytics and delivery. Aulendorf, Germany: Editio Cantor Verlag; 2009. 192–220.

55. Rosenberg E, Hepbildikler S, Kuhne W, Winter G. Ultrafiltration concentration of monoclonal antibody solutions: development of an optimized method minimizing aggregation. J Membr Sci 2009;342(1–2):50–59.

56. Thomas CR, Nienow AW, Dunnill P. Action of shear on enzymes: studies with alcohol dehydrogenase. Biotechnol Bioeng 1979;21(12):2263–2278.

57. Watterson JG, Schaub MC, Waser G. Shear-induced protein-protein interaction at the air-water interface. Biochim Biophys Acta 1974;356(2):133–143.

58. Katayama DS, Nayar R, Chou DK, Valente JJ, Cooper J, Henry CS, Vander Velde DG, Villarete L, Liu CP, Manning MC. Effect of buffer species on the thermally induced aggregation of interferon-tau. J Pharm Sci 2006;95(6):1212–1226.

59. Chi EY, Krishnan S, Randolph TW, Carpenter JF. Physical stability of proteins in aqueous solution: mechanism and driving forces in nonnative protein aggregation. Pharm Res 2003;20(9):1325–1336.

60. Le Brun V, Friess W, Schultz-Fademrecht T, Muehlau S, Garidel P. Lysozyme-lysozyme self-interactions as assessed by the osmotic second virial coefficient: impact for physical protein stabilization. Biotechnol J 2009;4(9):1305–1319.

61. Wang W. Protein aggregation and its inhibition in biopharmaceutics. Int J Pharm 2005;289:1–30.

62. Hall D, Minton AP. Macromolecular crowding: qualitative and semiquantitative successes, quantitative challenges. Biochim Biophys Acta 2003;1649:127–139.

63. Zimmerman SB, Minton AP. Macromolecular crowding: biochemical, biophysical, and physiological consequences. Annu Rev Biophys Biomol Struct 1993;22:27–65.

64. Dathe M, Gast K, Zirwer D, Welfle H, Mehlis B. Insulin aggregation in solution. Int J Pept Protein Res 1990;36:344–349.

65. Kendrick BS, Li T, Chang BS. Physical stabilization of proteins in aqueous solution. In: Carpenter JF, Manning MC, (editors. Rational design of stable protein formulations: theory and practice. New York: Kluwer Academic/Plenum Publishers; 2002. 61–84.

66. Kanai S, Liu J, Patapoff TW, Shire SJ. Reversible self-association of a concentrated monoclonal antibody solution mediated by Fab-Fab interaction that impacts solution viscosity. J Pharm Sci 2008;97(10):4219–4227.

67. Shire SJ, Liu J, Friess W, Jörg S, Mahler H-C. Considerations of high concentration antibody formulations. Jameel F, Hershenson S, editors. Formulation and process development strategies for manufacturing of a biopharmaceutical. New York, USA: John Wiley & Sons; 2010. 349–381.

68. Harris RJ, Shire SJ, Winter C. Commercial manufacturing scale formulation and analytical characterization of therapeutic recombinant antibodies. Drug Dev Res 2004;61(3):137–154.

69. Matheus S, Friess W, Mahler HC. Liquid high concentration IgG1-antibody formulations. Poster AAPS National Biotechnology Conference, San Francisco, USA; 2005.

70. Brange J Physical stability of proteins. In: Frokjaer S, Hovgaard L, editors. Pharmaceutical formulation development of peptides and proteins. London: Taylor and Francis; 2000. 89–112.

71. Bajaj H, Sharma VK, Kalonia DS. A high-throughput method for detection of protein self-association and second virial coefficient using size-exclusion chromatography through simultaneous measurement of concentration and scattered light intensity. Pharm Res 2007;24(11):2071–2083.

72. Costantino HR. Excipients for use in lyophilized pharmaceutical peptide, protein, and other bioproducts. In: Pikal MJ, Costantino HR, editors. Lyophilization of biopharmaceuticals. Arlington (VA): : AAPS Press; 2004. 139–228.

73. Crowe JH, Crowe LM, Carpenter JF. Preserving dry biomaterials: the water replacement hypothesis. Part 1. Biopharmacology 1993;6(3):28–33.

74. Andya JD, Hsu CC, Shire SJ. Mechanisms of aggregate formation and carbohydrate excipients stabilization of lyophlized monoclonal antibody formulations. APPS Pharm Sci 2003;5(2):1–11. Article 10.

75. Cleland J, Lam X, Kendrick B, Yang J, Yang T-H, Overcashier D, Brooks D, Hsu C, Carpenter JF. A specific molar ratio of stabilizer to protein is required for storage stability of a lyophilized monoclonal antibody. J Pharm Sci 2001;90:310–321.

76. Carpenter JF, Crowe JH. An infrared spectroscopic study of the interactions of carbohydrates with dried proteins. Biochemistry 1989;28(9):3916–3922.

77. Pikal MJ, Dellerman KM, Roy ML, Riggin RM. The effects of formulation variables on the stability of freeze-dried human growth hormone. Pharm Res 1991;8(4):427–436.

78. Prestrelski SJ, Tedeschi N, Arakawa T, Carpenter JF. Dehydration-induced conformational transitions in proteins and their inhibition by stabilizers. Biophys J 1993;65(2):661–671.

79. Prestrelski S, Pikal MJ, Katherine A, Arakawa T. Optimization of lyophilization conditions for recombinant human interleukin-2 by dried-state conformational analysis using Fourier-transform infrared spectroscopy. Pharm Res 1995;12(9):1250–1259.

80. Yoshioka, S. Molecular mobility of freeze-dried formulations as determined by NMR relaxation and its effect on storage stability. In: Rey L, May JC, editors. Freeze-drying/lyophilization of pharmaceutical and biological products. 2nd ed. New York, USA: Marcel Dekker Inc; 2007. 187–212.

81. Roy ML, Pikal MJ, Rickard EC, Maloney AM. The effects of formulation and moisture on the stability of a freeze-dried monoclonal antibody-vinca conjugate: a test of the WLF glass transition theory. Dev Biol Stand 1992;74:323–340.

82. Yoshioka S, Aso Y, Nakai Y, Kojima S. Effect of high molecular mobility of poly(vinyl alcohol) on protein stability of lyophilized gamma-globulin formulations. J Pharm Sci 1998;87(2):147–151.

83. Pikal MJ, Rigsbee DR, Roy ML. Solid state chemistry of proteins: I. Glass transition behavior in freeze dried disaccharide formulations of human growth hormone (hGH). J Pharm Sci 2007;96(10):2765–2776.

84. Pikal MJ, Rigsbee D, Roy ML, Galreath D, Kovach KJ, Wang B, Carpenter JF, Cicerone MT. Solid state chemistry of proteins: II. The correlation of storage stability of freeze-dried human growth hormone (hGH) with structure and dynamics in the glassy solid. J Pharm Sci 2008;97(12):5106–5121.

85. Pikal MJ, Rigsbee D, Roy ML. Solid state stability of proteins III: Calorimetric (DSC) and spectroscopic (FTIR) characterization of thermal denaturation in freeze dried human growth hormone (hGH). J Pharm Sci 2008;97(12):5122–5131.

86. Pikal MJ, Rigsbee D, Akers MJ. Solid state chemistry of proteins IV. What is the meaning of thermal denaturation in freeze dried proteins?. J Pharm Sci 2009;98(4):1387–1399.

87. Dixon D, Tchessalov S, Barry A, Warne N. The impact of protein concentration on mannitol and sodium chloride crystallinity and polymorphism upon lyophilization. J Pharm Sci 2009;98(9):3419–3429.

88. Schersch K. Effect of collapse on pharmaceutical protein lyophilisates [PhD thesis]. University of Munich, Germany;2009. 260–268.

INDEX

Analysis of Aggregates and Particles in Protein Pharmaceuticals, First Edition.
Edited by Hanns-Christian Mahler, Wim Jiskoot.
© 2012 John Wiley & Sons, Inc., Published 2012 by John Wiley & Sons, Inc.

Calcium phosphate, in controlling/monitoring aggregate level during protein purification, 339, 340
Calibration
  of dynamic light scattering, 322
  of ESZ-based techniques, 97, 99, 100
  for macro-IMS analysis, 137
  of MFI instrumentation, 153
  of microscopic particle count test, 95–96
  PSL spheres in, 105
Calibration constant, in ESZ measurements, 99
Calibration curves
  for light-obscuration particle count test apparatus, 89, 90, 91
  in stand-alone SLS system, 103
Cantilever, in atomic force microscopy, 284
Cao, Shawn, ix, 85
Capillaries
  in macro-IMS analysis of monoclonal antibodies, 140
  in macro-IMS analysis of virus-like particles, 150
  in particulate studies, 121
  in Taylor dispersion, 75
Capillary electrophoresis (CE), 313. *See also* CE-SDS methods
  in online detection methods, 65
  Taylor dispersion and, 75–76
Capillary electrophoresis technology, 29–30
Capillary occlusion, 108
Capillary tubes, for macro-IMS analysis, 137, 138
Carbohydrates, freeze-thaw and, 357
Carbon dioxide (CO_2), rotational and vibrational molecular motions of, 228–229
Carbon monoxide (CO), molecular vibrational motion of, 228
Carpenter, John F., ix, 1
Cassegrain objective, in infrared microscopy, 291, 292, 294, 295
Cation–π interactions, in protein dynamic property studies, 183–184
Cation exchange (CEX) chromatography
  for controlling/monitoring aggregate level during protein purification, 338, 339, 343
  in virus inactivation/removal, 351, 352
Cations, as extrinsic UV chromophores, 176
Cavitation, protein aggregation resulting from, 11
CCD (charge-coupled device) camera
  in nanoparticle tracking analysis, 158, 160
  in single-particle tracking, 219
  in transmission electron microscopy, 281
Cell assembly, for analytical ultracentrifuges, 16–17, 18

Cell culture media components, as protein drug impurity, 336
Cell debris, as protein drug impurity, 336
Cell holder, in spectrophotometer, 173
Cellulose, Raman microscopy and contamination by, 261–263
Centerpiece, in analytical ultracentrifuges, 16–17, 18, 19
Centrifugal field strength, in analytical ultracentrifugation, 16
Centrifugation. *See also* Analytical ultracentrifugation (AUC)
  dynamic light scattering and, 321
  enhancing light scattering techniques with, 49
  in identifying particulate matter, 119–120
  of protein precipitates, 243–244
  for studying biologics molecules, 61
Centrifuges, high-speed, 16–17, 19
Ceramic hydroxyapatite (CHT®), in controlling/monitoring aggregate level during protein purification, 339, 340
CE-SDS methods, 29–30, 31. *See also* Capillary electrophoresis (CE); Sodium dodecyl sulfate-polyacrylamide gel electrophoresis (SDS-PAGE)
  reducing and nonreducing, 32
  traditional gel electrophoresis *vs.*, 29–30
Channel flow, in field-flow fractionation, 24
Channel flow rate, in protein separation by flow FFF method, 26
Channels, in macro-IMS analysis of monoclonal antibodies, 138
Chaotropic agents, in difference spectroscopy, 178
Chaperone GroEL, nano-ESI mass spectrometry of, 78
Chaperones
  protein pharmaceutical mechanical stress stability and, 373–374
  protein refolding and, 355
Characteristic X-ray emission, in scanning electron microscopy, 282
Characterization
  with infrared microscopy, 295, 297
  of soluble aggregates, 305–333
Charge-reduced ions, in macro-IMS, 135–136
Charge-reduced nanoelectrospray unit, 137
Chemical bonds, infrared spectroscopy and, 227, 228. *See also* Hydrogen bonds
Chemical degradation, of therapeutic protein aggregates, 1, 2
Chemical denaturants, protein refolding and, 355
Chemical fingerprints, in micro-Raman setup, 258